I0066423

Total Knee Arthroplasty: Modern Techniques in Orthopedic Surgery

Total Knee Arthroplasty: Modern Techniques in Orthopedic Surgery

Edited by Jasper Max

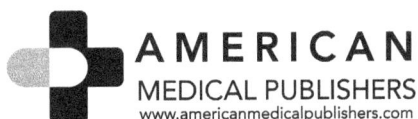

AMERICAN
MEDICAL PUBLISHERS
www.americanmedicalpublishers.com

American Medical Publishers,
41 Flatbush Avenue,
1st Floor, New York,
NY 11217, USA

Visit us on the World Wide Web at:
www.americanmedicalpublishers.com

© American Medical Publishers, 2022

This book contains information obtained from authentic and highly regarded sources. Copyright for all individual chapters remain with the respective authors as indicated. All chapters are published with permission under the Creative Commons Attribution License or equivalent. A wide variety of references are listed. Permission and sources are indicated; for detailed attributions, please refer to the permissions page and list of contributors. Reasonable efforts have been made to publish reliable data and information, but the authors, editors and publisher cannot assume any responsibility for the validity of all materials or the consequences of their use.

ISBN: 978-1-63927-405-5

Trademark Notice: Registered trademark of products or corporate names are used only for explanation and identification without intent to infringe.

Cataloging-in-Publication Data

Total knee arthroplasty : modern techniques in orthopedic surgery / edited by Jasper Max.
p. cm.
Includes bibliographical references and index.
ISBN 978-1-63927-405-5
1. Total knee replacement. 2. Knee--Surgery. 3. Arthroplasty. I. Max, Jasper.
RD561 .T68 2022
617.582--dc23

Table of Contents

Preface

Knee arthroplasty or knee replacement surgery is a procedure which is aimed at the replacement of the damaged surfaces of the knee joint with an artificial prosthesis to relieve pain and disability. It is performed when the knee joint is affected by osteoarthritis, psoriatic arthritis and rheumatoid arthritis. Knee arthroplasty can be total or partial. Total knee arthroplasty is intended to correct bone and knee joint trauma, or correct varus deformity or mild valgus. Obesity is often seen to present complications in total knee arthroscopy, and therefore bariatric surgery is recommended in morbidly obese patients. This book elucidates the concepts and innovative models around the techniques of total knee arthroplasty. It strives to provide a fair idea about this operative procedure and to help develop a better understanding of the complications involved in this surgery, and their management strategies. For all readers who are interested in orthopedics and orthopedic surgery, the case studies included in this book will serve as an excellent guide to develop a comprehensive understanding.

This book is a result of research of several months to collate the most relevant data in the field.

When I was approached with the idea of this book and the proposal to edit it, I was overwhelmed. It gave me an opportunity to reach out to all those who share a common interest with me in this field. I had 3 main parameters for editing this text:

1. Accuracy – The data and information provided in this book should be up-to-date and valuable to the readers.

2. Structure – The data must be presented in a structured format for easy understanding and better grasping of the readers

3. Universal Approach – This book not only targets students but also experts and innovators in the field, thus my aim was to present topics which are of use to all

Thus, it took me a couple of months to finish the editing of this book.

I would like to make a special mention of my publisher who considered me worthy of this opportunity and also supported me throughout the editing process. I would also like to thank the editing team at the back-end who extended their help whenever required.

Editor

Local anesthetic infusion pump for pain management following total knee arthroplasty

Yeying Zhang[1], Ming Lu[2] and Cheng Chang[3*]

Abstract

Background: We performed a systematic review and meta-analysis of randomized controlled trials (RCTs) were to evaluate the effect and safety of local anesthetic infusion pump versus placebo for pain management following total knee arthroplasty (TKA).

Methods: In September 2016, a systematic computer-based search was conducted in the Pubmed, ISI Web of Knowledge, Embase, Cochrane Database of Systematic Reviews. Randomized controlled trials of patients prepared for primary TKA that compared local anesthetic infusion pump versus placebo for pain management following TKA were retrieved. The primary endpoint was the visual analogue scale (VAS) with rest or mobilization at 24, 48 and 72 h and morphine consumption at 24 and 48 h. The second outcomes are range of motion, length of hospital stay (LOS) and complications (infection, deep venous thrombosis (DVT), prolonged drainage and postoperative nausea and vomiting (PONV)).

Results: Seven clinical studies with 587 patients were included and for meta-analysis. Local anesthetic infusion pump are associated with less pain scores with rest or mobilization at 24 and 48 h with significant difference. However, the difference was likely no clinical significance. There were no significant difference between the LOS, the occurrence of DVT, prolonged drainage and PONV. However, local anesthetic infusion pump may be associated with more infection.

Conclusion: Based on the current meta-analysis, we found no evidence to support the routine use of local anesthetic infusion pump in the management of acute pain following TKA. More RCTs are still need to identify the pain control effects and optimal dose and speed of local anesthetic pain pump.

Keywords: Local anesthesia, Infusion pump, Total knee arthroplasty, Meta-analysis

Background

The number of primary total knee arthroplasty (TKA) procedures will be reached at 3.48 million in 2030 in the United States and the number will be as eight-fold to the year of 2005 [1]. TKA was associated with moderate to severe postoperative pain. It is reported that approximately 60% of patients have severe pain and 30% of patients have moderate pain after TKA [2]. The pain has follow specific characteristics: the occurrence in mobilization is higher than in rest; and pain intensity always peaking at 3 to 6 h after TKA and continuing for the following 72 h [3]. Achievement of pain relief after TKA is necessary and early pain control after TKA can increasing patients satisfaction and reducing the length of hospital stay [4, 5]. Several effective modalities are available, but each has its own drawbacks. These modalities including oral opiates, femoral nerve block (FNB) and local infiltration anesthesia [6, 7]. FNB may weaken the quadriceps strength and increase the occurrence of fall. Oral opiates will increase the complications such as the postoperative nausea and vomiting (PONV).

Local infiltration anesthesia (LIA) has been identified a successful and easy way to management postoperative pain, and promote early mobilization after TKA [8]. A

* Correspondence: scitougao007@qq.com
[3]Department of anesthesiology, School of Medicine, Hangzhou Normal University, the affiliated Hospital of Hangzhou Normal University, 16 Xuelin St, Xiasha Higher Education Campus, Hangzhou, Zhejiang 310036, China
Full list of author information is available at the end of the article

meta-analysis indicated that LIA shows better pain control than FNB, which is considered to be the gold standard anesthesia method [9]. However, the anesthetic effects of LIA disappears within the first 24 h, attempts have been made to prolong the anesthetic effect using infusion pump for continuous local infiltration anesthesia (CLIA) [10]. There have been controversies about the effects of CLIA with infusion pump after TKA [11, 12]. Thus, we carried a systematic review and meta-analysis to re-assess the efficacy and safety of pain control of CLIA for pain control after TKA.

Methods

Search strategies

Two reviewers independently retrieved randomized controlled trials of CLIA for pain control in patients after TKA from PubMed, EMBASE, and the Cochrane Library. The search was last performed on August 23, 2016. There was no language restriction. The keywords and Mesh terms used in the search included "Arthroplasty, Replacement, Knee"[Mesh], "total knee arthroplasty", "total knee replacement", "TKA", "TKR", "Anesthesia, Local"[Mesh], "local infiltration anesthesia". We selected local infiltration anesthesia for avoiding leave out relevant studies. The Boolean operators "AND" and "OR" were used to connect these terms. The bibliographies of all included studies and other relevant publications, including systematic reviews and meta-analyses, were traced to identify the missed relevant reports. Based on the titles and abstracts, 2 reviewers selected the potential eligible studies. And then the full text of the remaining articles was examined for eligibility.

Inclusion and exclusion criteria

Inclusion criteria: Participants, patients with osteoarthritis or rheumatoid arthritis who prepared for primary TKA. Intervention and comparison-intervention group was continuous local infiltration anesthesia via infusion pump and the comparison group was placebo alone; Outcomes-The visual analogue scale (VAS) with rest or mobilization at 12, 24, 48 and 72 h. Study-Only randomized controlled trials were included in this study. Exclusion criteria: Participants, who underwent revision TKA; non-RCTs, comments, incomplete data for meta-analysis and letters.

Data extraction and outcome measures

Two independent reviewers selected the eligible studies and extracted the following data from the included publication: the first author, year of publication, geographical location, number of patients, intervention and comparison, duration of the treatment, follow-up, patient characteristics, and study type. We contacted the first or the corresponding author for detailed study information. Any discrepancies between the 2 reviewers were resolved by an additional investigator.

The primary outcomes were the VAS with rest at 24, 48 and 72 h, VAS with mobilization at 24, 48 and 72 h and total morphine consumption. The secondary outcomes were range of motion (ROM) of knee at 6 month, length of hospital stay (LOS), and the complications (infection, deep venous thrombosis (DVT), prolonged drainage and postoperative nausea and vomiting (PONV)). We chose the longest time point to measure the range of motion of knee.

When standard deviations (SD) were not provided in a study, standard error of the mean (SEM) was transferred into SD. If necessary, the means, SD, or SEM were extracted from the available diagrams and tables by the software of "GetData Graph Digitizer".

Risk of bias assessment

The risk of bias tool was used to estimate the quality by using Review Manager, version 5.3 (The Nordic Cochrane Centre, The Cochrane Collaboration, Copenhagen, 2014). The sequence generation, allocation concealment, blinding of participants and personnel, blinding of outcome assessment, incomplete outcome data, selective outcome reporting, and other biases (baseline balance and fund) was measured and the risk of bias results was exported from Review Manager, version 5.3. Two authors independently assessed the quality of the studies, and disagreements were resolved via a discussion with a third author. And the level of agreement between the 2 reviewers was assessed with the Cohen kappa statistic and set the acceptable threshold value as 0.61 [13, 14].

Statistical analysis

The meta-analysis was performed on the eligible data using Stata12.0 (Stata Corp, College Station, TX). The relative risk (RR) with 95% confidential intervals (CIs) was calculated for the dichotomous outcomes, and the mean difference (MD) with 95% CIs was calculated for the continuous outcomes. The I^2 statistic was used to test the heterogeneity between studies. Heterogeneity was considered statistically significant if the I^2 value was >50%. To assess the reliability of the results, a sensitivity analysis was performed by sequentially removing individual studies and recalculating the results. $P < 0.05$ was considered statistically significant and reported as a 2-sided test. Egger linear regression test and funnel plots would be implemented to estimate the publication bias.

Results

Search results and quality assessment

The initial search yielded 213 citations, of which, 48 duplicates were removed using Endnote software. After reading the titles and abstracts, 49 studies were excluded according to the inclusion criteria. Finally, 7 RCTs [10–18] with 587 TKAs were identified in our study (Fig. 1). The characteristics of the included studies are presented in Table 1.

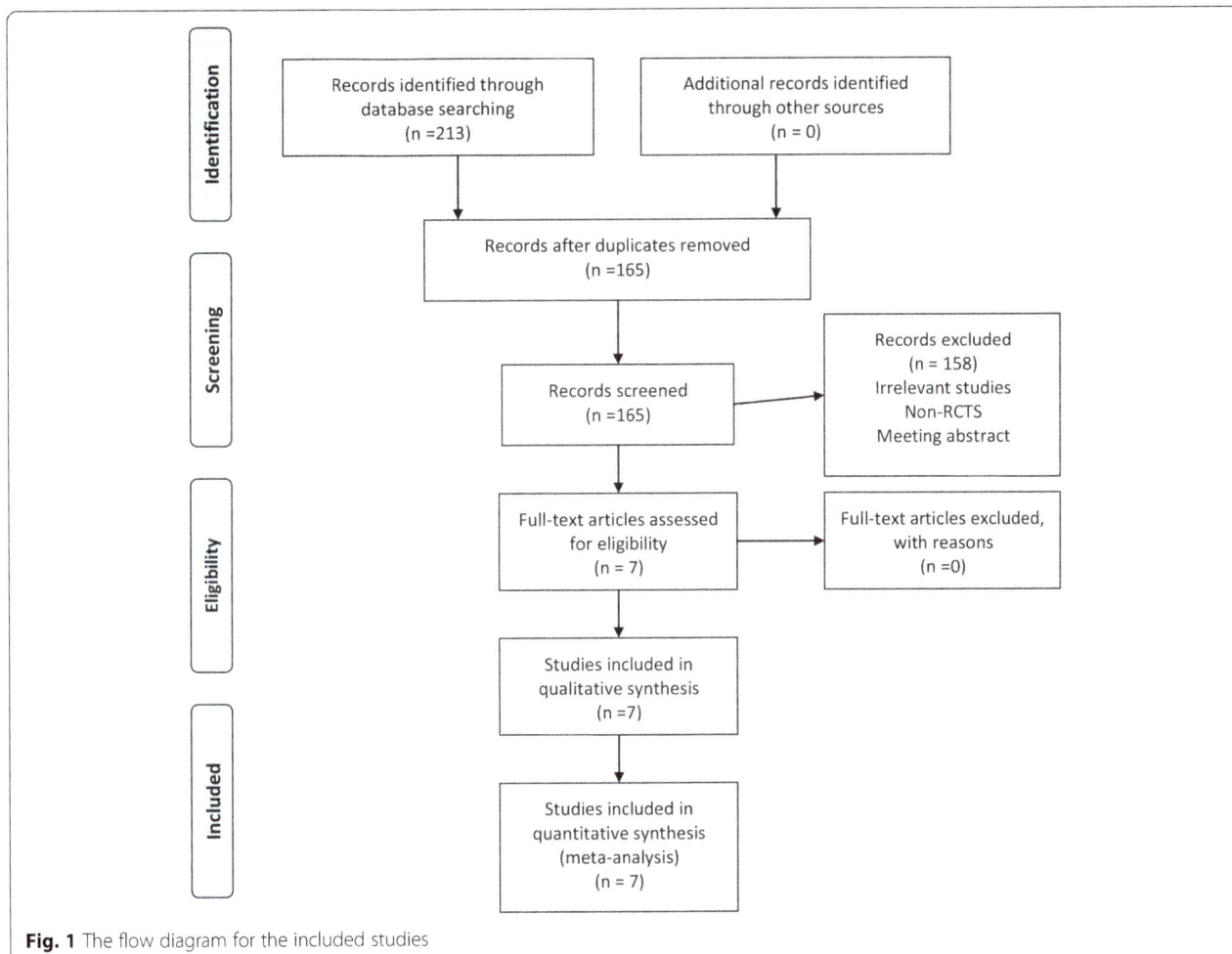

Fig. 1 The flow diagram for the included studies

Table 1 The general characteristic for the included studies, 1 VAS with rest at 12 h, 2 VAS with rest at 24 h, 3 VAS with rest at 48 h, 4, VAS with rest at 72 h, 5, VAS with mobilization at 12 h, 6, VAS with mobilization at 24 h, 7, VAS with mobilization at 48 h, 8, VAS with mobilization at 72 h; 9, length of hospital stay; 10, morphine consumption at 24 h; 11, morphine consumption at 48 h; 12, the occurrence of infection; 13, nausea, 14; postoperative nausea and vomiting; 15, range of motion; 16, total morphine consumption

Reference	No. of patients		Male, %	Mean age, year	Intervention		Outcomes	Study design	Follow up
	CLIA	C			CLIA	C			
Nechleba 2005 [15]	14	16	63.3	65	200 cc 0.25% bupivacaine at 4.16 cc	200 cc Saline	2 3 11 12	RCT	6 week
Reeves 2009 [16]	31	30	41	69	240 cc 0.2% ropivacaine or 0.375% ropivacaine at 5 cc/h	240 cc Saline	2 3 6 7 8 11	RCT	2 day
Gomez-Cardero 2011	25	25	38	71	300 cc 0.2% ropivacaine at a speed of 5 cc/h	300 cc Saline	12	RCT	1 month
Zhang 2011 [12]	27	26	47.2	67	199 cc 2 mg/ml ropivacaine plus 2 ml 2 mg/ml ketorolac at 4 cc/h	199 cc saline	1 2 3 5 6 7 9 10 11 12 14	RCT	3 month
Goyal 2013 [10]	75	75	45.3	63	300 cc 0.5% bupivacaine	300 cc Saline	6 7 8 9 10 11 12	RCT	6 week
Williams 2013 [11]	26	25	41.2	67	0.5% bupivacaine at 2 cc/h	Saline	2, 3 9 13 9 10 14	RCT	1 y
Ali 2015 [18]	97	95	36.5	69	100 cc 7.5 mg/ml ropivacaine at 2 cc/h	100 cc Saline	2 3 4 7 10 11 12 13	RCT	3 m

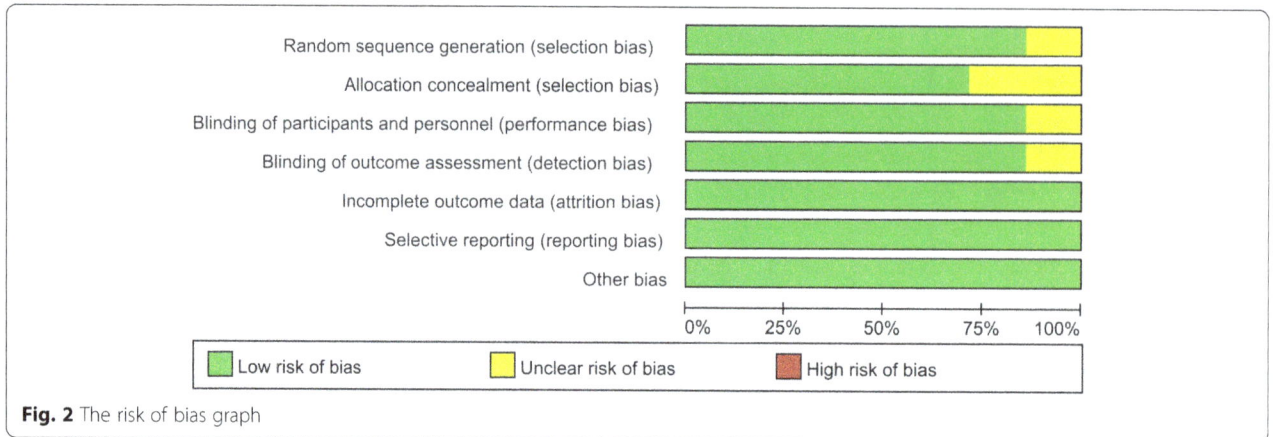

Fig. 2 The risk of bias graph

The included studies were published from the year of 2005 to 2015. The sample of patients ranged from14 to 97. The mean age of patients ranging from 63 to 71. And the volume of pain pump ranging from 100 to 300 ml. The delivery speed from 2 to 5 ml/h. Only one study did not state the delivery speed [10].

The quality assessment results can be seen in Figs. 2 and 3. Only 1 study did not state the random sequence generation [15]. The other studies are all give appropriate random sequence generation. The allocation concealment are not clear in 2 studies [15, 16]. Blinding of participants and outcome assessment are unclear in 1 study [15]. The other bias are all with low bias. The agreement between the reviewers for risk of bias, based on kappa statistic, was 0.90.

Results of the meta-analysis
VAS with rest at 24, 48 and 72 h

Five studies, including 384 patients, provided data for the VAS with rest at 24 h. The CLIA group was associated with a significant decrease in the VAS with rest at 24 h compared with the controls (MD = −11.09, 95% CI: −18.17–4.00, $P = 0.002$; $I^2 = 75.1\%$, Fig. 4). The data on the VAS with rest at 48 h and at 72 h were available from 5 studies and 2 studies respectively. There was no significant difference between the VAS with rest at 48 h (MD = −5.55, 95% CI: −16.30–5.20, $P = 0.311$; $I^2 = 91.5\%$, Fig. 4) and 72 h (MD = 0.53, 95% CI: −5.65–6.72, $P = 0.866$; $I^2 = 38.4\%$, Fig. 4) between CLIA group with control group. Egger's test was performed to test the publication bias between the included studies. Results indicated that there was no publication bias between the studies ($P = 1.000$, Fig. 5).

VAS with mobilization at 24, 48 and 72 h

Three studies ($n = 263$) contributed to the analysis of the VAS with mobilization at 24 h. The VAS with mobilization at 24 h was significantly decreased in the CLIA group compared with the controls (MD = −13.94, 95% CI: −17.31– −10.57, $P = 0.000$; $I^2 = 0.0\%$, Fig. 6).

The data on the VAS with mobilization at 48 h were available in 3 studies, the pooled results indicated that CLIA can reduce VAS with mobilization at 48 h for a mean of 9.50 (95% CI: −15.20– −10.56, $P = 0.001$, Fig. 6). There was no significant difference between the VAS with mobilization at 72 h (MD = −1.33, 95% CI: −16.95–14.30, $P = 0.868$; $I^2 = 86.9\%$, Fig. 6).

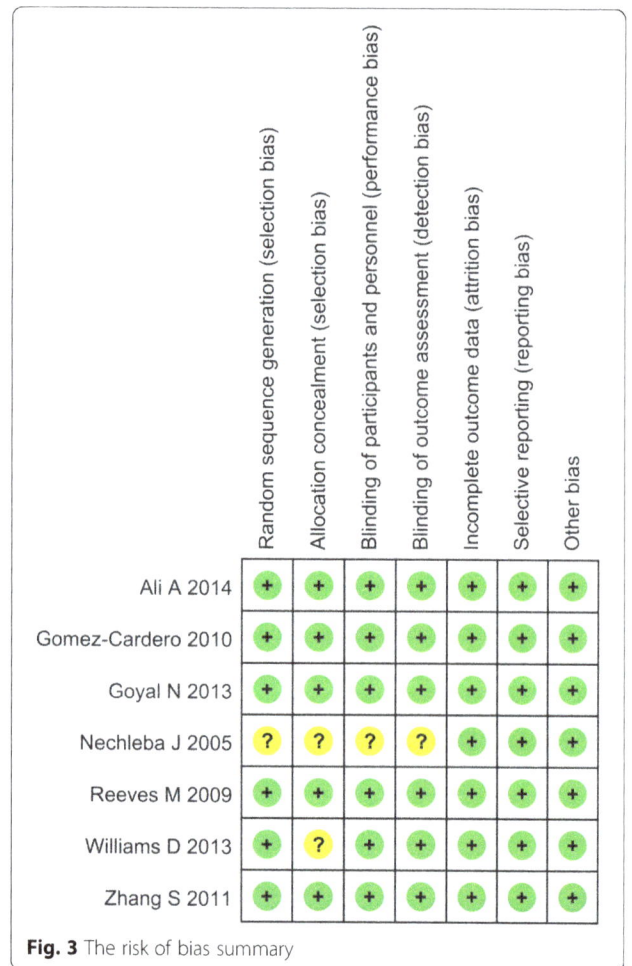

Fig. 3 The risk of bias summary

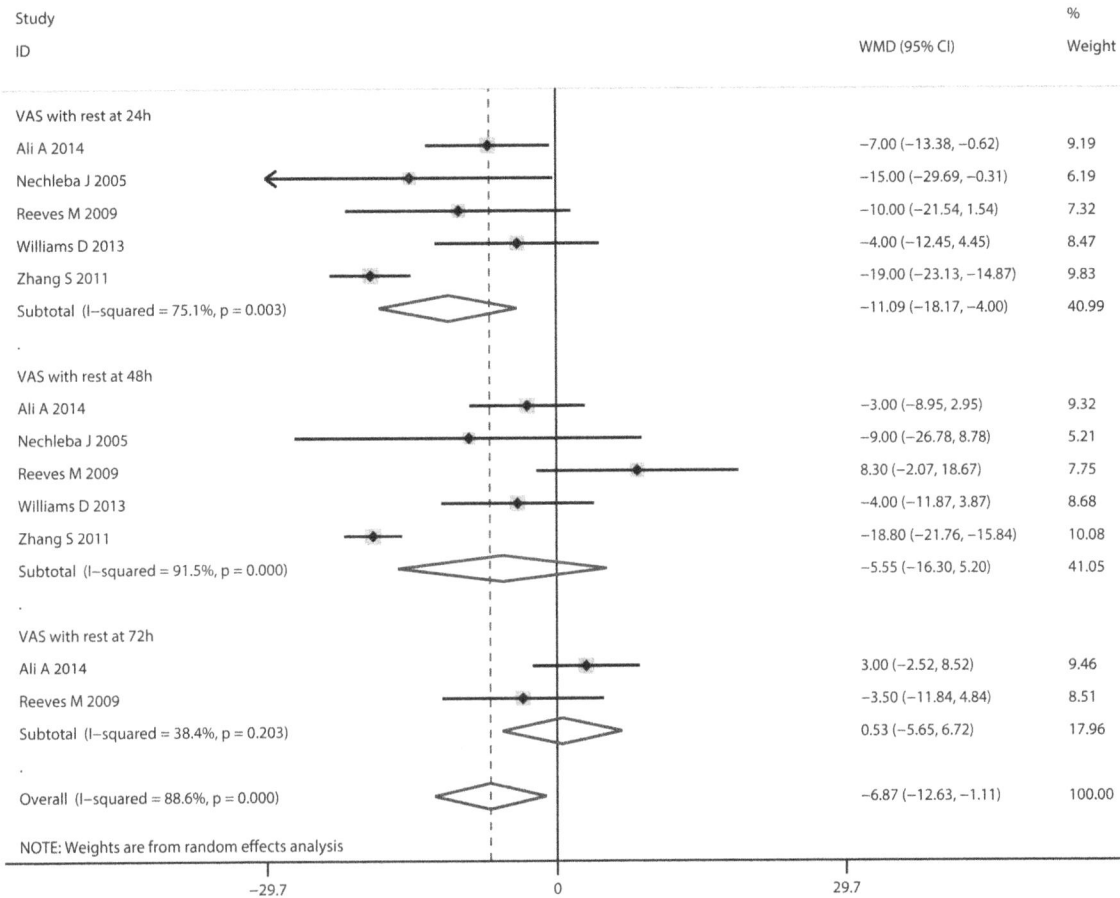

Fig. 4 Forest plot comparing VAS with rest at 24, 48 and 72 h

Total morphine consumption

In 3 studies ($n = 296$), provided the data for the total morphine consumption between the CLIA group with controls. Pooled results indicated that there was no significant difference between the morphine consumption between CLIA group with controls (SMD = −0.64, 95% CI: −0.88− −0.40, $P = 0.000$; $I^2 = 90.3$%, Fig. 7).

ROM of knee at 6 month after TKA

Four studies with 324 patients reported the relevant data of ROM of knee at 6 month after TKA. Pooled results indicated that, compared with control group, CLIA can increase the ROM of knee at 6 month after TKA (MD = 5.26, 95% CI: 3.63~6.89, $P = 0.000$, Fig. 8).

LOS

Three studies ($n = 411$) contributed to the analysis of LOS. We observed similar LOS when comparing the CLIA group with the control group (MD = 0.05, 95% CI: −0.20~0.30, $P = 0.086$, Fig. 9).

Complications

Four common complications (infection, DVT, prolonged drainage and PONV) were compared between the included studies. Results indicated that there was no significant difference between the occurrence of DVT (RR = 1.01, 95% CI :0.30~3.41, $P = 0.987$, Fig. 10), prolonged drainage (RR = 1.67, 95% CI :0.23~12.33, $P = 0.617$, Fig. 10) and the occurrence of PONV (RR = 1.27, 95% CI :0.77~2.12, $P = 0.255$, Fig. 10). However CLIA increase the occurrence of infection (RR = 3.45, 95% CI :1.16~10.33, $P = 0.027$, Fig. 10).

Subgroup analysis

The results of VAS with rest has large heterogeneity between the included studies. Subgroup analysis was conducted according to the delivery speed (<2 cc/h or >2 cc/h) and the type of anesthesia drug (ropivacaine or bupivacaine). Pooled results indicated that local infiltration anesthesia with pain pump with a high speed (>2 cc/h) associated with less VAS with rest at 24 and 48 h than the low speed (<2 cc/h). And the local

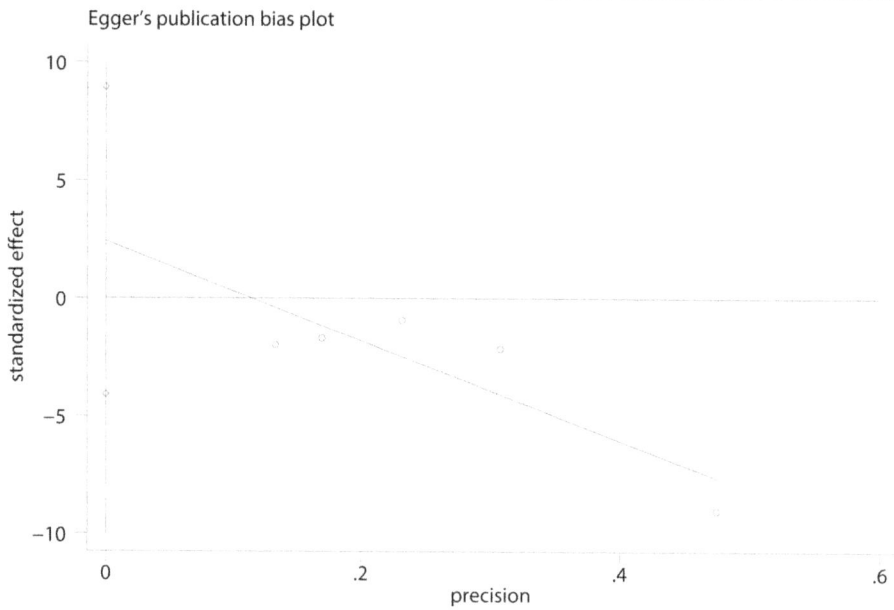

Fig. 5 Egger's test for publication bias for VAS with rest at 24 h

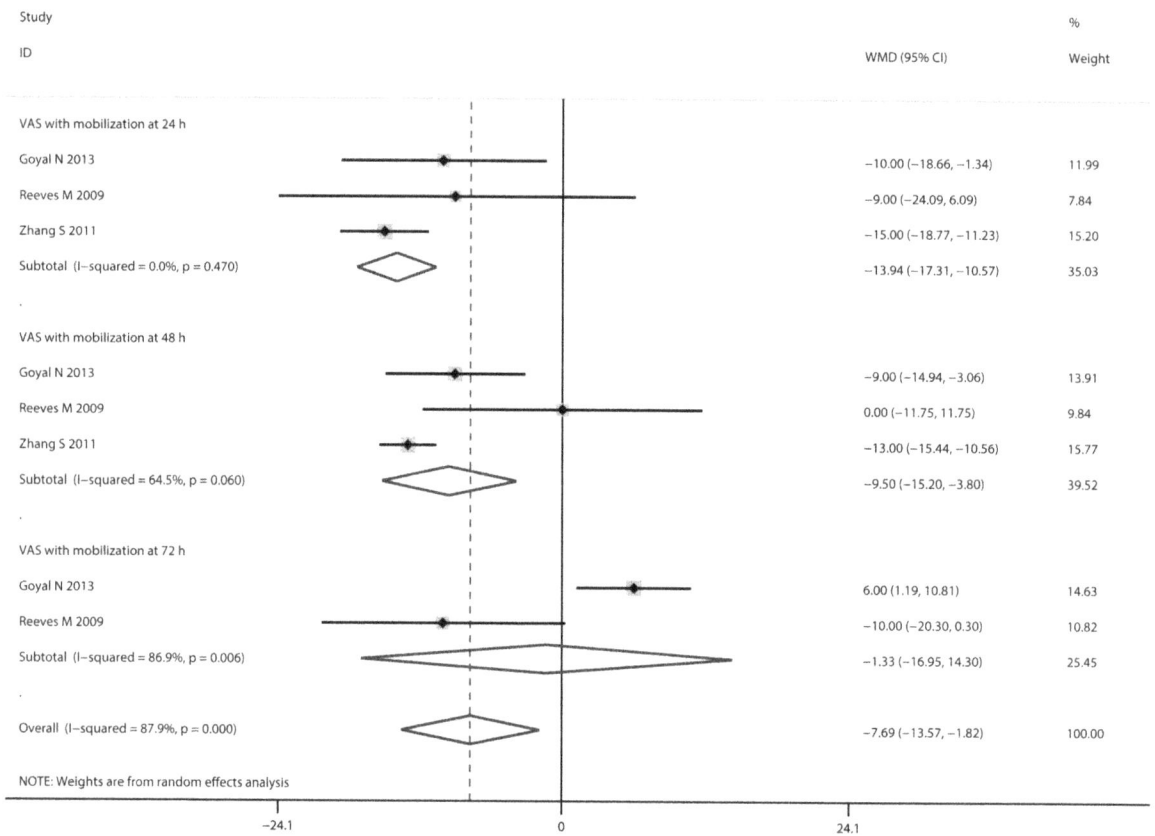

Fig. 6 Forest plot comparing VAS with mobilization at 24, 48 and 72 h

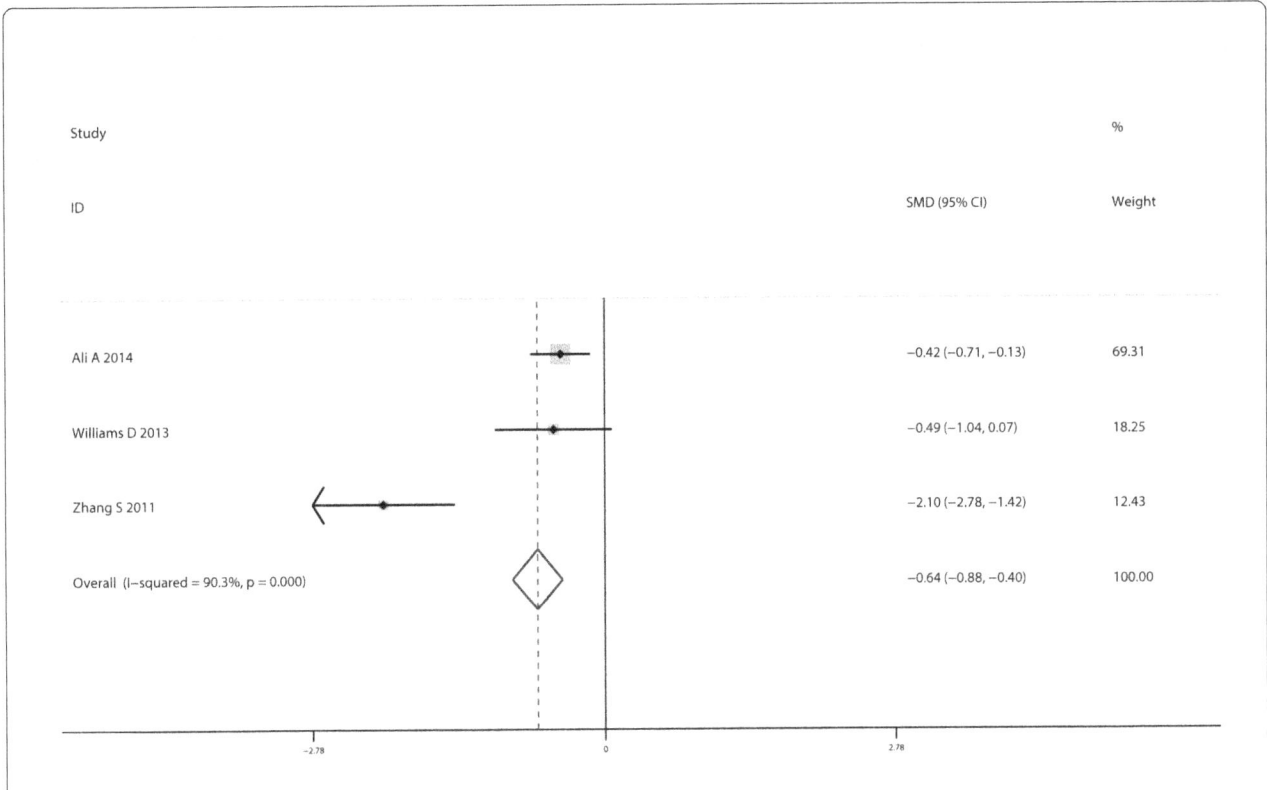

Fig. 7 Forest plot comparing total morphine consumption between the two groups

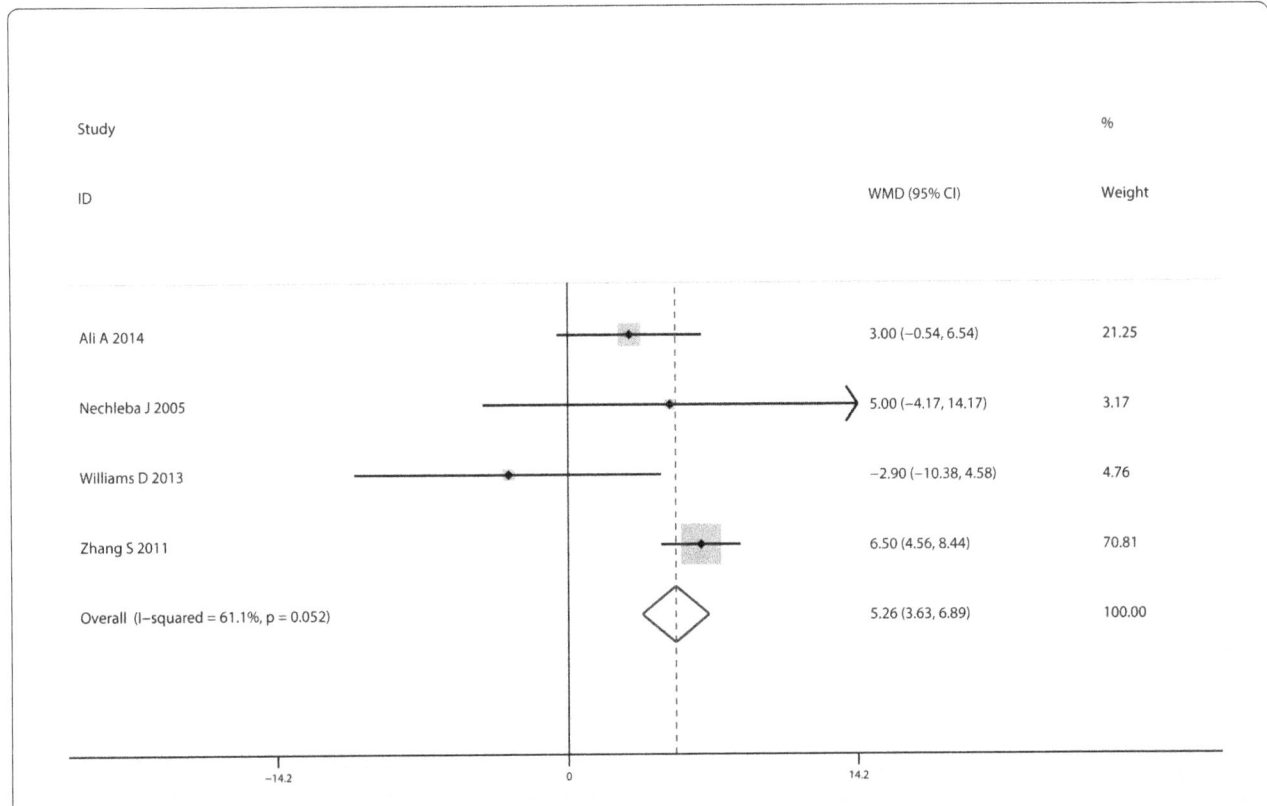

Fig. 8 Forest plot comparing range of motion between the two groups

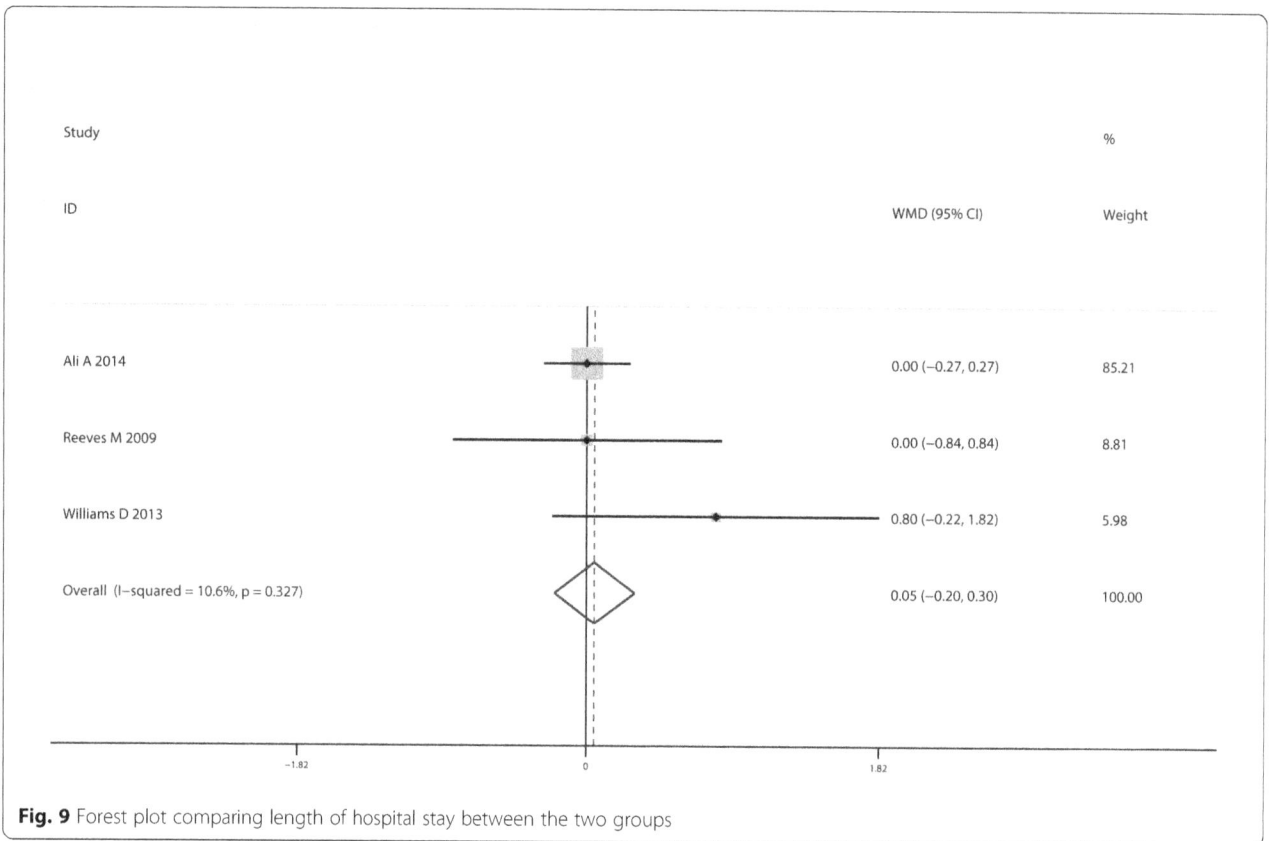

Fig. 9 Forest plot comparing length of hospital stay between the two groups

infiltration with ropivacaine is better than bupivacaine for reducing VAS with rest at 24 and 48 h (Table 2).

Discussion

This is the first systematic review and meta-analysis that compared local anesthetic infusion pump versus placebo for pain management following TKA. The pooled results indicated that administration with local anesthetic infusion pump can reduce pain intensity with mobilization and morphine consumption. The pain control and morphine consumption were likely of no clinical importance. There was no significant difference between the CLIA group versus placebo group in terms of LOS and complications such as PONV, DVT and prolonged drainage. However, the occurrence of infection in local anesthetic infusion pump group is higher than in placebo group. Though there was significant difference between pain score at 24 h with rest or mobilization, the clinical effects was limited. Thus, more RCTs for comparing local anesthetic infusion pump versus placebo after TKA are still need to identify the clinical value for pain control after TKA.

For this meta-analysis, we only included RCTs for meta-analysis, the quality of the included studies are all high and comparable. Only one study did not state the random sequence generation and the rest studies are all referenced the random sequence generation. All included studies all showed comparable characteristic and intent to treatment. The local infiltration drugs and drug delivery speed were different with each other. However, the half-time of all the local infiltration drugs were very nearly the same. The half-lives of bupivacaine was 3.5 h and ropivacaine was 2 to 6 h [19]. Thus, subgroup analysis was conducted to independent analysis the ropivacaine and bupivacaine for the VAS with rest at 24 and 48 h. Indirect comparison shown that the pain-sparing effects was better in ropivacaine group than in bupivacaine group. What's more, the local infiltration anesthesia with a high speed is better than low speed group.

Pain control after TKA is always associated with the functional recovery and patients satisfaction [20]. An option that has gained popularity is peri-articular infiltration anesthesia or intra-articular anesthesia with pain pump for continuous infiltration. There is no consistent conclusion about the efficacy and safety of local anesthetic infusion pump for pain control after TKA [11, 12]. Williams et al. [11] conducted a RCT and found that pain score and morphine consumption are not significantly reduced when adding 48 h of 0.5% bupivacaine infiltration with pain pump. Ali et al. [18] also performed a RCT about CLIA with placebo for pain control after TKA and found that CLIA has no relevant clinical effect on VAS pain and does

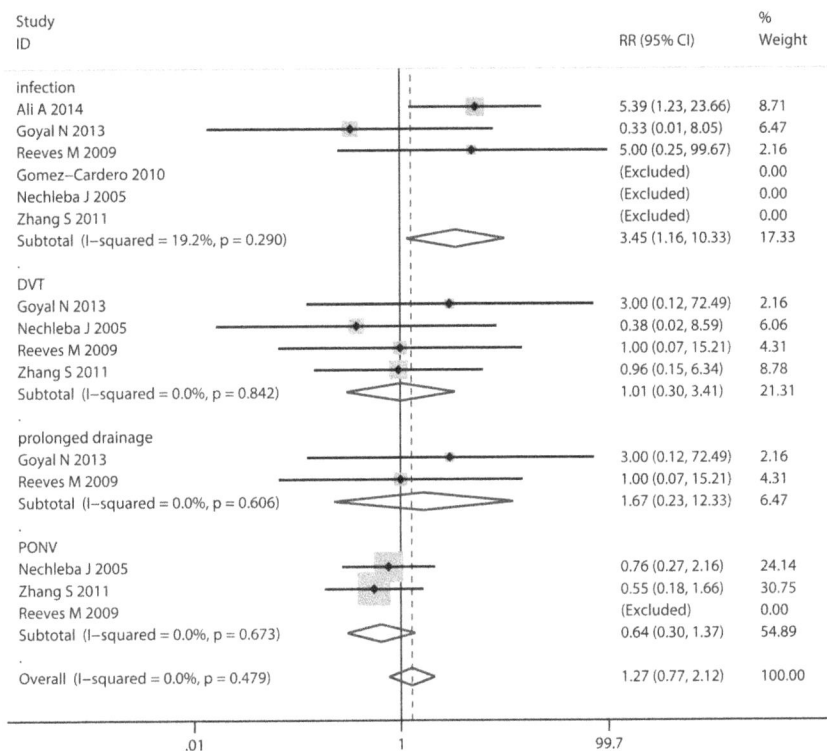

Fig. 10 Forest plot comparing the complications between the two groups

not affect LOS, morphine consumption but with a higher risk of wound-healing complications: deep infections. In this meta-analysis, the pain score was reduced 11.09 score with rest at 24 h and 13.94 score at 24 h with mobilization. This effect was likely of clinical importance. With time going on, the pain score was reduced 5.55 with rest at 48 h and 9.50 with mobilization at 48 h. The VAS with mobilization at 48 h was likely clinical importance. For VAS with rest or mobilization at 72 h, there were no

clinical importance for these outcomes. Indeed, the attempts that administration with pain pump for prolong the analgesic effect still need for more studies to identify. The development of portable elastomeric infusion pumps can make the infusion of postoperative local anesthetic more easily available. However, if the pain control was limited in the first 24 h after TKA. The local infiltration anesthesia with long action bupivacaine can also reach the same effects. The costs and the operating time will be

Table 2 The subgroup analysis for the VAS with rest or mobilization at 24 and 48 h

Outcome	Studies	Overall effects			Heterogeneity	
		Effect estimate	95% CI	P value	I² (%)	P value
VAS with rest at 24 h						
low speed	2	−5.91	−11.00, −0.82	0.000	0.0	0.579
high speed	3	−17.78	−21.54, −14.02	<0.001	9.9	0.330
ropivacaine	3	−15.00	−18.32, −11.68	0.000	80.7	0.006
bupivacaine	2	−6.74	−14.06, −0.59	0.072	38.2	0.203
VAS with rest at 48 h						
low speed	2	−3.36	−8.11, 1.38	0.165	0.0	0.843
high speed	3	−17.79	−20.59, −14.98	0.000	56.5	0.100
ropivacaine	3	−15.22	−17.78, −12.66	0.000	91.5	0.000
bupivacaine	3	−4.82	−12.02, 2.38	0.189	0.0	0.614

increased correspondingly. Zhang et al. [12] compared single-injection versus CLIA for pain control after TKA and found that CLIA provided prolonged superior analgesia and was associated with more functional recovery compared with single-injection local anesthesia. Wu et al. [21] conducted a meta-analysis to compare local anesthetic infusion pump for pain management following open inguinal hernia repair and found local anesthetic infusion pump was more efficacious for reducing postoperative pain than a placebo. The patients with different surgery type may suffer from variable pain intensity.

For morphine consumption, though CLIA can decrease the morphine consumption, however, only 0.64 mg was saved. The saving effects was found to be small of clinical effects. Thus, the effects of CLIA for morphine-saving is limited. For knee function, 4 studies with 324 patients perform range of motion of knee and pooled results indicated that CLIA can increase the ROM of knee for a mean of 5.26°. A total of 324 patients analyzed the ROM of the knee and thus further studies are needed to enhance the strength of the evidence presented. As for the complications, local anesthetic infusion pump are associated with more patients subjected to infection. Though the difference is statistically significant, the clinical significance worth deep research.

Our study has several limitations. First, the studies contain small samples, ranging from 14 to 75 patients per group, which might detract from the statistical power of the results. Second, several studies did not report the details of the generation and concealment of the allocation, and displayed other bias risks, such as the undetermined number of surgeons involved in the study. Finally, several of our primary and secondary outcomes were variably reported, thus potentially limiting the inferences based on our analysis.

Conclusions

In conclusion, the results of our meta-analysis revealed that applying a local anesthetic infusion pump following TKA reduced postoperative pain compared to the placebo treatments during postoperative day 1 to day 2. However, the findings were based on a small body of evidence in which the methodological quality was not high. And the difference seems to be small of clinical effects. Based on the current evidence, we did not recommend routinely administration with local anesthetic infusion pump. Further research involving high quality RCTs might be warranted.

Abbreviations

CIs: Confidential intervals; CLIA: Continuous local infiltration anesthesia; DVT: Deep venous thrombosis; FNB: Femoral nerve block; LIA: Local infiltration anesthesia; LOS: Length of hospital stay; MD: Mean difference; PONV: Postoperative nausea and vomiting; RCTs: Randomized controlled trials; RR: Relative risk; SD: Standard deviation; SEM: Standard error of the mean; TKA: Total knee arthroplasty; VAS: Visual analogue scale

Acknowledgements
Not applicable.

Funding
No funding was obtained for this study.

Authors' contributions
YYZ conceived the study design. ML and CC performed the study, collected the data and contributed to the study design. YYZ prepared the manuscript. ML and CC edited the manuscript. All authors read and approved the final manuscript.

Competing interests
The authors declare that they have no competing interests.

Consent for publication
Not applicable.

Author details
[1]Department of Anesthesiology, the Affiliated Hospital of Hangzhou Normal University, 126 Wenzhou Road, Hangzhou, Zhejiang 310015, China. [2]Department of Cardiology, Second Affiliated Hospital of Zhejiang Chinese Medical University, Hangzhou, Zhejiang 310005, China. [3]Department of anesthesiology, School of Medicine, Hangzhou Normal University, the affiliated Hospital of Hangzhou Normal University, 16 Xuelin St, Xiasha Higher Education Campus, Hangzhou, Zhejiang 310036, China.

References
1. Kurtz S, Ong K, Lau E, et al. Projections of primary and revision hip and knee arthroplasty in the United States from 2005 to 2030. J Bone Joint Surg Am. 2007;89(4):780–5.
2. Sun XL, Zhao ZH, Ma JX, et al. Continuous local infiltration analgesia for pain control after total knee arthroplasty: a meta-analysis of randomized controlled trials. Medicine (Baltimore). 2015;94(45):e2005.
3. Beaussier M. Frequency, intensity, development and repercussions of postoperative pain as a function of the type of surgery. Ann Fr Anesth Reanim. 1998;17(6):471–93.
4. Dong J, Li W, Wang Y. The effect of pregabalin on acute postoperative pain in patients undergoing total knee arthroplasty: a meta-analysis. Int J Surg. 2016;34:148–60.
5. Hamilton TW, Strickland LH, Pandit HG. A meta-analysis on the use of gabapentinoids for the treatment of acute postoperative pain following total knee arthroplasty. J Bone Joint Surg Am. 2016;98(16):1340–50.
6. Sakai N, Nakatsuka M, Tomita T. Patient-controlled bolus femoral nerve block after knee arthroplasty: quadriceps recovery, analgesia, local anesthetic consumption. Acta Anaesthesiol Scand. 2016;60(10):1461–9.
7. Chan EY, Fransen M, Parker DA, et al. Femoral nerve blocks for acute postoperative pain after knee replacement surgery. Cochrane Database Syst Rev. 2014;5:CD009941.
8. Seangleulur A, Vanasbodeekul P, Prapaitrakool S, et al. The efficacy of local infiltration analgesia in the early postoperative period after total knee arthroplasty: a systematic review and meta-analysis. Eur J Anaesthesiol. 2016; 33(11):816–31.
9. Fan L, Yu X, Zan P, et al. Comparison of local infiltration analgesia with femoral nerve block for total knee arthroplasty: a prospective, randomized clinical trial. J Arthroplasty. 2016;31(6):1361–5.
10. Goyal N, McKenzie J, Sharkey PF, et al. The 2012 Chitranjan Ranawat award: intraarticular analgesia after TKA reduces pain: a randomized, double-blinded, placebo-controlled, prospective study. Clin Orthop Relat Res. 2013; 471(1):64–75.

11. Williams D, Petruccelli D, Paul J, et al. Continuous infusion of bupivacaine following total knee arthroplasty: a randomized control trial pilot study. J Arthroplasty. 2013;28(3):479–84.
12. Zhang S, Wang F, Lu ZD, et al. Effect of single-injection versus continuous local infiltration analgesia after total knee arthroplasty: a randomized, double-blind, placebo-controlled study. J Int Med Res. 2011;39(4):1369–80.
13. Landis JR, Koch GG. An application of hierarchical kappa-type statistics in the assessment of majority agreement among multiple observers. Biometrics. 1977;33(2):363–74.
14. Landis JR, Koch GG. The measurement of observer agreement for categorical data. Biometrics. 1977;33(1):159–74.
15. Nechleba J, Rogers V, Cortina G, et al. Continuous intra-articular infusion of bupivacaine for postoperative pain following total knee arthroplasty. J Knee Surg. 2005;18(3):197–202.
16. Reeves M, Skinner MW. Continuous intra-articular infusion of ropivacaine after unilateral total knee arthroplasty. Anaesth Intensive Care. 2009;37(6):918–22.
17. Gomez-Cardero P, Rodriguez-Merchan EC. Postoperative analgesia in TKA: ropivacaine continuous intraarticular infusion. Clin Orthop Relat Res. 2010; 468(5):1242–7.
18. Ali A, Sundberg M, Hansson U, et al. Doubtful effect of continuous intraarticular analgesia after total knee arthroplasty: a randomized double-blind study of 200 patients. Acta Orthop. 2015;86(3):373–7.
19. Ong JC, Chin PL, Fook-Chong SM, et al. Continuous infiltration of local anaesthetic following total knee arthroplasty. J Orthop Surg (Hong Kong). 2010;18(2):203–7.
20. Wu ZQ, Min JK, Wang D, et al. Liposome bupivacaine for pain control after total knee arthroplasty: a meta-analysis. J Orthop Surg Res. 2016;11(1):84.
21. Wu CC, Bai CH, Huang MT, et al. Local anesthetic infusion pump for pain management following open inguinal hernia repair: a meta-analysis. Int J Surg. 2014;12(3):245–50.

2

Peri-articular tranexamic acid injection in total knee arthroplasty

P Pinsornsak[*], S Rojanavijitkul and S Chumchuen

Abstract

Background: Intravenous tranexamic acid (IV TXA) is one of the most effective agents in use for reducing blood loss following total knee arthroplasty (TKA) but its safety regarding venous thromboembolic events (VTEs) remains in question. The direct, local application of TXA may reduce systemic toxicity whilst maintaining good or better bleeding control compared to IV TXA. The topical application of TXA via Hemovac drains has been reported previously with good results. However, there are no data on peri-articular TXA injections during TKA.

Methods: We conducted an open randomized, pilot study of peri-articular vs. IV TXA in 60 patients undergoing TKA. 30 patients received either: (i) 750 mg peri-articular TXA into the medial, lateral capsules and the quadriceps tendon prior to capsular closure and tourniquet deflation (group1), or (ii) 750 mg of IV TXA just before tourniquet deflation. Blood loss in the hemovac drain and hemoglobin (Hb) concentrations were measured at 24 and 48 h (h), and the number of blood transfusions and leg circumference measurements were recorded.

Results: At 48 h, the total blood loss in the hemovac drain was 445 mL in group 1 vs. 520 mL in group 2 ($p = 0.081$) and the corresponding declines in Hb were 1.85 g/dL vs. 1.87 g/dL ($p = 0.84$). 16 patients received blood transfusions: 9 vs. 7 in groups 1 and 2, respectively ($p = 0.928$). There were no differences in thigh and lower leg circumferences, pain scores, knee flexion at discharge date and lengths of hospital stay. There were no clinically detected venous thromboembolic events.

Conclusion: This pilot study has shown promising results for peri-articular TXA during TKA. Additional, larger studies are needed to confirm our results and be powered to show differences in efficacy and safety of peri-articular vs. IV TXA.

Keywords: Tranexamic acid, Peri-articular injection, Total knee arthroplasty, Blood loss

Background

Postoperative bleeding in total knee arthroplasty (TKA), which can result in hypovolemic shock and the need for allogenic blood transfusions, is a major concern for orthopedic surgeons. Several strategies are used to reduce postoperative blood loss, including preoperative autologous blood transfusions, hemoglobin raising agents, intraoperative tourniquets, cell savers, intravenous (IV), and topical tranexamic acid (TXA) [1–7]. TXA is an antifibrinolytic agent that inhibits the conversion of plasminogen to

plasmin and also acts as a plasmin inhibitor. This results in inhibition of the breaking down of fibrin blood clots (fibrinolysis) [8] and fibrin clot stabilization rather than the promotion of clot aggregation [9, 10]. Plasmin activation due to tissue trauma increases after release of the surgical tourniquet and increased fibrinolysis [8, 11, 12].

IV TXA is commonly used intravenously for reducing blood loss and blood transfusions following TKA. Blood loss reduction varies from 10 % to 70 % compared to control groups not receiving TXA [13–15]. However, there are reports of thrombus formation associated with IV TXA [16, 17]. Topical TXA applications have been reported as another method to reduce blood loss and

---

* Correspondence: pinpiya2003@yahoo.com
Department of Orthopaedic Surgery, Thammasat University, 99 Moo 18, Khlong Nueng, Khlong Luang, Pathumthani, Thailand12120

are associated with fewer systemic side effects compared to IV TXA [6, 7, 18–21]. Topical TXA is usually applied by soaking TXA in the operating field and washed after period of time or left to drain out following wound closure and drain insertion. Topical TXA is only has superficial contact with the bleeding surface and for a limited period of time. We do not know the effect of topical TXA on polyethylene and this needs the further study.

Another approach could be peri-articular TXA injections which would act directly on the injured tissue and for a longer duration compared to topical and IV TXA. This may result in better reduced blood loss comparable or better than topical or IV TXA but without the potential systemic toxicity of IV TXA [22, 23].

Given the lack of data on peri-articular TXA, we evaluated the benefits and toxicity of peri-articular TXA compared to standard IV TXA and report the results, herein.

Methods

This prospective, randomized trial was conducted from October 2012 to October 2013, and approved by the Ethics Committee, Institutional Review Board of Thammasat University (Registry #MTU-EC-OT-0-096/54). All patients had been provided with written, informed consent prior to their participation in the study.

The study inclusion criteria were adult patients with osteoarthritis in need of a TKA.

The exclusion criteria were the patients with inflammatory arthritis, post-traumatic arthritis, a history of or current venous thromboembolic disease, any underlying disease of haemostasis, cirrhosis, chronic renal failure, patients on anticoagulants or strong antiplatelet drugs (e.g. warfarin, clopidogrel), know allergy to TXA, defective color vision, and a preoperative hemoglobin <10 g/dL or a platelet count < 140,000 /uL^3.

Study conduct

All patients underwent routine preoperative preparations. Patients on aspirin were asked to stop them at least 7 days before the operation. The surgeries were performed by a single surgeon (P.P.). The same surgical technique was used throughout the study. After the tourniquet was inflated, a limited medial parapatellar skin incision (~10 cm length) was made beginning 2 cm proximal to the superior pole of the patella and passing along the medial border of the patella to the medial border of the tibial tubercle. A medial parapatellar approach was used in all cases. Routine femoral (intramedullary guide) and tibial (extramedullary guide) preparations were carried out and the TKAs were performed using the standard measured-resection technique. A cemented, posterior stabilized, fixed bearing TKA prosthesis was used in all cases (Nexgen®; Zimmer,

Warsaw, IN, USA). No patellae were resurfaced but were all denervated by electro cautery. Ten minutes prior to deflating the tourniquet, sealed envelopes were opened containing the randomized the allocated treatment. In group 1, patients received 750 mg of peri-articular TXA (Transamin®; OLIC Thailand Ltd, Bangkok, Thailand; 250 mg/5 mL, 15 cc total volume, Fig. 1) injection into the soft tissue around medial capsule (5 ml), lateral capsule (5 ml) and around the quadriceps muscle (5 ml). In group 2, the patients received 750 mg of IV TXA (250 mg/5 ml, 15 cc total volume, keeping within the therapeutic range of 10–15 mg/kg/dose). One drain (Privac®; Primed Halberstadt Medizintechnik GmbH, Halberstadt, Germany) was positioned in the lateral gutter (Fig. 1) and the wound closed. The tourniquet was deflated following skin closure. The drain was clamped and reopened three hours postoperatively. The drain output was recorded at 24 and 48 h (post skin closure) and removed at 48 h in all patients. Hemoglobin and hematocrit levels were recorded at 24 and 48 h postoperatively. The criteria for blood transfusion were a hemoglobin concentration < 10 g/dL or if patients had any signs of anemia (e.g. chest pain that suggested from cardiac origin, congestive heart failure, and unexplained tachycardia or hypotension unresponsive to fluid replacement) at 24 or 48 h. One unit of packed red cells was transfused per 1 g/dL of hemoglobin drop. No anticoagulant agents were used but postoperative foot pump exercises and early ambulation were encouraged for all patients. Patients with clinically suspected deep vein thrombosis or a pulmonary venous thromboembolic event (VTE) were sent for further investigation. Patients were discharged when they were able to walk with walking aid more than 10 m, pain was controlled by oral analgesics and there was no continuous bleeding or oozing from the wound.

The primary outcomes were: the volume of postoperative blood loss in the drain, changes in hemoglobin concentrations, and the necessity for a blood transfusion. As for secondary outcomes, we measured knee diameter for swelling, local soft tissue complications, skin necrosis, and clinically confirmed VTEs, and pain, using a Visual Analogue Scales (VAS, 0 = no pain, 10 = the worst imaginable pain), knee flexion at discharge and the length of hospital stay.

Knee swelling was measured circumferentially at the thigh (taken at 10 cm above the upper pole of the patella) and the lower leg (taken at 10 cm below the lower pole of the patella), and calculated as the differences in the circumferences pre- and 48-h post-operation.

Sample size

The sample size was calculated based on the measured postoperative blood loss. We assumed an alpha error of

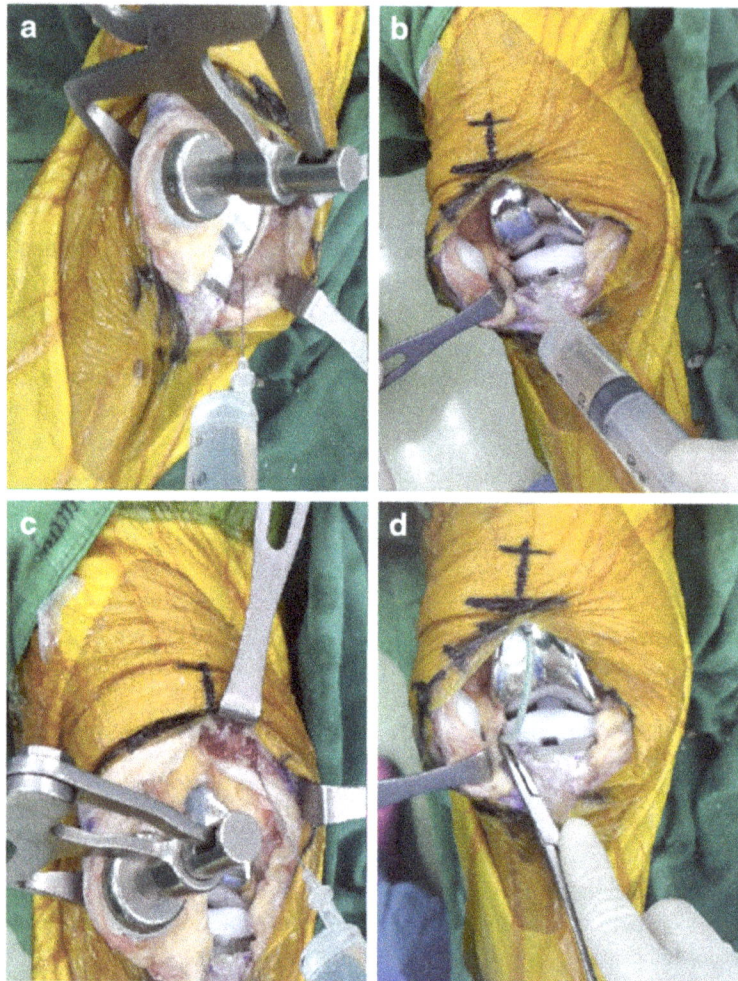

Fig. 1 Peri-articular tranexamic acid injection (right knee) at **a** the medial gutter and medial capsule, **b** the lateral gutter and lateral capsule and **c** around the quadriceps muscle. **d** One drain (Privac®; Primed Halberstadt Medizintechnik GmbH, Halberstadt, Germany) was positioned at the lateral gutter

0.05 and applied an allocation ratio of 1. A sample size of 30 participants, which allowed with a dropout rate of 10 % (3 participants), was calculated to provide a 80 % power in detecting a difference of 150 mL or reducing postoperative blood loss by 30 % in favour of the peri-articular TXA injection (from 10 patients of our earlier pilot study); we considered these parameters to be clinically relevant [24]. All statistical analyses were performed using SPSS software version 17.0 (SPSS Inc, Chicago, IL, USA). Differences in categorical variables were analyzed by chi squared or Fisher's exact test, as necessary, and the unpaired 't' test was used for normally distributed, continuous variables.

Results

Of the 63 patients seen, two were diagnosed with inflammatory arthritis and one patient with post-traumatic arthritis and so were excluded from the study. A total 60 patients were recruited, underwent a unilateral TKA and

completed the study. Half received either peri-articular (group 1) or IV (group 2) TXA. Their ages ranged from 50–80 years. There were no significant differences preoperative Body Mass Index (BMI), hemoglobin, and hematocrit level between the two groups (Table 1).

Blood loss measured in the drain postoperatively was less in group 1 at both time points but the difference was not statistically significant (Table 2). The changes in hemoglobin and hematocrit were small and similar between both groups as was the number of blood transfusions.

The postoperative leg, thigh swelling also showed no significant differences (Table 3).

VAS for pain at the 24 and 48 h assessments, postoperative knee flexion at discharge and hospital lengths of stay were similar (Table 4).

No patients had clinical evidence of tense hemarthroses, subcutaneous hematomas, peroneal nerve palsies, surgical wound infections, skin necrosis or symptomatic VTEs up to 14 days following the surgery.

Table 1 Patient characteristics at baseline

	Peri-articular group (n = 30)	Intravenous group (n = 30)	P value*
Sex (male/female)	5/25	7/23	-
Age (y)	67.63 (+/− 7.96)	69.97 (+/− 7.55)	0.248
Weight (kg)	66.88 (+/− 11.29)	65.14 (+/− 9.32)	0.517
Height (cm)	155.73 (+/− 6.59)	156.77 (+/− 6.39)	0.539
BMI (kg/m^2)	27.96 (+/− 4.99)	26.52 (+/− 3.71)	0.208
Hemoglobin (g/dL)	12.01 (+/− 1.27)	12.27 (+/− 1.30)	0.436
Hematocrit (%)	36.58 (+/− 3.63)	37.58 (+/− 3.49)	0.283

Values are number or mean (+/−Standard deviation = SD)
*P < 0.05 considered significant

Table 3 Thigh and leg circumferences (centimeters)

	Peri-articular group (n = 30)	Intravenous group (n = 30)	P value*
Thigh (cm)			
Preoperative	44.25 (+/− 6.61)	43.63 (+/− 4.24)	0.627
Postoperative	46.30 (+/− 7.03)	45.10 (+/− 4.21)	0.398
Difference	2.05 (+/− 1.47)	1.47 (+/− 1.19)	0.093
Leg (cm)			
Preoperative	35.20 (+/− 3.88)	33.57 (+/− 2.97)	0.069
Postoperative	36.57 (+/− 3.96)	34.70 (+/− 3.37)	0.052
Difference	1.39 (+/− 1.27)	1.16 (+/− 1.08)	0.491

Values are number or mean (+/−Standard deviation = SD)
*P < 0.05 considered significant

Discussion

TXA has been shown to be an effective antifibrinolytic agent for reducing blood loss following TKA [8, 10]. However, IV TXA is a systemic therapy and requires systemic distribution to exert its antibleeding effects. Peri-articular TXA injection could, theoretically, be more effective and cause less systemic toxicity like thrombosis and systemic hypersensitivity reactions [25]. Given the lack of data, a randomized trial was needed comparing peri-articular with the current standard treatment of IV TXA.

Our study has demonstrated that the 750 mg of peri-articular TXA injection group had less blood loss in the drain and lower decreases in hemoglobin concentration but a slight increase in the number of blood transfusion rates which would be from lower initial hemoglobin level

in the peri-articular TXA injection group. Although none of these differences were statistically significant, the data hint that the antibleeding effects may have been roughly similar. This was a pilot study using a "best guess" dose. No dose ranging studies have been conducted to determine the optimal peri-articular dose and this is an area of future research.

There are the case reports of VTEs associated with IV TXA administration which is concern to the surgeon [16, 17]. Two recent meta-analyses of IV TXA in TKA was unable to conclude definitively on its safety because the studies were underpowered [26, 27]. Our study found no VTE in either group but our patient numbers were very small. The peri-articular TXA injection group did not show signs of drug toxicity as evidenced by the

Table 2 Blood loss and blood transfusions

Variable	Group 1: Peri-articular group (n = 30)	Group 2: Intravenous group (n = 30)	P value*
Blood in Hemovac drain(ml)			
24-h postoperative	300 (+/− 128)	334 (+/− 124)	0.279
48-h postoperative	145 (+/− 92)	186 (+/− 106)	0.094
Total	445 (+/− 158)	520 (+/− 175)	0.081
Hematocrit (%)			
Preoperative	36.4 (+/− 3.6)	37.6 (+/− 3.5)	0.226
24-h postoperative	29.7 (+/− 3.4)	30.4 (+/− 4.0)	0.550
48-h postoperative	31.0 (+/− 2.7)	31.8 (+/− 3.4)	0.352
Total Hct change (%) (pre op − 48 hr)	−5.4 (+/− 3.1)	−5.8 (+/− 4.4)	0.730
Hemoglobin (g/dL)			
preoperative	12.01 (+/− 1.27)	12.27 (+/− 1.30)	0.628
24-h postoperative	9.69 (+/− 1.19)	10.09 (+/− 1.50)	0.215
48-h postoperative	10.16 (+/− 0.98)	10.40 (+/− 1.28)	0.693
Total Hb change (g/dL) (pre op − 48 hr)	−1.85 (+/− 0.95)	−1.87 (+/− 1.37)	0.840
Total blood transfusion (PRC in unit)	12	8	-
Number of patients with blood transfusion	9	7	0.928

Values are number or mean (+/−Standard deviation = SD)
*P < 0.05 considered significant

Table 4 Visual Analogue score (VAS) for pain, knee flexion at discharge, and length of hospital stay

	Peri-articular group (n = 30)	Intravenous group (n = 30)	P value*
VAS (0–10)			
24-h postoperative	3.8 (+/− 2.48)	3.70 (+/− 2.44)	0.889
48-h postoperative	3.56 (+/− 1.89)	3.43 (+/− 1.67)	0.724
Knee flexion at discharge	97° (+/− 10.87°)	90° (+/− 17.41°)	0.087
Hospital stay(Days)	5.7 (+/− 1.46)	5.3 (+/− 0.84)	0.276

Values are number or mean (+/−Standard deviation = SD)
*P < 0.05 considered significant

lack of local physical signs, like excess bleeding, swelling, and wound infections. This is a promising finding but more studies are needed, including dose ranging studies to ascertain if toxicity is dose related. Trying to detect if there might be differences in risk of VTEs between peri-articular and IV TXA would require very large sample sizes and is best left to pharmacovigilance if peri-articular TXA becomes an established practice. We acknowledge our study's limitations. The sample size was small and so we were underpowered to detect uncommon events like VTEs. Moreover, we were guided by symptoms and signs of VTEs and did not actively seek asymptomatic VTEs. A lack of resources precluded the monitoring of serum TXA concentrations which could have suggested under or over exposure of IV TXA. We did not establish placebo group in the study, since the administration of IV TXA is a standard protocol for our patients and possible problem with ethical issues. The previous prospective randomized controlled trial study comparing IV TXA with placebo in the patients undergone TKA found significantly lower blood loss in IV TXA group [13].

Conclusions

Our small pilot study has shown promising initial results regarding peri-articular TXA injection. This, in primary TKA, peri-articular TXA injection could be an alternative route of TXA administration. More research is needed to determine the optimal TXA dose and define better the risks and benefits.

Abbrevations

BMI, body mass index; TKA, total knee arthroplasty; VAS, visual analogue scales for pain; VTE, venous thromboembolic event

Acknowledgements

We thank Thananit Sangkomkamhang, MD, for help with the statistical analysis and Dr. Bob Taylor for reviewing the manuscript. We also thank all study participants.

Funding

The study has not received any external funding.

Authors' contributions

PP participated in the design, performed the surgeries, analysis and interpretation of the data and manuscript writing. SR participated in the design, gathered data of patients, analysis and interpretation of the data and manuscript writing. SC participated in the analysis and interpretation of the data and manuscript writing or revising it critically for important intellectual content. All authors read and approved the final manuscript.

Competing interests

The authors declare that they have no competing interests.

Consent for publication

Not applicable.

References

1. Sinclair KC, Clarke HD, Noble BN. Blood management in total knee arthroplasty: a comparison of techniques. Orthopedics. 2009;32:19.
2. Gonzalez-Porras JR, Colado E, Conde MP, Lopez T, Nieto MJ, Corral M. An individualized pre-operative blood saving protocol can increase pre-operative haemoglobin levels and reduce the need for transfusion in elective total hip or knee arthroplasty. Transfus Med. 2009;19:35–42.
3. Parvizi J, Diaz-Ledezma C. Total knee replacement with the use of a tourniquet: more pros than cons. Bone Joint J. 2013;95-B(Supple A):133–4.
4. Sabatini L, Trecci A, Imarisio D, Uslenghi MD, Bianco G, Scagnelli R. Fibrin tissue adhesive reduces postoperative blood loss in total knee arthroplasty. J Orthop Traumatol. 2012;13:145–51.
5. Pitta M, Zawadsky M, Verstraete R, Rubinstein A. Intravenous administration of tranexamic acid effectively reduces blood loss in primary total knee arthroplasty in a 610-patient consecutive case series. Transfusion. 2016;56(2):466–71.
6. Wong J, Abrishami A, El Beheiry H, Mahomed NN, Roderick Davey J, Gandhi R, et al. Topical application of tranexamic acid reduces postoperative blood loss in total knee arthroplasty: a randomized, controlled trial. J Bone Joint Surg Am. 2010;92:2503–13.
7. Aggarwal AK, Singh N, Sudesh P. Topical vs Intravenous Tranexamic Acid in Reducing Blood Loss After Bilateral Total Knee Arthroplasty: A Prospective Study. J Arthroplasty. 2015 Dec 21. doi:10.1016/j.arth.2015.12.033. [Epub ahead of print]
8. Benoni G, Lethagen S, Fredin H. The effect of tranexamic acid on local and plasma fibrinolysis during total knee arthroplasty. Thromb Res. 1997;85:195–206.
9. Dunn CJ, Goa KL. Tranexamic acid: a review of its use in surgery and other indications. Drugs. 1999;57:1005–32.
10. Eubanks JD. Antifibrinolytics in major orthopaedic surgery. J Am Acad Orthop Surg. 2010;18:132–8.
11. Kluft C, Verheijen JH, Jie AF, Rijken DC, Preston FE, Sue-Ling HM, et al. The postoperative fibrinolytic shutdown: a rapidly reverting acute phase pattern for the fast-acting inhibitor of tissue-type plasminogen activator after trauma. Scand J Clin Lab Invest. 1985;45:605–10.

10. Eubanks JD. Antifibrinolytics in major orthopaedic surgery. J Am Acad Orthop Surg. 2010;18:132–8.

11. Kluft C, Verheijen JH, Jie AF, Rijken DC, Preston FE, Sue-Ling HM, et al. The postoperative fibrinolytic shutdown: a rapidly reverting acute phase pattern for the fast-acting inhibitor of tissue-type plasminogen activator after trauma. Scand J Clin Lab Invest. 1985;45:605–10.

12. Murphy WG, Davies MJ, Eduardo A. The haemostatic response to surgery and trauma. Br J Anaesth. 1993;70:205–13.

13. Charoencholvanich K, Siriwattanasakul P. Tranexamic acid reduces blood loss and blood transfusion after TKA: a prospective randomized controlled trial. Clin Orthop Relat Res. 2011;469:2874–80.

14. Orpen NM, Little C, Walker G, Crawford EJ. Tranexamic acid reduces early postoperative blood loss after total knee arthroplasty; a prospective randomized controlled trial of 29 patients. Knee. 2006;13:106–10.

15. Ortega-Andreu M, Pérez-Chrzanowska H, Figueredo R, Gómez-Barrena E. Blood loss control with two doses of tranexamic Acid in a multimodal protocol for total knee arthroplasty. Open Orthop J. 2011;5:44–8.

16. Mannucci PM. Hemostatic drugs. N Engl J Med. 1998;339:245–53.

17. Mannucci PM. Prevention and treatment of major blood loss. N Engl J Med. 2007;356:2301–11.

18. Ishida K, Tsumura N, Kitagawa A, Hamamura S, Fukuda K, Dogaki Y, et al. Intra-articular injection of tranexamic acid reduces not only blood loss but also knee joint swelling after total knee arthroplasty. Int Orthop. 2011;35:1639–45.

19. Maniar RN, Kumar G, Singhi T, Nayak RM, Maniar PR. Most effective regimen of tranexamic acid in knee arthroplasty: a prospective randomized controlled study in 240 patients. Clin Orthop Relat Res. 2012;470:2605–12.

20. Roy SP, Tanki UF, Dutta A, Jain SK, Nagi ON. Efficacy of intra-articular tranexamic acid in blood loss reduction following primary unilateral total knee arthroplasty. Knee Surg Sports Traumatol Arthrosc. 2012;20:2494–501.

21. Wang H, Shen B, Zeng Y. Blood Loss and Transfusion After Topical Tranexamic Acid Administration in Primary Total Knee Arthroplasty. Orthopedics. 2015;38(11):e1007–16. doi:10.3928/01477447-20151020-10.

22. Spreng UJ, Dahl V, Hjall A, Fagerland MW, Ræder J. High-volume local infiltration analgesia combined with intravenous or local ketorolac + morphine compared with epidural analgesia after total knee arthroplasty. Br J Anaesth. 2010;105:675–82.

23. Manor D, Sadeh M. Muscle fiber necrosis induced by intramuscular injection of drugs. Br J Exp Pathol. 1989;70:457–62.

24. Pinsornsak P, Chumchuen S. Can a modified Robert Jones bandage after knee arthroplasty reduce blood loss? A prospective randomized controlled trial. Clin Orthop Relat Res. 2013;471(5):1677–81.

25. Kagoma YK, Crowther MA, Douketis J, Bhandari M, Eikelboom J, Lim W. Use of antifibrinolytic therapy to reduce transfusion in patients undergoing orthopedic surgery: a systematic review of randomized trials. Thromb Res. 2009;123:687–96.

26. Alshryda S, Sarda P, Sukeik M, Nargol A, Blenkinsopp J, Mason JM. Tranexamic acid in total knee replacement: a systematic review and meta-analysis. J Bone Joint Surg (Br). 2011;93:1577–85.

27. Gandhi R, Evans HM, Mahomed SR, Mahomed NN. Tranexamic acid and the reduction of blood loss in total knee and hip arthroplasty: a meta-analysis. BMC Res Notes. 2013;6:184.

3

The efficacy and safety of tranexamic acid in revision total knee arthroplasty

Peng Tian[1†], Wen-bin Liu[2†], Zhi-jun Li[3], Gui-jun Xu[1], Yu-ting Huang[4] and Xin-long Ma[1*]

Abstract

Background: There is no consistent conclusion regarding the efficacy and safety of the intravenous administration of tranexamic acid (TXA) for reducing blood loss in revision total knee arthroplasty (TKA). We performed a meta-analysis of comparative trials to evaluate the efficacy and safety of TXA in revision TKA.

Methods: We conducted a search of PubMed, EMBASE, The Cochrane Library and Web of Science for randomized controlled trials (RCTs) and non-RCTs. Two authors selected the studies, extracted the data, and assessed the risk of bias independently. A pooled meta-analysis was performed using RevMan 5.3 software.

Results: Four non-RCTs met the inclusion criteria. The meta-analysis indicated that the use of TXA was related to significantly less transfusion requirements (RD = −0.25; 95% CI: -0.43 to −0.08; P = 0.005), drainage volume (MD = −321.07; 95% CI: -445.13 to −197.01, P = 0.005), hemoglobin reduction (MD = −0.52; 95% CI: -0.79 to −0.25, P = 0.0001), and length of hospital stay (MD = −2.36; 95% CI: -4.00 to −0.71, P = 0.005). No significant differences in the incidence of deep venous thrombosis (DVT) or pulmonary embolism (PE) were noted.

Conclusions: The use of TXA for patients undergoing revision TKA may reduce blood loss and transfusion requirements without increasing the risk of postoperative venous thromboembolism. Due to the limited quality of the currently available evidence, more high-quality RCTs are required.

Keywords: Knee, Arthroplasty, Revision, Tranexamic acid, Meta-analysis

Background

Total knee arthroplasty (TKA) is a common surgical method for the treatment of end-stage knee disease, which could effectively relieve knee pain and greatly improve patient quality of life [1, 2]. A substantial increase in the prevalence of TKA over time and a shift to younger ages was noted [3], such that the number of revision TKAs has increased annually [4]. The common causes of revision TKA include infection, mechanical loosening, and pain and knee instability [5]. Compared with primary TKA, revision TKA may be challenging due to longer operative time and more blood loss [6]. Controlling blood loss and reducing transfusion rates are problems that clinical orthopedic surgeons face.

Tranexamic acid (TXA) has been widely used to reduce blood loss and transfusion requirements in primary TKA [7–9]. However, little is known about the efficacy and safety of the use of TXA in revision TKA. Recently, several published studies have demonstrated that TXA could safely and effectively reduce blood loss and transfusion rates in revision TKA [10–13]. However, some of these studies have been criticized for poor design, low power, inconclusive results and small sample size. It is imperative to clarify whether the use of TXA is effective in revision TKA. Thus, we conducted a meta-analysis to ascertain whether the application of TXA would reduce blood loss and transfusion requirements in revision TKA.

* Correspondence: maxinlong868686@163.com
†Equal contributors
[1]Department of Orthopedics, Tianjin Hospital, No. 406, Jiefang Nan Road, Tianjin 300211, People's Republic of China
Full list of author information is available at the end of the article

Methods

This meta-analysis was performed in accordance with the Preferred Reporting Items for Systematic Reviews and Meta-Analyses reporting guidelines for the meta-analysis of intervention trials.

Inclusion and exclusion criteria

Studies were included if the following criteria were met: (1) study design: comparative studies (randomized controlled trials, RCTs or non-RCTs); (2) study subjects: adult patients with indications for revision TKA; (3) operative intervention: patients in the TXA group received intravenous TXA and patients in the control group received placebo or nothing; (4) outcome measures: the primary outcomes included calculated total blood loss, hidden blood loss, transfusion rate, and postoperative complications. Secondary outcomes included hemoglobin reduction, surgical duration, and length of hospital stay.

Articles that reported at least one outcome were included, and those without the outcome measures of interest were excluded. Letters, comments, editorials, reviews and practice guidelines were excluded. Any controversy was cross-checked and resolved by a third author to reach a final consensus.

Search strategy

PubMed, Medline, Embase, Web of Science and the Cochrane Library were searched up to October 2016 for comparative studies involving TXA for reducing blood loss in patients undergoing revision TKA. The search terms were as follows: "tranexamic acid", "knee arthroplasty", "knee replacement" and "revision". The language for the publications was limited to English. The titles and abstracts of studies identified in the search were reviewed to exclude clearly irrelevant studies. The reference lists of all eligible studies and relevant reviews were searched manually for additional trials. The search for titles and abstracts was conducted independently by two reviewers. Disagreements were resolved by consulting a third reviewer.

Quality assessment

Two authors independently assessed the risk of bias of the included studies. RCTs were assessed with the RCT bias risk assessment tools of the Cochrane Handbook Version 5.3 [14]. Non-RCTs were assessed with the Methodological Index for Non-randomized Studies (MINORS) [15]. Disagreement was resolved by the third author.

Data extraction

For each eligible study, both reviewers extracted all the relevant data independently. Data available in articles or tracked by e-mail were extracted independently by two authors. The following variables were recorded: name of the first author, year of publication, sample size, participant sex and age, revision reason, surgical approach, anesthesia and outcome measurements. Data in other forms (i.e., median, interquartile range, and mean ± 95% confidence interval (CI)) were converted to mean ± standard deviation (SD) according to the Cochrane Handbook. If data were not reported numerically, we extracted them by manual measurements from published figures.

Data analysis and statistical methods

All statistical analyses were performed with Review Manager (version 5.3 for Windows, The Cochrane Collaboration, The Nordic Cochrane Centre, Copenhagen, 2008). The mean difference (MD) with a 95% CI was calculated for continuous data. The risk difference (RD) with 95% CI was calculated for dichotomous data. Heterogeneity among studies was estimated using the I^2 statistic; substantial heterogeneity was represented by $I^2 > 50\%$. A random effects model was used if the heterogeneity test was not significant ($I^2 > 50\%$; $P < 0.1$). Otherwise, we adopted the fixed-effects model, and $P < 0.05$ was considered significant. Subgroup analysis was performed to explore the impact of an individual study by removing one study from the analysis each time.

Results

Study characteristics

The search process is shown in Fig. 1. Table 1 summarizes the characteristics of the four included studies, which were published between 2012 and 2016. The studies' sample size was 47–422 patients. All of the trials involved revision TKA. Baseline characteristics between the two groups in each study were well matched. All included studies reported the use of a tourniquet and chemoprophylaxis for deep venous thrombosis (DVT) or pulmonary embolism (PE). All included studies reported no differences in preoperative hemoglobin between the two groups. All studies described an indication for transfusion associated with a reduction in hemoglobin level or hematocrit and clinical symptoms. Thromboembolic complications, such as DVT or PE, were reported in three studies [10, 12, 13]. Two included studies reported that revision components were implanted in both the femur and the tibia [10, 11]. The other two studies stated patients were undergoing revision of two components, revision of one component, or an isolated liner exchange.

Risk of bias assessment

Four included studies were non-RCTs, and the MINORS scores were 18–20 for the retrospectively controlled trials. The methodological quality assessment is presented in Table 2.

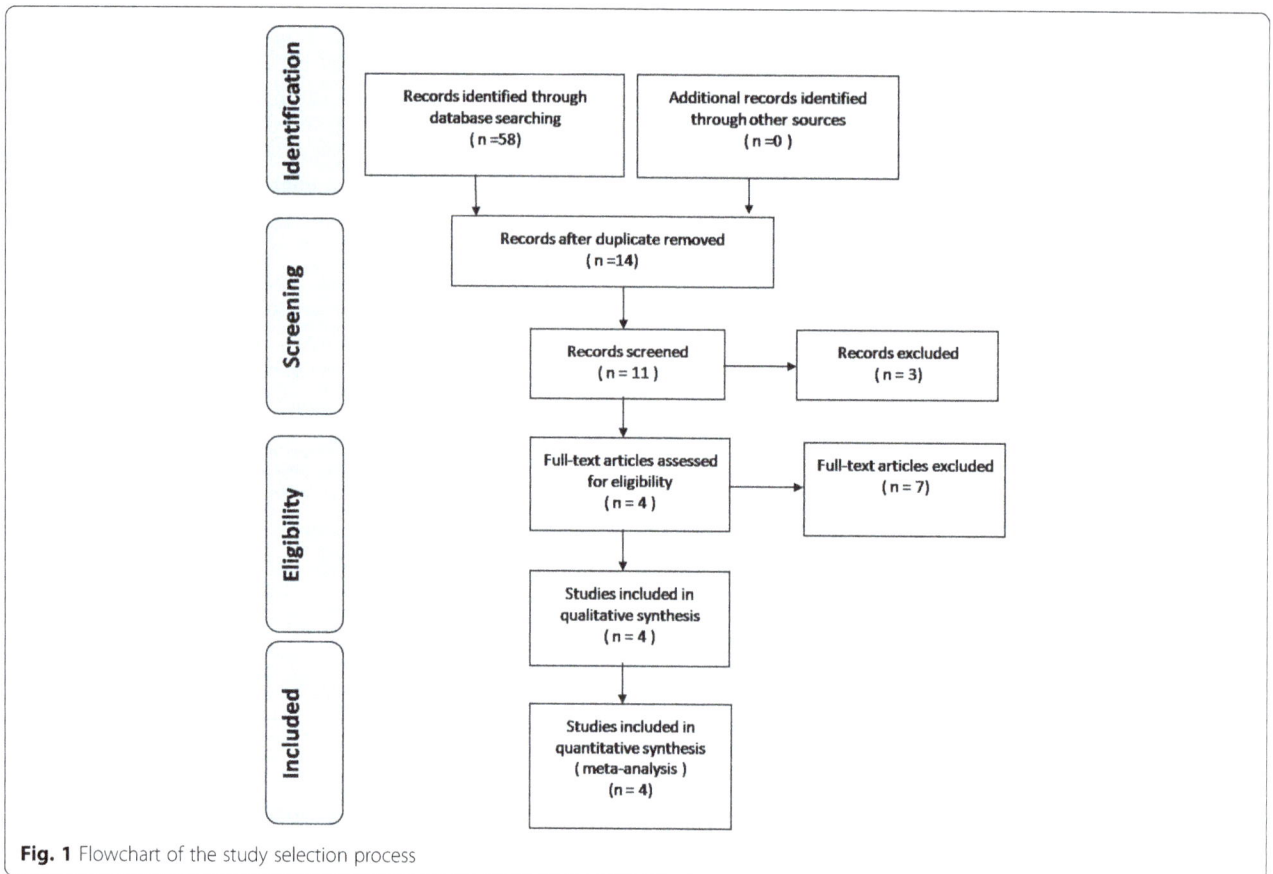

Fig. 1 Flowchart of the study selection process

Outcomes of the meta-analysis
Transfusion requirements
Four studies involving 667 patients were used to perform a meta-analysis on the requirements of blood transfusion [10–13]. The transfusion rate was 14.5% and 33.8% in the TXA (51 patients) and control groups (107 patients), respectively. Significant heterogeneity was observed, and a random effects model was used ($I^2 = 85\%$, $P = 0.0002$). The meta-analysis revealed significant differences in transfusion requirements between the two groups (RD = −0.25; 95% CI: -0.43 to −0.08; $P = 0.005$, Table 3).

Drainage volume
Data from two studies involving 135 patients were available to examine drainage volume [10, 11]. No significant heterogeneity was observed, and a fixed effects model was used ($I^2 = 0\%$, $P = 0.68$). The application of TXA in revision TKA produced significantly less drainage

Table 1 Characteristics of included studies

Study	Group	Simple size	Age (Y)	Gender (M/F)	Preoperative hemoglobin (g/l)	Intervention	Diagnosis
Aguilera 2012 [10]	TXA	19	75	2/17	132	1 g	Aseptic loosening
	Control	28	74	9/19	134		
Ortega-Andreu 2016 [11]	TXA	44	68.8	12/32	141	two doses of 15 mg/kg per dose	Aseptic loosening; Pain; Polyethylene wear; Prosthesis malposition; Fracture
	Control	43	74.2	11/32	138		
Samujh 2014 [12]	TXA	43	65.4	14/19	132	15 mg/Kg	NS
	Control	68	64.7	29/39	135		
Smit 2013 [13]	TXA	246	68.9	121/125	132.1	20 mg/Kg	Loosening; Infection; Polywear; Instability; Stiffness; Malalignment; Patellar problems; Pain
	Control	178	69.8	87/91	129.9		

Table 2 Quality assessment for non-randomized trials

Quality assessment for non-randomized trials	Aguilera 2012 [10]	Ortega-Andreu 2016 [11]	Samujh 2014 [12]	Smit 2013 [13]
A clearly stated aim	2	2	2	2
Inclusion of consecutive patients	2	2	2	2
Prospective data collection	2	2	2	2
Endpoints appropriate to the aim of the study	2	2	2	2
Unbiased assessment of the study endpoint	0	0	0	0
A follow-up period appropriate to theaims of study	2	2	2	2
Less than 5% loss to follow-up	2	2	2	2
Prospective calculation of the sample size	0	0	0	0
An adequate control group	2	2	2	2
Contemporary groups	0	2	1	2
Baseline equivalence of groups	2	2	2	2
Adequate statistical analyses	2	2	2	2
Total score	18	20	19	20

volume compared with the control group (MD = −321.07; 95% CI: -445.13 to −197.01, P = 0.005, Table 3).

Hemoglobin reduction

Two studies involving 511 patients reported hemoglobin reduction after revision TKA [11, 13]. No significant heterogeneity was observed, and a fixed effects model was used (I^2 = 62%, P = 0.11). A significant difference was observed between the two groups regarding the amount of hemoglobin reduction after revision TKA (MD = −0.52; 95% CI: -0.79 to −0.25, P = 0.0001, Table 3).

Length of hospital stay

Data were available from three studies involving 558 patients [10, 11, 13]. Significant heterogeneity was observed, and a random effects model was used (I^2 = 70%, P = 0.04). A statistically significant difference in the length of hospital stay was noted between the two groups (MD = −2.36; 95% CI: -4.00 to −0.71, P = 0.005, Table 3).

Deep venous thrombosis

Three studies reported the post-operative incidence of DVT [10, 12, 13]. No significant heterogeneity was

observed, and a fixed effects model was used (I^2 = 0%, P = 0.97). The meta-analysis revealed no significant difference in the post-operative incidence of DVT between the two groups (MD = 0.00, 95% CI: -0.01 to 0.02, P = 0.69, Table 3).

Pulmonary embolism

Two studies reported the post-operative incidence of PE [12, 13]. No significant heterogeneity was observed, and a fixed effects model was used (I^2 = 0%, P = 0.89). The meta-analysis revealed no significant difference in the post-operative incidence of PE between two groups (MD = −0.01, 95% CI: -0.03 to 0.01, P = 0.18, Table 3).

Discussion

Although the patients with TKA can experience good functional outcomes and long-term implant survivorship [2], TKA failure and revision TKA continue to be a significant clinical challenge for orthopedic surgeons. Revision TKA could produce more blood loss and higher transfusion rates compared with primary TKA [16]. Perioperative blood loss is an inevitable

Table 3 Meta-analysis results

Outcome	Studies	Groups (TXA/Placebo)	Overall effect			Heterogeneity	
			Effect estimate	95% CI	p-Value	I^2(%)	p-Value
Transfusion requirements	4	352/317	−0.25	−0.43, −0.08	0.005	85	0.0002
Drainage volume	2	63/72	−321.07	−445.13, −197.01	0.005	0	0.68
Hb reduction	2	290/221	−0.52	−0.79, −0.25	0.0001	62	0.11
Length of hospital stay	3	309/249	−2.36	−4.00, −0.71	0.005	70	0.04
Deep venous thrombosis	3	308/274	0.00	−0.01, 0.02	0.69	0	0.97
Pulmonary embolism	2	289/246	−0.01	−0.03, 0.01	0.18	0	0.89

TXA tranexamic acid, *CI* confidence interval

complication of revision TKA, which could lead to anemia. Effective blood management can minimize blood loss and transfusions such that patients achieve better results. TXA, an antifibrinolytic agent, could be effective and safe in reducing blood loss in primary TKA. The main applications of TXA are intravenous or intra-articular injection. However, there is relatively little research on the role and dosing regimen of TXA in revision TKA.

The most important findings of the present meta-analysis are that the application of intravenous TXA for patients undergoing revision TKA may reduce the transfusion rate, drainage volume, hemoglobin reduction and length of hospital stay without increasing the risks of DVT or PE. To our knowledge, this is the first meta-analysis of comparative trials to evaluate the efficacy and safety of TXA in revision TKA.

To date, the efficacy and safety of intravenous TXA for reducing blood loss and transfusion rates in revision TKA remains controversial. Many scholars continue to explore the strategy of intravenous TXA administration in revision TKA. In revision TKA, preoperative hemoglobin could be an important factor to avoid transfusion. All included studies indicated no differences from preoperative hemoglobin between two groups. The present meta-analysis demonstrated that hemoglobin reduction was reduced in the TXA group compared with the control group.

The pooled results demonstrated significant differences in the transfusion rate between the TXA group and the control group. The transfusion rate was 14.5% and 33.8% in the TXA group and the control group, respectively. Aguilera et al. [10] first evaluated the effectiveness of TXA in revision TKA and provided evidence that the early administration of TXA could decrease the transfusion rate of the patients with revision TKA. Ortega-Andreu et al. [11] confirmed that a two-dose intravenous administration of TXA in revision TKA was effective in decreasing hemoglobin loss and the transfusion rate. Although all included studies described an indication for transfusion associated with a reduction in hemoglobin level or hematocrit and clinical symptoms, the outcome of units transfused was reported in two studies that were not analyzed owing to insufficient data.

The application of TXA could reduce postoperative drainage volume and earlier drainage tube removal, which could be helpful for rapid recovery [11]. TXA could also be associated with shortening the length of hospital stay [13]. The present meta-analysis revealed that the application of TXA could significantly reduce the average length of hospital stay and drainage in patients undergoing revision TKA. Reducing transfusion rates and minimizing the average length of hospital stay could reduce financial burden. According to the cost savings calculation [17], there would be a potential yearly cost savings of $22,300 with the application of TXA in revision TKA [13].

The application of TXA did not increase the incidence of DVT and PE in patients undergoing primary TKA. Therefore, the application of TXA is mainly concerned about the incidence of thromboembolic events in revision TKA. In the present meta-analysis, no significant differences in the incidence of DVT or PE were noted between the TXA group and the control group.

It is imperative to acknowledge some potential limitations in our meta-analysis: (1) the sample sizes of the included studies were relatively small, (2) the methodologies of the included studies have their own limitations, and (3) there were some differences in TXA and dosing regimen. Given the above defects and deficiencies, the pooled estimates should be explored with caution.

Conclusion

The application of intravenous TXA for patients undergoing revision TKA may reduce transfusion rate, drainage volume, hemoglobin reduction and length of hospital stay without increasing the risks of DVT or PE. Due to the limited quality and data from the studies currently available, more high-quality randomized controlled trials are required.

Abbreviations
CI: Confidence intervals; DVT: Deep venous thrombosis; MD: Mean difference; MINORS: Methodological Index for Non-randomized Studies; PE: Pulmonary embolism; RD: Risk difference; SD: Standard deviation; TKA: Total knee arthroplasty; TXA: Tranexamic acid

Acknowledgements
We would like to acknowledge all authors of the original studies included in this meta-analysis.

Funding
This work was supported by funding from National Natural Science Foundation of China (no. 81572154; no. 81401792).

Authors' contributions
PT, WBL and XLM conceived of the design of the study. PT, YTH, GJX and ZJL performed and collected the data and contributed to the design of the study. PT, ZJL and XLM prepared and revised the manuscript. All authors read and approved the final content of the manuscript.

Authors' information
The author information can be found in the title page.

Competing interests
The authors declare that they have no competing interests.

Consent for publication
Not applicable.

Author details
[1]Department of Orthopedics, Tianjin Hospital, No. 406, Jiefang Nan Road, Tianjin 300211, People's Republic of China. [2]Department of Joint Surgery, Tianjin Hospital, No. 406, Jiefang Nan Road, Tianjin 300211, People's Republic of China. [3]Department of Orthopedics, General Hospital of Tianjin Medical University, No. 154, Anshan Road, Tianjin 300052, People's Republic of China. [4]Cancer & Immunology Research, Children's Research Institute, Children's National Medical Center, 111 Michigan Avenue, NW, Washington, DC 20010, USA.

References
1. De Martino I, D'Apolito R, Sculco PK, Poultsides LA, Gasparini G. Total knee Arthroplasty using Cementless porous tantalum Monoblock Tibial component: a minimum 10-year follow-up. J Arthroplast. 2016;31(10):2193–8.
2. Keating EM, Meding JB, Faris PM, Ritter MA. Long-term followup of nonmodular total knee replacements. Clin Orthop Relat Res. 2002;404:34–9.
3. Maradit Kremers H, Larson DR, Crowson CS, Kremers WK, Washington RE, Steiner CA, et al. Prevalence of Total hip and knee replacement in the United States. J Bone Joint Surg Am. 2015;97(17):1386–97.
4. Patel A, Pavlou G, Mujica-Mota RE, Toms AD. The epidemiology of revision total knee and hip arthroplasty in England and Wales: a comparative analysis with projections for the United States. A study using the National Joint Registry dataset. Bone Joint J. 2015;97-B(8):1076–81.
5. Bozic KJ, Kurtz SM, Lau E, Ong K, Chiu V, Vail TP, et al. The epidemiology of revision total knee arthroplasty in the United States. Clin Orthop Relat Res. 2010;468(1):45–51.
6. Hamilton DF, Howie CR, Burnett R, Simpson AH, Patton JT. Dealing with the predicted increase in demand for revision total knee arthroplasty: challenges, risks and opportunities. Bone Joint J. 2015;97-B(6):723–8.
7. Alshryda S, Sarda P, Sukeik M, Nargol A, Blenkinsopp J, Mason JM. Tranexamic acid in total knee replacement: a systematic review and meta-analysis. J Bone Joint Surg Br. 2011;93(12):1577–85.
8. Tan J, Chen H, Liu Q, Chen C, Huang W. A meta-analysis of the effectiveness and safety of using tranexamic acid in primary unilateral total knee arthroplasty. J Surg Res. 2013;184(2):880–7.
9. Yang ZG, Chen WP, Wu LD. Effectiveness and safety of tranexamic acid in reducing blood loss in total knee arthroplasty: a meta-analysis. J Bone Joint Surg Am. 2012;94(13):1153–9.
10. Aguilera X, Videla S, Almenara M, Fernandez JA, Gich I, Celaya F. Effectiveness of tranexamic acid in revision total knee arthroplasty. Acta Orthop Belg. 2012;78(1):68–74.
11. Ortega-Andreu M, Talavera G, Padilla-Eguiluz NG, Perez-Chrzanowska H, Figueredo-Galve R, Rodriguez-Merchan CE, et al. Tranexamic acid in a multimodal blood loss prevention protocol to decrease blood loss in revision Total knee Arthroplasty: a cohort study. Open Orthop J. 2016;10:439–47.
12. Samujh C, Falls TD, Wessel R, Smith L, Malkani AL. Decreased blood transfusion following revision total knee arthroplasty using tranexamic acid. J Arthroplast. 2014;29(9 Suppl):182–5.
13. Smit KM, Naudie DD, Ralley FE, Berta DM, Howard JL. One dose of tranexamic acid is safe and effective in revision knee arthroplasty. J Arthroplast. 2013;28(8 Suppl):112–5.
14. Li ZJ, Wang Y, Zhang HF, Ma XL, Tian P, Huang Y. Effectiveness of low-level laser on carpal tunnel syndrome: a meta-analysis of previously reported randomized trials. Medicine (Baltimore). 2016;95(31):e4424.
15. Slim K, Nini E, Forestier D, Kwiatkowski F, Panis Y, Chipponi J. Methodological index for non-randomized studies (minors): development and validation of a new instrument. ANZ J Surg. 2003;73(9):712–6.
16. Cankaya D, Della Valle CJ. Blood loss and transfusion rates in the revision of Unicompartmental knee Arthroplasty to Total knee Arthroplasty are similar to those of primary Total knee Arthroplasty but are lower compared with the revision Total knee Arthroplasty. J Arthroplast. 2016;31(1):339–41.
17. Ralley FE, Berta D, Binns V, Howard J, Naudie DD. One intraoperative dose of tranexamic acid for patients having primary hip or knee arthroplasty. Clin Orthop Relat Res. 2010;468(7):1905–11.

The efficacy and safety of autologous blood transfusion drainage in patients undergoing total knee arthroplasty

Jian-ke Pan[1†], Kun-hao Hong[2†], Hui Xie[1†], Ming-hui Luo[1], Da Guo[1] and Jun Liu[1*]

Abstract

Background: Autologous blood transfusion drainage (ABTD) has been used for many years to reduce blood loss in total knee arthroplasty (TKA). We evaluate the current evidence concerning the efficiency and safety of ABTD used in TKA compared with conventional suction drainage (CSD).

Methods: We performed a systematic literature search of the PubMed, Embase, Cochrane Library and four Chinese databases. All randomized controlled trials (RCTs) that compared the effects of ABTD versus CSD in TKA were included in the meta-analysis.

Results: Sixteen RCTs involving 1534 patients who compared the effects of ABTD versus CSD were included. Five of the RCTs were performed in Asia, ten in Europe, and one in North America. Patients in the ABTD group had a lower blood transfusion rate (OR: 0.25 [0.13, 0.47]; $Z = 4.27$, $P < 0.0001$) and fewer units transfused per patient (WMD: -0.68 [-0.98, -0.39]; $Z = 4.52$, $P < 0.00001$) than did patients in the CSD group. Wound complications, deep vein thrombosis, febrile complications, post-operative hemoglobin days 5–8, drainage volume, and length of hospital stay did not differ significantly between the two types of drainage systems.

Conclusion: This meta-analysis suggests that ABTD is a safe and effective method that yields a lower blood transfusion rate and fewer units transfused per patient in TKA compared with CSD.

Keywords: Autologous blood transfusion drainage, Total knee arthroplasty, Meta-analysis, Randomized controlled trials

Background

Total knee arthroplasty (TKA) can result in significant blood loss [1, 2]. One study estimated the average blood loos in TKA to be 1500 mL [3]. The average reduction in Hb concentration after TKA has been estimated to be 3.85 g/dL [4]. Blood transfusion may be considered necessary in some patients to avoid symptomatic anemia and subsequent delays in postoperative rehabilitation [5]. The blood transfusion rate in TKA reach 39 % [2, 6, 7].

Conventional suction drainage (CSD) is used worldwide for postoperative wound blood collection in TKA [8]. Formerly, CSD was believed to be effective in decreasing hematoma formation [9–11] and potentially able to decrease postoperative pain, swelling, and the incidence of infection [12]. However, a closed suction drainage system increases bleeding because it eliminates the tamponade effect of a closed, undrained wound [8]. Surgeons use adjunctive measures such as autologous blood transfusion drainage (ABTD) to reduce excessive blood loss from the drain [13], and recent studies have shown that ABTD can decrease the rate of blood transfusion [14–16].

The efficacy and safety of ABTD in the management of a patient's blood during TKA surgery was assessed in a previous meta-analysis of eight randomized controlled trials (RCTs) [17]. The meta-analysis showed that ABTD was superior to CSD with respect to the blood

* Correspondence: liujun.gdtcm@hotmail.com
[†]Equal contributors
[1]Department of Orthopedics, Second Affiliated Hospital of Guangzhou University of Chinese Medicine (Guangdong Provincial Hospital of Chinese Medicine), No 111 Dade Road, Guangzhou, Guangdong 510120, China
Full list of author information is available at the end of the article

transfusion rate (OR: 0.25 [0.13, 0.47]; $P < 0.0001$), the number of units transfused per patient (WMD: -0.84 [-1.13, -0.56]; $P < 0.0001$), and the length of hospital stay (WMD: -0.25 [-0.48, -0.01]; $P = 0.04$). However, data extraction errors involving the number of patients requiring homologous blood transfusion occurred with two of the studies [18, 19] included in the meta-analysis. Furthermore, the meta-analysis did not employ intention-to-treat (ITT) analysis, which may have led to anti-conservative estimates of treatment effectiveness. In addition, systematic reviews that fail to search non-English databases may miss relevant studies and cause selection bias [20]. As trials with statistically significant results are more likely to be published in English than are those with non-significant results [21], systematic reviews that include studies published only in English might overestimate true effects, In addition, the previous meta-analysis did not evaluate the outcomes of additional measures such as wound complications (including wound infection, wound abscess, wound dehiscence, and wound hematoma) and febrile complications.

In recent years, several studies comparing ABTD and CSD have reported conflicting outcomes [1, 22–24]. Whether the benefits of ABTD are limited to the reduction of the blood transfusion rate is unclear. Therefore, we comprehensively searched several bibliographic databases to identify RCTs conducted to date. We then analyzed the clinical evidence to evaluate the effectiveness and safety of ABTD relative to CSD. We also investigated the potential benefits of ABTD.

Methods

In accordance with Preferred Reporting Items for Systematic Reviews and Meta-analysis [25], we made a prospective protocol of objectives, literature-search strategies, inclusion and exclusion criteria, outcome measurements, and methods of statistical analysis before the research began.

Data sources and search strategies

A systematic literature search of the Pubmed (1950–February 2016), Embase (1974–February 2016), Cochrane Library (February 2016 Issue 2), Chinese Biomedical Literature (CBM) (1990 to February 2016), China National Knowledge Infrastructure (CNKI) (1979 to February 2016), Chinese Scientific Journals (VIP) (1989 to February 2016) and Wanfang (1982 to February 2016) databases was conducted. The following MeSH terms or Emtree terms and their combinations were searched in [Title/Abstract]: "Drainage", "Suction", "Blood Transfusion, Autologous", "Operative Blood Salvage", "Arthroplasty, Replacement, Knee" or "wound drainage", "closed

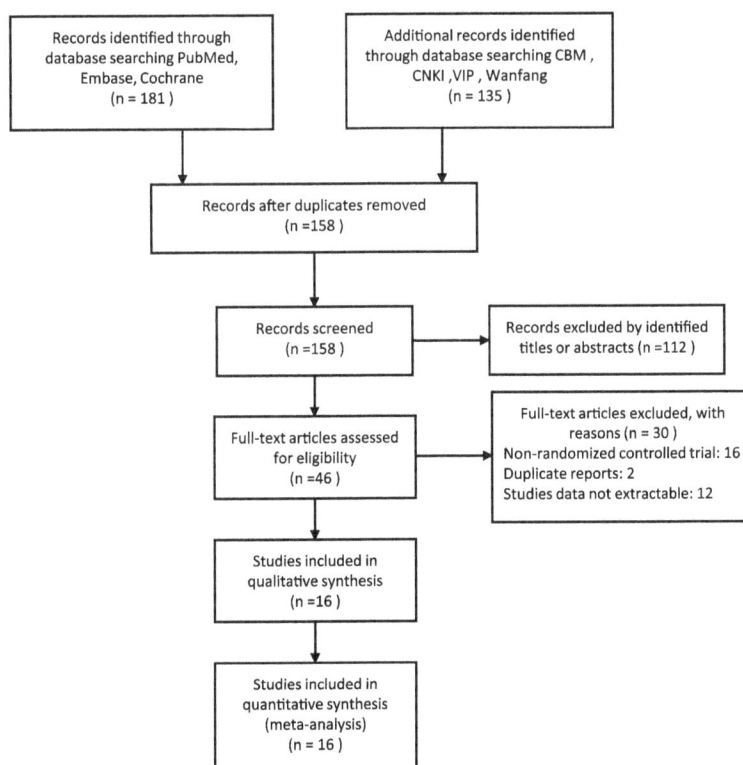

Fig. 1 Flow diagram of studies identified, included, and excluded

Table 1 Characteristics of the included studies

Study	Country	Jadad score	Patients, no.		Surgical method	Age[a]		M:F ratio		Pre-op Hb[a]	
			ABTD	CSD		ABTD	CSD	ABTD	CSD	ABTD	CSD
Deng YJ 2015 [40]	China	1	11	12	B-TKA	57.7 ± 16.3	60.7 ± 17.3	5:6	5:7	13.4 ± 3.6	13.5 ± 3.7
Jin CH 2014 [42]	China	1	70	70	SU-TKA	66 ± 4	64 ± 4	12:58	13:57	13.1 ± 1.3	13. 2 ± 1. 4
Sun YT 2014 [39]	China	1	72	60	SU-TKA	65.3	64.7	15:57	13:47	13.1 ± 1.4	13.4 ± 2.0
Amin A 2008 [29]	UK	2	92	86	SU-TKA	70.3	70.4	43:49	39:47	13.2 ± 1.2	13.4 ± 1.3
Shen Y 2007 [41]	China	0	60	60	SU-TKA	NA	NA	NA	NA	NA	NA
Zacharopoulos A 2007 [30]	Greece	1	30	30	SU-TKA	69.2	70.2	6:24	7:23	NA	NA
Abuzakuk T 2007 [31]	UK	2	52	52	SU-TKA	NA	NA	21:31	22:30	13.6 ± 1.5	13.5 ± 1.2
Kirkos JM 2006 [32]	Greece	0	78	77	SU-TKA	69.1 ± 5.5	68.9 ± 5.1	18:60	10:67	13.0 ± 1.4	13.1 ± 1.4
Dramis A 2006 [33]	UK	1	25	24	SU-TKA	NA	NA	NA	NA	NA	NA
Cheng SC 2005 [34]	China	2	26	34	SU-TKA	72	69.6	6:20	12:22	12.4	12.8
Thomas D 2001 [35]	UK	2	115	116	SU-TKA	NA	NA	44:71	55:61	NA	NA
Breakwell LM 2000 [36]	UK	1	14	19	B-TKA	66.8	73.7	8:6	8:11	12.9	12.8
Adalberth G 1998 [18]	Sweden	3	30	30	SU-TKA	71 ± 5.4	72 ± 8.0	NA	NA	13.8 ± 1.1	14.3 ± 1.3
Newman J 1997 [37]	UK	2	35	35	SU-TKA	NA	NA	NA	NA	13.4 ± 1.2	13.2 ± 1.4
Heddle NM 1992 [19]	Canada	3	39	40	SU-TKA	69.3 ± 6.9	71.0 ± 9.0	25:14	26:14	NA	NA
Majkowski RS 1991 [38]	UK	1	20	20	SU-TKA	71.3	70.3	6:14	6:14	13.2	12.7

SU-TKA selective unilateral total knee replacement, *B-TKA* bilateral total knee replacement, *ABTD* autologous blood transfusion drainage, *CSD* conventional suction drain, *NA* data not available, *M* male, *F* female, *Pre-op Hb* pre-operative hemoglobin
[a]Mean or Mean ± SD

drainage", "drainage catheter", "drainage tube", "suction drain", "surgical drainage", "drain", "wound drain", "blood autotransfusion", "autotransfusion unit", "blood salvage", "knee arthroplasty". (See Additional file 1 for details on the search strategies.) Only articles that were originally written in English or Chinese or that had been translated into English were considered. Unpublished trials were not included. When multiple reports describing the same population were published, the most recent or complete report was used. Additional eligible studies were sought by searching the reference lists of primary articles and relevant reviews.

Inclusion criteria

All available RCTs that compared ABTD with CSD in TKA and for which one or more comparable quantitative outcomes (the quantitative data must be presented as means and standard deviations or 95 % confidence intervals) could be extracted and analyzed were included.

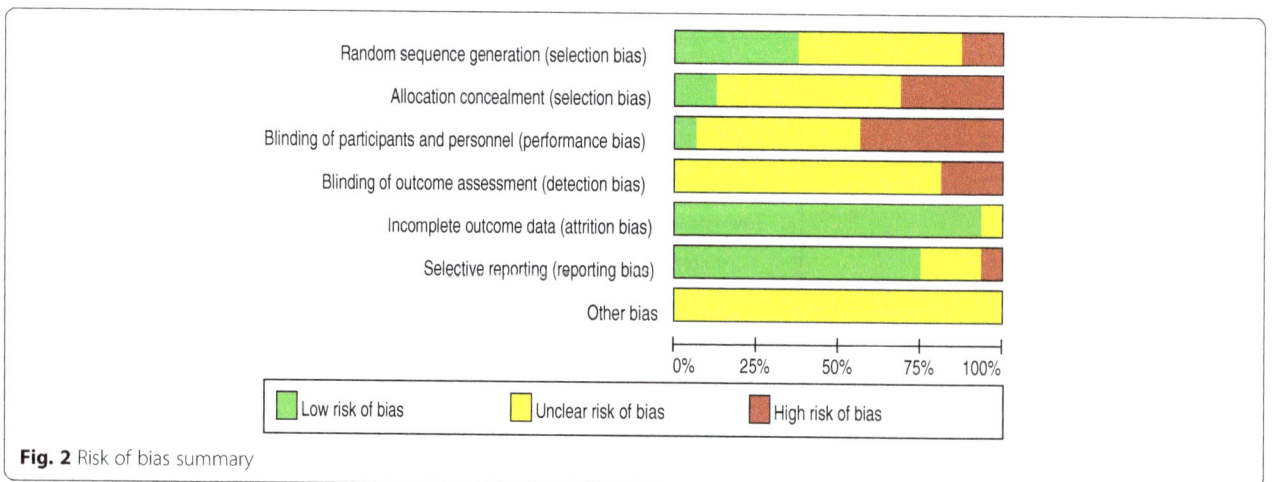

Fig. 2 Risk of bias summary

The efficacy and safety of autologous blood transfusion drainage in patients undergoing total knee...

27

Exclusion criteria

We excluded case reports, non-original research (e.g., review articles, editorials, letters to the editor), non-human animal studies, and duplicate publications.

Data extraction and analysis

Data abstraction was conducted by two authors (Hong and Xie) independently. In cases of disagreement, consensus was established through discussion with two other experienced authors (Pan and J. Liu).

The primary outcomes were blood transfusion rate, mean number of units transfused per patient, wound complications, and deep vein thrombosis.

The secondary outcomes were febrile complications, post-operative hemoglobin on days 5–8, drainage volume, and length of hospital stay.

Quality assessment

The Jadad quality scale [26] and the Cochrane risk of bias tool [27] were used to assess the methodological quality of the included RCTs. Studies with a Jadad score ≥ 3 were considered high quality, and those with a Jadad score ≤2 were considered low quality.

Data synthesis and analysis

We based our analysis on intent-to-treat (ITT) or modi-fied ITT data. Review Manager 5.3.5 (Cochrane) was employed for the meta-analysis. Odds ratios (ORs) and 95 % confidence intervals (CIs) were calculated for blood transfusion rate, wound complications, deep vein thrombosis and febrile complications. Weighted mean differences (WMDs) and 95 % CIs were calculated for the mean number of units transfused per patient, post-operative hemoglobin on days 5–8, drainage volume, and length of hospital stay. We regarded the volume of one unit of transfused blood as approximately 300 mL [18, 28]. When continuous data from the included studies were presented as means and 95 % confidence intervals, standard deviations were calculated by using Review Manager 5.3.5 (Cochrane).

Heterogeneity among the studies was assessed using the I-square test. Where heterogeneity ($I^2 > 50$ %) was detected, a random-effects model was applied; otherwise, a fixed-effects model was applied [27]. For outcome measures with I^2 values greater than 50 %, we conducted sensitivity analyses to determine the source. Funnel plots were inspected visually to assess the possibility of publication bias.

Results

Study selection

Sixteen [18, 19, 29–42] studies including 1534 cases (769 cases for ABTD and 765 cases for CSD) met the inclusion criteria and were included in the final analysis

(Fig. 1). Search of the reference lists revealed no additional studies that met the inclusion criteria.

Characteristics of the included studies

The characteristics of the included studies are summarized in Table 1. Four studies [39–42] were identified from Chinese databases, and 12 studies [18, 19, 29–38] were identified from international databases. Geographically, five RCTs were performed in Asia, 10 in Europe, and one in North America.

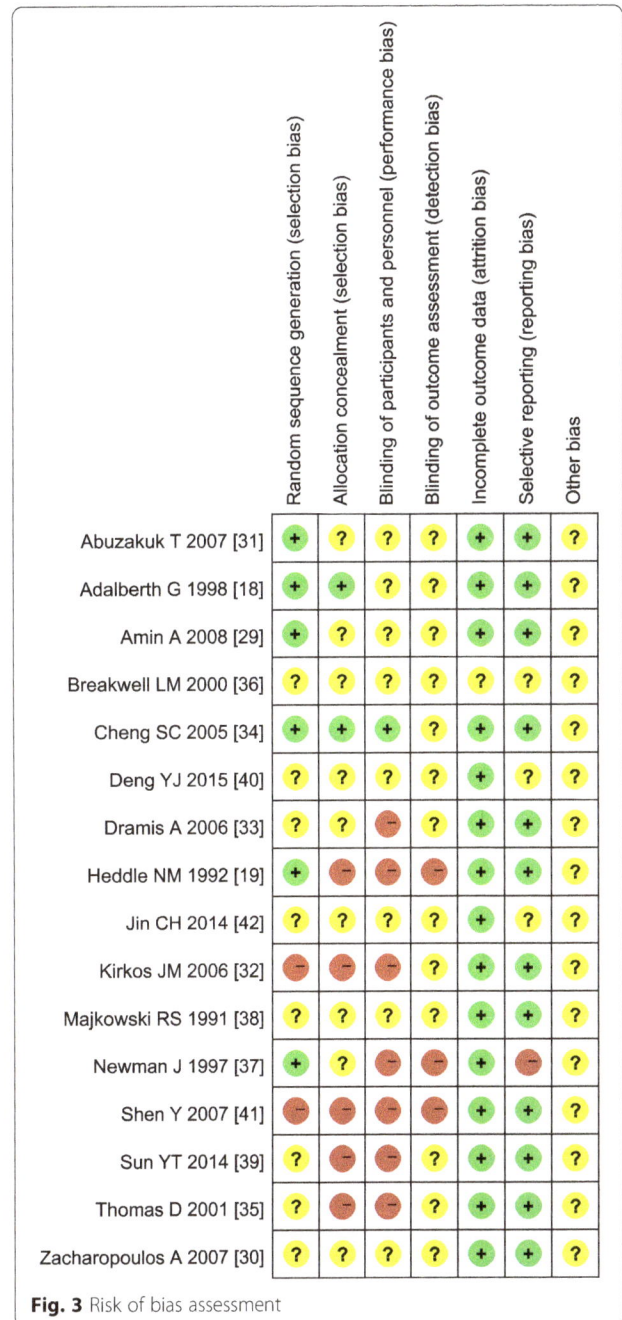

Fig. 3 Risk of bias assessment

Study or Subgroup	Experimental Events	Total	Control Events	Total	Weight	Odds Ratio M-H, Random, 95% CI
Abuzakuk T 2007 [31]	13	52	12	52	9.3%	1.11 [0.45, 2.73]
Adalberth G 1998 [18]	8	30	10	30	8.5%	0.73 [0.24, 2.21]
Amin A 2008 [29]	12	92	13	86	9.5%	0.84 [0.36, 1.96]
Cheng SC 2005 [34]	4	26	13	34	7.9%	0.29 [0.08, 1.05]
Dramis A 2006 [33]	3	25	10	24	7.2%	0.19 [0.04, 0.82]
Heddle NM 1992 [19]	10	39	27	40	9.0%	0.17 [0.06, 0.44]
Jin CH 2014 [42]	9	70	19	70	9.4%	0.40 [0.16, 0.95]
Majkowski RS 1991 [38]	7	20	19	20	4.8%	0.03 [0.00, 0.26]
Newman J 1997 [37]	3	35	28	35	7.2%	0.02 [0.01, 0.10]
Sun YT 2014 [39]	14	72	48	60	9.4%	0.06 [0.03, 0.14]
Thomas D 2001 [35]	12	115	33	116	9.9%	0.29 [0.14, 0.60]
Zacharopoulos A 2007 [30]	5	30	10	30	8.0%	0.40 [0.12, 1.36]
Total (95% CI)		**606**		**597**	**100.0%**	**0.25 [0.13, 0.47]**
Total events	100		242			

Heterogeneity: Tau² = 0.94; Chi² = 48.42, df = 11 (P < 0.00001); I² = 77%
Test for overall effect: Z = 4.27 (P < 0.0001)

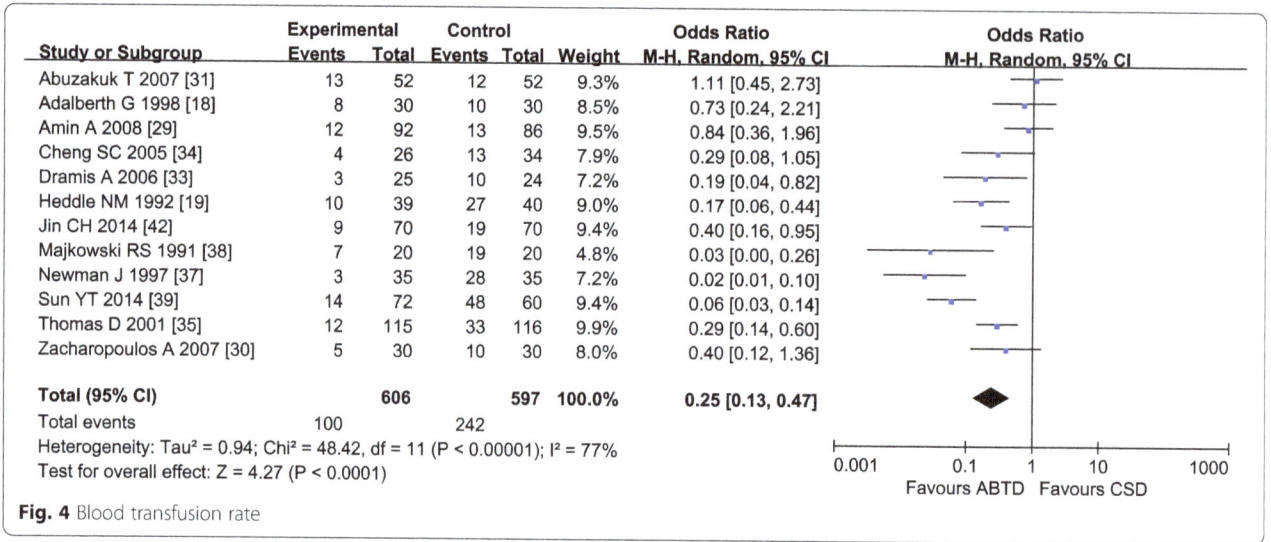

Fig. 4 Blood transfusion rate

We evaluated the methodological quality of all of the included studies using the Jadad quality scale and Cochrane risk of bias criteria (Table 1, Figs. 2 and 3). The Jadad scores ranged from 0 to 3 points, with an average score of 1.4. Only two RCTs [18, 19] were of high quality. Six studies [18, 19, 29, 31, 34, 37] reported a method of randomization, and two studies [32, 41] used a method of quasi-randomization. The remaining eight studies [30, 33, 35, 36, 38–40, 42] did not report the method of randomization. None of the included studies used the double-blinded method. The two RCTs [18, 19] of high quality described the number of cases and the reasons for drop-out in detail. Two studies [18, 34] reported the method of allocation concealment. One study [34] provided information regarding the blinding method. None of the 16 studies [18, 19, 29–42] reported the method of blinding outcome assessment. Fifteen studies [18, 19, 29–35, 37–42] reported the complete analysis. One study [37] was at high risk of selective reporting.

Patients in 14 studies [18, 19, 29–35, 37–39, 41, 42] were undergoing selective unilateral TKA, and those

of the remaining two [36, 40] were undergoing bilateral TKA.

The majority of the RCTs reviewed in this meta-analysis were of low quality. All of the included studies reported that the baseline characteristics of the study groups, including age, gender and pre-operative hemoglobin, were comparable, as shown in Table 1.

Primary outcomes

Blood transfusion rate

Twelve trials [18, 19, 29–31, 33–35, 37–39, 42] compared ABTD with CSD in the number of patients requiring homologous blood transfusion. Ten trials [18, 19, 29–31, 33–35, 37–39, 42] showed substantial heterogeneity in the trial results (chi-square = 48.42, P < 0.00001; I² = 77 %). Therefore, a random effects model was used for statistical analysis. The meta-analysis showed a significant beneficial effect of ABTD compared with CSD on blood transfusion rate (16.50 and 40.54 %, respectively; OR: 0.25 [0.13, 0.47]; Z = 4.27, P < 0.0001) (Fig. 4). Due to marked heterogeneity in the blood transfusion rate data, sensitivity analysis was conducted by excluding

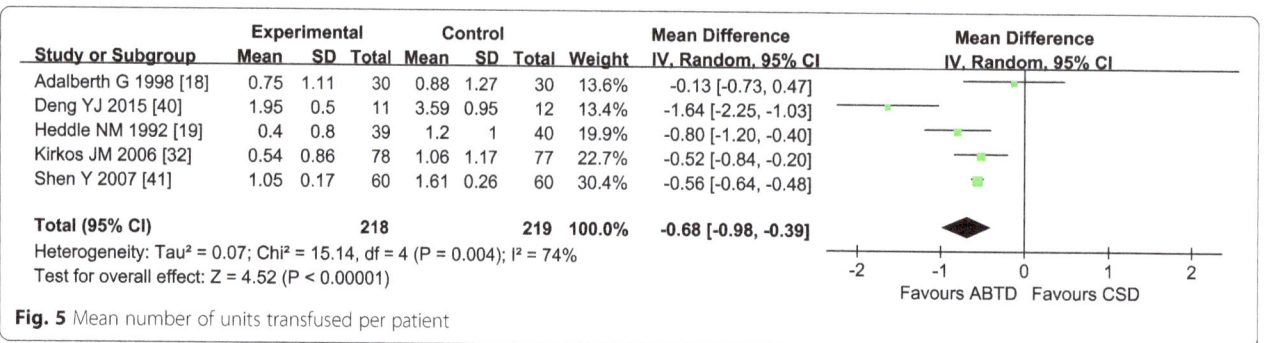

Study or Subgroup	Experimental Mean	SD	Total	Control Mean	SD	Total	Weight	Mean Difference IV, Random, 95% CI
Adalberth G 1998 [18]	0.75	1.11	30	0.88	1.27	30	13.6%	-0.13 [-0.73, 0.47]
Deng YJ 2015 [40]	1.95	0.5	11	3.59	0.95	12	13.4%	-1.64 [-2.25, -1.03]
Heddle NM 1992 [19]	0.4	0.8	39	1.2	1	40	19.9%	-0.80 [-1.20, -0.40]
Kirkos JM 2006 [32]	0.54	0.86	78	1.06	1.17	77	22.7%	-0.52 [-0.84, -0.20]
Shen Y 2007 [41]	1.05	0.17	60	1.61	0.26	60	30.4%	-0.56 [-0.64, -0.48]
Total (95% CI)			**218**			**219**	**100.0%**	**-0.68 [-0.98, -0.39]**

Heterogeneity: Tau² = 0.07; Chi² = 15.14, df = 4 (P = 0.004); I² = 74%
Test for overall effect: Z = 4.52 (P < 0.00001)

Fig. 5 Mean number of units transfused per patient

Study or Subgroup	Experimental Events	Total	Control Events	Total	Weight	Odds Ratio M-H, Fixed, 95% CI	Odds Ratio M-H, Fixed, 95% CI
Amin A 2008 [29]	4	92	2	86	20.1%	1.91 [0.34, 10.70]	
Majkowski RS 1991 [38]	4	20	5	20	40.6%	0.75 [0.17, 3.33]	
Thomas D 2001 [35]	3	115	4	116	39.4%	0.75 [0.16, 3.43]	
Total (95% CI)		227		222	100.0%	0.98 [0.40, 2.38]	
Total events	11		11				

Heterogeneity: Chi² = 0.82, df = 2 (P = 0.66); I² = 0%
Test for overall effect: Z = 0.04 (P = 0.97)

0.001   0.1   1   10   1000
Favours ABTD   Favours CSD

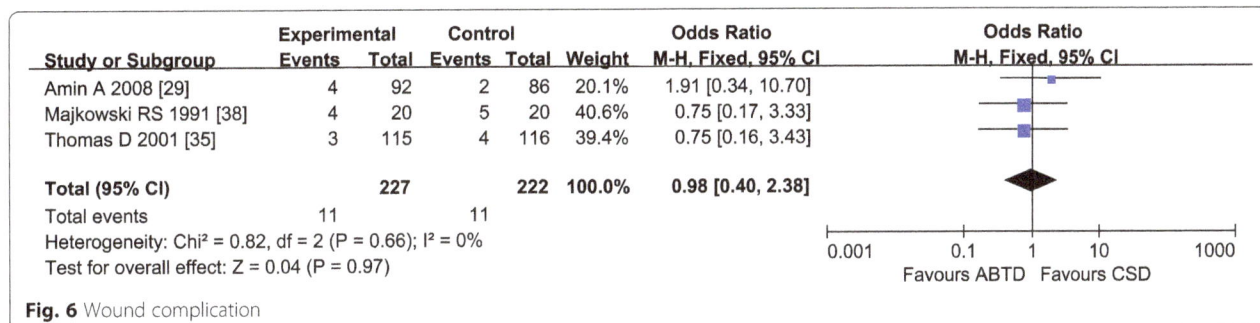

Fig. 6 Wound complication

one study randomly. Dropping any one study did not reduce the heterogeneity, suggesting that the result was robust against the heterogeneity.

Mean number of units transfused per patient

Five trials [18, 19, 32, 40, 41] that included a total of 437 patients reported the mean number of units transfused per patient (Fig. 5). These five trials [18, 19, 32, 40, 41] showed moderate heterogeneity in the results (chi-square = 15.14, $P = 0.004$; $I^2 = 74$ %). Therefore, a random effects model was used for statistical analysis. The meta-analysis showed a significant beneficial effect of ABTD compared with CSD; i.e., a lower mean number of units transfused per patient (WMD: −0.68 [−0.98, −0.39]; $Z = 4.52$, $P < 0.00001$). Due to marked heterogeneity in blood transfusion rate, sensitivity analysis was conducted by excluding one study [40] of lower quality, which reduced the heterogeneity ($I^2 = 12$ %, $P = 0.33$). The random effects model also showed a significant beneficial effect of ABTD relative to CSD (WMD: −0.56 [−0.68, −0.44]; $Z = 9.39$, $P < 0.00001$). Dropping any one study did not influence the qualitative result.

Wound complications

The analysis of data extracted from three studies [29, 35, 38] that assessed wound complications in 449 patients revealed no significant difference between the ABTD and CSD groups (4.85 and 4.95 %, OR: 0.98 [0.40, 2.38]; $Z = 0.04$, $P = 0.97$). No significant heterogeneity was detected ($P = 0.66$, $I^2 = 0$ %) (Fig. 6).

Deep vein thrombosis

Data extracted from four studies [18, 29, 35, 38] that assessed deep vein thrombosis in 509 patients showed no significant difference between the ABTD and CSD groups (1.56 and 2.38 %, OR: 0.69 [0.21, 2.24]; $Z = 0.61$, $P = 0.54$). No significant heterogeneity was detected ($P = 0.64$, $I^2 = 0$ %) (Fig. 7).

Secondary outcomes
Febrile complications

Six trials [19, 31, 32, 34, 36, 37] compared ABTD with CSD with respect to febrile complications. These six trials showed substantial heterogeneity in the results (chi-square = 11.28, $P = 0.05$; $I^2 = 56$ %); therefore, a random effects model was used. The meta-analysis showed no significant difference between the two groups (20.49 and 25.68 %, OR: 0.78 [0.25, 2.40]; $Z = 0.43$, $P = 0.67$) (Fig. 8). Due to marked heterogeneity in the febrile complications data, sensitivity analysis was conducted by excluding one study [37] of lower quality, which reduced the heterogeneity ($I^2 = 30$ %, $P = 0.22$). The random effects model also showed no significant difference between the ABTD and CSD groups (21.01 and 22.52 %, OR: 1.21 [0.39, 3.68]; $Z = 0.33$, $P = 0.74$). Dropping any one study did not qualitatively alter the result.

Post-operative hemoglobin on days 5–8

Four studies [18, 31, 37, 42] reported post-operative hemoglobin on days 5–8. Among these studies, one [31]

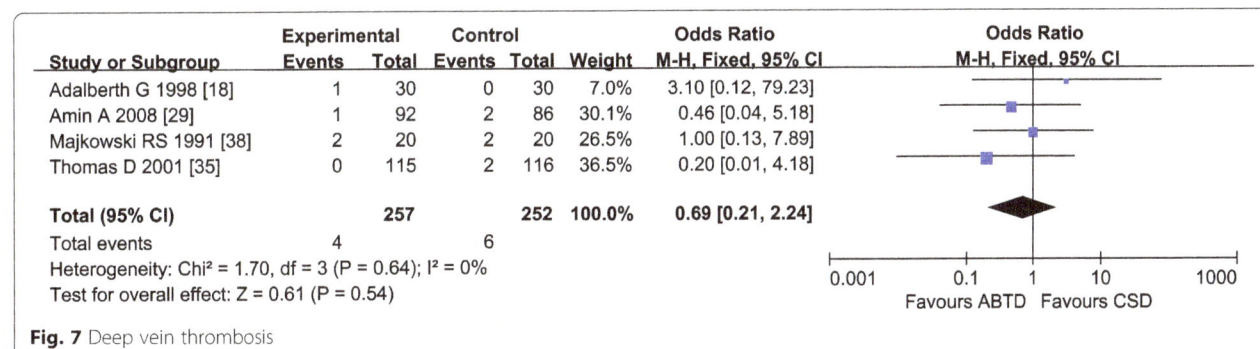

Study or Subgroup	Experimental Events	Total	Control Events	Total	Weight	Odds Ratio M-H, Fixed, 95% CI	Odds Ratio M-H, Fixed, 95% CI
Adalberth G 1998 [18]	1	30	0	30	7.0%	3.10 [0.12, 79.23]	
Amin A 2008 [29]	1	92	2	86	30.1%	0.46 [0.04, 5.18]	
Majkowski RS 1991 [38]	2	20	2	20	26.5%	1.00 [0.13, 7.89]	
Thomas D 2001 [35]	0	115	2	116	36.5%	0.20 [0.01, 4.18]	
Total (95% CI)		257		252	100.0%	0.69 [0.21, 2.24]	
Total events	4		6				

Heterogeneity: Chi² = 1.70, df = 3 (P = 0.64); I² = 0%
Test for overall effect: Z = 0.61 (P = 0.54)

0.001   0.1   1   10   1000
Favours ABTD   Favours CSD

Fig. 7 Deep vein thrombosis

Study or Subgroup	Experimental		Control		Weight	Odds Ratio M-H. Random, 95% CI	Odds Ratio M-H. Random, 95% CI
	Events	Total	Events	Total			
Abuzakuk T 2007 [31]	2	52	0	52	9.8%	5.20 [0.24, 110.95]	
Breakwell LM 2000 [36]	0	14	2	19	9.6%	0.24 [0.01, 5.44]	
Cheng SC 2005 [34]	2	26	1	34	13.2%	2.75 [0.24, 32.10]	
Heddle NM 1992 [19]	3	39	0	40	10.1%	7.77 [0.39, 155.50]	
Kirkos JM 2006 [32]	39	78	47	77	32.2%	0.64 [0.34, 1.21]	
Newman J 1997 [37]	4	35	16	35	25.1%	0.15 [0.04, 0.53]	
Total (95% CI)		**244**		**257**	**100.0%**	**0.78 [0.25, 2.40]**	
Total events	50		66				
Heterogeneity: Tau² = 0.92; Chi² = 11.28, df = 5 (P = 0.05); I² = 56%							
Test for overall effect: Z = 0.43 (P = 0.67)							

0.001   0.1   1   10   1000
Favours ABTD   Favours CSD

Fig. 8 Febrile complications

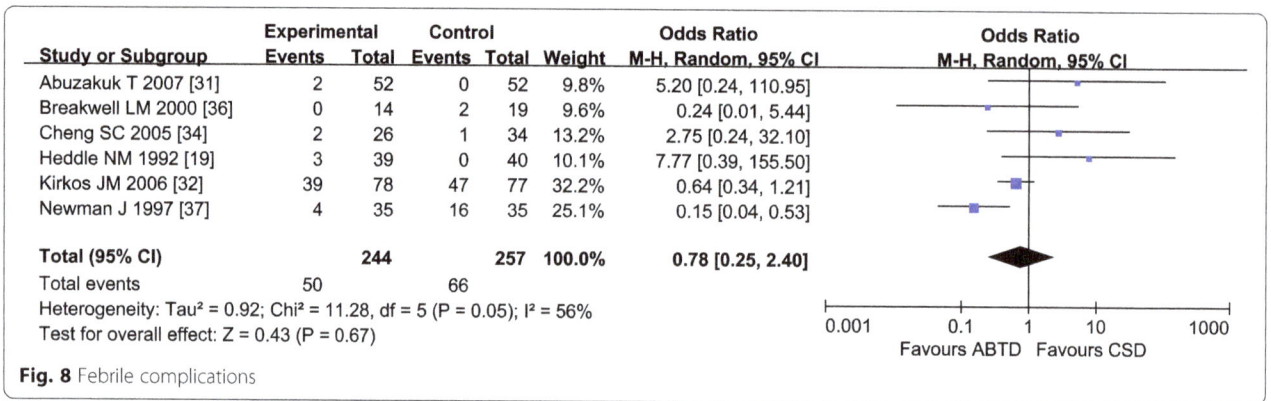

reported hemoglobin on the fifth day post-operation, one [18] reported hemoglobin on the eighth day post-operation, and the remaining two [37, 42] reported hemoglobin on the seventh day post-operation. Because the four studies [18, 31, 37, 42] showed moderate heterogeneity in the results (chi-square = 5.74, $P = 0.13$; $I^2 = 48$ %), a fixed effects model was used. The meta-analysis showed a significant beneficial effect of CSD compared with ABTD on post-operative hemoglobin on days 5–8 (WMD: 0.21 [–0.07, 0.48]; $Z = 1.47$, $P = 0.14$) (Fig. 9).

Drainage volume

Seven studies [18, 19, 31, 37–39, 41] reported post-operative drainage volume. These seven studies showed moderate heterogeneity in the results (chi-square = 9.03, $P = 0.17$; $I^2 = 34$ %); therefore, a fixed effects model was used. Pooling and analysis of the data of the 605 patients from the seven studies revealed no significant difference between the ABTD and CSD groups (WMD: –2.91 [–43.50, 37.68]; Z =0.14, $P = 0.89$) (Fig. 10).

Length of hospital stay

Three trials [18, 31, 37] compared ABTD with CSD in length of hospital stay. The three trials [18, 31, 37] showed substantial heterogeneity in the results (chi-square = 4.14, $P = 0.13$; $I^2 = 52$ %); therefore, a random effects model was used. The meta-analysis showed no significant difference in length of hospital stay between the ABTD and CSD groups (WMD: –0.96 [–2.09, 0.17]; $Z = 1.67$, $P = 0.10$)

(Fig. 11). Due to marked heterogeneity in length of hospital stay, sensitivity analysis was conducted by excluding one study [37] of lower quality, resulting in no significant heterogeneity detected ($P = 0.32$, $I^2 = 0$ %). The random effects model also showed no significant difference between the two groups in length of hospital stay (WMD: –0.52 [–1.30, 0.25]; $Z = 1.33$, $P = 0.18$).

Publication bias

The funnel plot of blood transfusion rate (Fig. 12) showed a markedly asymmetrical distribution of effect estimate, which indicated the presence of publication bias.

Discussion

The meta-analysis of 16 RCTs, including 1534 patients, suggested that ABTD is a safe system that yields a significantly reduced blood transfusion rate and fewer units of transfused blood per patient compared with CSD. We found no significant differences between the two drainage systems in wound complications, deep vein thrombosis, febrile complications, post-operative hemoglobin on days 5–8, drainage volume, or length of hospital stay.

TKA patients require post-operative allogenic blood transfusion, which was markedly reduced by using ABTD compared with CSD. Although allogenic transfusion remains the most popular method of compensating for blood loss in TKA patients, it can have potential deleterious effects, including transfusion-related infection, incompatibility-related transfusion reaction,

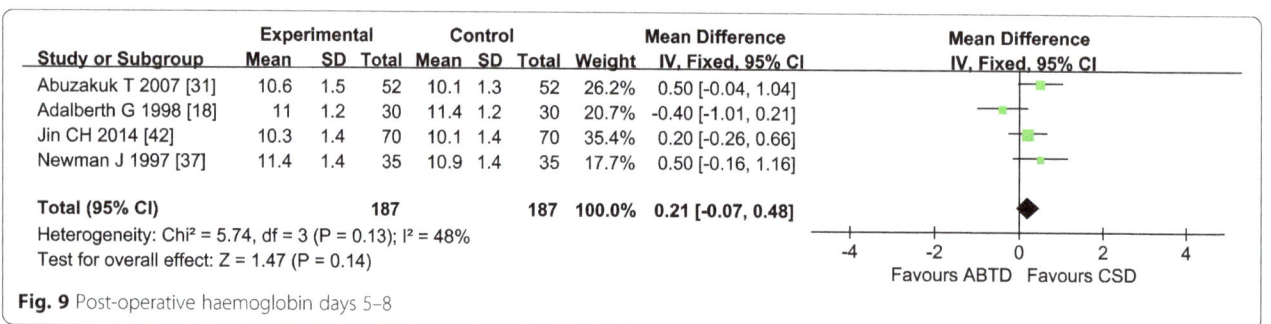

Study or Subgroup	Experimental			Control			Weight	Mean Difference IV. Fixed, 95% CI	Mean Difference IV. Fixed, 95% CI
	Mean	SD	Total	Mean	SD	Total			
Abuzakuk T 2007 [31]	10.6	1.5	52	10.1	1.3	52	26.2%	0.50 [–0.04, 1.04]	
Adalberth G 1998 [18]	11	1.2	30	11.4	1.2	30	20.7%	–0.40 [–1.01, 0.21]	
Jin CH 2014 [42]	10.3	1.4	70	10.1	1.4	70	35.4%	0.20 [–0.26, 0.66]	
Newman J 1997 [37]	11.4	1.4	35	10.9	1.4	35	17.7%	0.50 [–0.16, 1.16]	
Total (95% CI)			**187**			**187**	**100.0%**	**0.21 [–0.07, 0.48]**	
Heterogeneity: Chi² = 5.74, df = 3 (P = 0.13); I² = 48%									
Test for overall effect: Z = 1.47 (P = 0.14)									

-4   -2   0   2   4
Favours ABTD   Favours CSD

Fig. 9 Post-operative haemoglobin days 5–8

Study or Subgroup	Experimental			Control			Weight	Mean Difference IV, Fixed, 95% CI
	Mean	SD	Total	Mean	SD	Total		
Abuzakuk T 2007 [31]	673	355	52	867	434	52	7.1%	-194.00 [-346.40, -41.60]
Adalberth G 1998 [18]	881	403	30	737	417	30	3.8%	144.00 [-63.52, 351.52]
Heddle NM 1992 [19]	1,006	534	39	1,008	484	40	3.3%	-2.00 [-226.91, 222.91]
Majkowski RS 1991 [38]	1,020	540	20	1,140	513	20	1.5%	-120.00 [-446.43, 206.43]
Newman J 1997 [37]	896	545	35	891	401	35	3.3%	5.00 [-219.16, 229.16]
Shen Y 2007 [41]	605	168	60	590	106	60	65.2%	15.00 [-35.26, 65.26]
Sun YT 2014 [39]	639	286	72	656	308	60	15.8%	-17.00 [-119.17, 85.17]
Total (95% CI)			308			297	100.0%	-2.91 [-43.50, 37.68]

Heterogeneity: Chi² = 9.03, df = 6 (P = 0.17); I² = 34%
Test for overall effect: Z = 0.14 (P = 0.89)

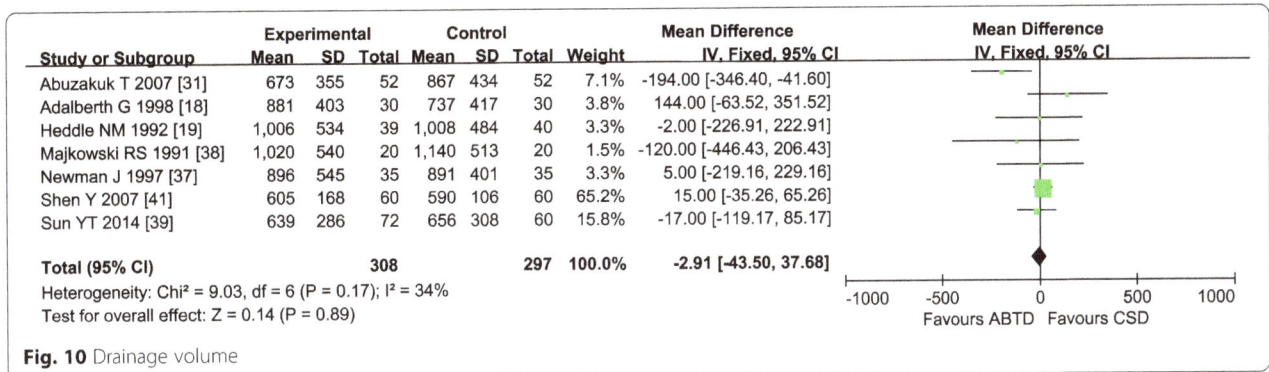

Fig. 10 Drainage volume

immune modulatory effects, and febrile complications [34]. These risks have led to use of autologous pre-donation blood, which also has drawbacks, e.g., difficulty of organizing patients for pre-donation and adherence to iron or erythropoietin therapy [43]. Studies have reported that nearly half of the autologous blood donated by patients for surgery is discarded [44, 45]. The use of autologous pre-donation blood is wasteful and costly [46]. Compared with the use of autologous pre-donation blood, ABTD has been found to be easier to perform, more cost-effective and able to lower the risks associated with allogenic blood use [47]. The present meta-analysis found that ABTD showed a significantly reduced blood transfusion rate and number of units transfused per patient; therefore, although the ABTD device is more expensive than CSD, a TKA patient using ABTD could spend 20 to 70 % less money on allogenic blood transfusion [30, 32, 34–36]. The procedures for setting up an ABTD system are similar to those for standard allogeneic blood transfusions [34] and require no additional medical personnel, but they do add staff time [31, 35]. The exact costs saved by using ABTD was not quantified in the present study because the unit cost of allogenic blood varies among regions.

Analysis of the extracted data on postoperative outcomes demonstrated that ABTD is safe and effective for TKA. There were no significant differences between ABTD and CSD in wound complications, deep vein thrombosis, and febrile complications. Kristiansson et al.

[48] found that hypercoagulability and high concentrations of IL-6 were present in drained blood. Some studies have reported that drained blood shows decreased platelet counts, pH levels, and clotting factor levels as well as increased fibrin degradation products [49, 50]. Hand et al. [51] identified low levels of methyl methacrylate monomers in filtered blood. Contra-indications to the use of unwashed shed blood have been formulated by the American Association of Blood Banks [52], who suggested that various cytokines are activated in drained blood and may be problematic for some patients if they increased to higher levels more than 6 h after bleeding [53]. In all of the studies included in the present meta-analysis, re-infusion was completed within 6 h post-operation. A lower rate of allogenic blood transfusion may help prevent febrile complications. Postoperative febrile complications were generally observed in the context of major orthopedic surgery, and it has been suggested that the rise in temperature is a response to the surgical procedure [54]. Some previous studies have also reported no difference between ABTD and CSD in the development febrile complications [55–57]. The absence of significant differences in wound complications, deep vein thrombosis, and febrile complications between ABTD and CSD indicate that ABTD is as safe as CSD.

Analysis of the pooled data revealed no significant difference in drainage volume, suggesting that ABTD is equally safe as CSD with respect to wound bleeding.

We found no significant differences between the two systems in post-operative hemoglobin on days 5–8. ABTD was found to be effective in reducing allogeneic

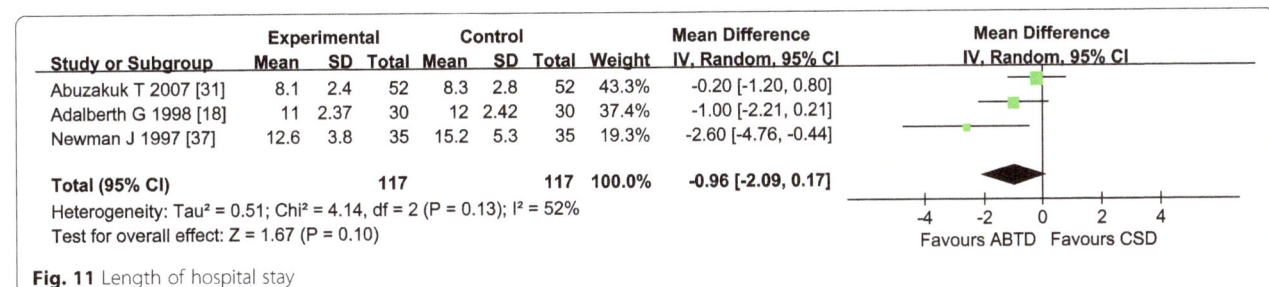

Study or Subgroup	Experimental			Control			Weight	Mean Difference IV, Random, 95% CI
	Mean	SD	Total	Mean	SD	Total		
Abuzakuk T 2007 [31]	8.1	2.4	52	8.3	2.8	52	43.3%	-0.20 [-1.20, 0.80]
Adalberth G 1998 [18]	11	2.37	30	12	2.42	30	37.4%	-1.00 [-2.21, 0.21]
Newman J 1997 [37]	12.6	3.8	35	15.2	5.3	35	19.3%	-2.60 [-4.76, -0.44]
Total (95% CI)			117			117	100.0%	-0.96 [-2.09, 0.17]

Heterogeneity: Tau² = 0.51; Chi² = 4.14, df = 2 (P = 0.13); I² = 52%
Test for overall effect: Z = 1.67 (P = 0.10)

Fig. 11 Length of hospital stay

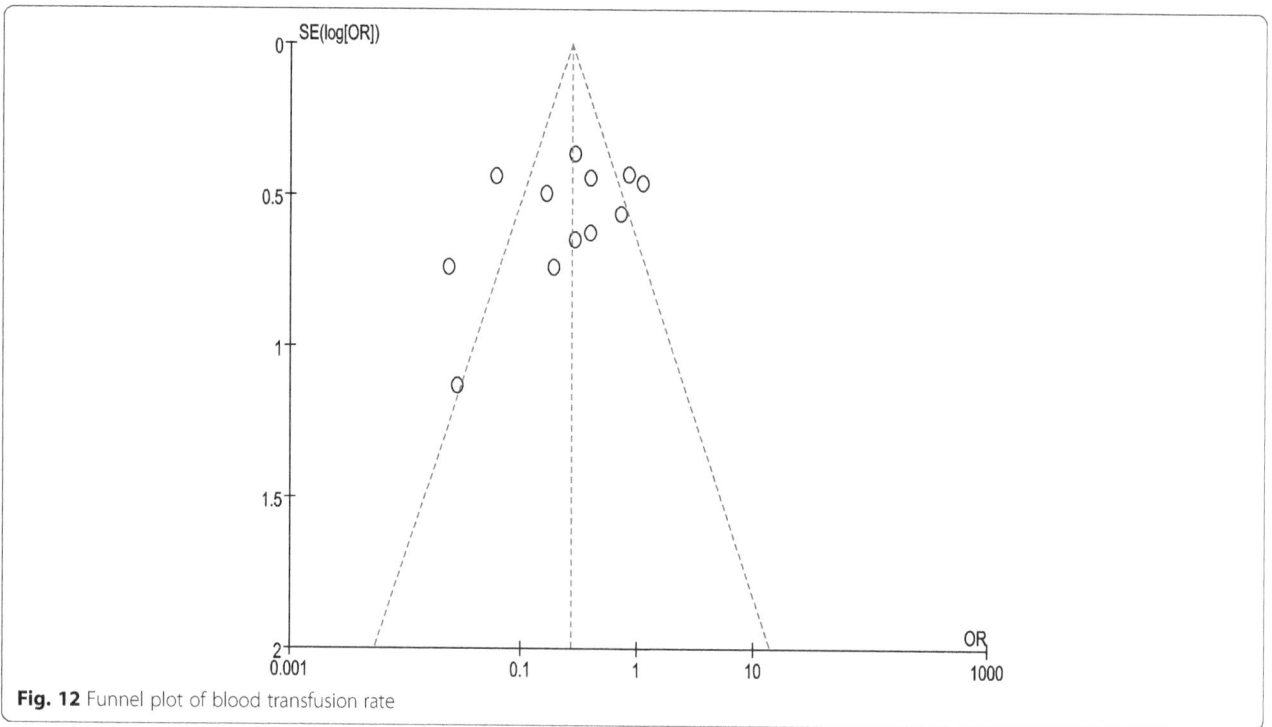

Fig. 12 Funnel plot of blood transfusion rate

blood transfusions but not in achieving high postoperative hemoglobin levels. A high postoperative hemoglobin level has been reported to be associated with better rehabilitation outcomes after TKA [58]. The present findings suggest that ABTD was not useful in achieving high postoperative hemoglobin levels to enhance rehabilitation, similar to the findings of other studies [57, 59].

The present meta-analysis revealed no significant difference in length of hospital stay between ABTD and CSD. However, the previous meta-analysis [17] found a longer length of hospital stay in the CSD group. The data on length of hospital stay in Amin A et al. [29] were presented as means and ranges, and we were unable to obtain the original data by contacting the corresponding author. Therefore, we excluded these data [29], which were included in the previous meta-analysis [17]. Due to country and regional variation in medical insurance policies and social support facilitating discharge, the length of hospital stay could not be used in the present study as a measure of cost [36].

Two studies [36, 40] on bilateral TKA reported different outcomes that could not be synthesized. Due to this limited number of studies and insufficient description of the study methods, the outcomes could not be analyzed in a subgroup analysis.

To assess the impact of one study on the effect estimates, we performed sensitivity analysis by excluding one study with a high weight or of lower quality. The results regarding blood transfusion rate, febrile complications, and length of hospital stay were qualitatively

unchanged by this analysis. However, as a result of the sensitivity analysis, the original result regarding postoperative hemoglobin on days 5–8 was changed to favor CSD, and the heterogeneity decreased from 48 to 0 % when the study by Adalberth et al. [18] was excluded. Analysis of the four studies [18, 31, 37, 42] reporting on pre-operative hemoglobin revealed no significant difference between the two systems (Heterogeneity: chi-square = 3.09, $P = 0.38$; $I^2 = 3$ %; WMD: −0.07 [−0.33, 0.20]; $Z = 0.49$, $P = 0.62$). Some non-RCT studies [43, 60] have similarly found no significant difference in hemoglobin levels before and after TKA between the ABTD and CSD groups. Another study [31] found that ABTD could prevent a rapid decrease in hemoglobin level during the early postoperative period, although this benefit was no longer present by post-operative day 5. Because only three studies [18, 31, 37] included in this meta-analysis reported on post-operative hemoglobin, further studies are needed to evaluate the benefit of ABTD with respect to post-operative hemoglobin.

Limitations

This meta-analysis has limitations. We used the Jadad quality scale [26] and the Cochrane risk of bias tool [27] to assess the methodological quality of the included RCTs. According to the Jadad quality scale, the average score of the included studies was 1.4, and only two RCTs [18, 19] were of high quality. The Jadad score places more emphasis on reporting rather than performance, and its advantage is its simplicity and easy implementation.

The Jadad score was used in this study because it makes it easy for readers to comprehend the quality of the included studies. Although a lack of adequate allocation concealment have been found in Jadad scores, this domain was assessed using criteria adopted from the Cochrane Handbook. The more important evaluation method used in this study is the Cochrane risk of bias tool.

The majority of the included RCTs were of moderate quality, and their sample sizes were comparatively small. In addition, it appears that the lack of random sequence generation increased the risk of bias.

Another limitation is that adequate information concerning each final outcome was not consistently provided among the 16 studies included. Furthermore, a prerequisite for the initial meta-analysis was the assumption of similarity between the two kinds of surgeries (SU-TKA and B-TKA), which enabled them to be evaluated together.

Fortunately, the results of the sensitivity analyses were similar to those of the original analyses. Another limitation of the present study is the heterogeneity among the included studies, which may reflect inter-study differences in analysis methodology, surgical method (SU-TKA vs. B-TKA), country and racial type. Future systematic reviews should assess different surgical methods, countries and racial types individually when sufficient high-quality RCT data become available. Surgeon experience in various TKA surgical approaches might also influence the results. Finally, as few of the included studies involving long-term follow-up, long-term outcomes could not be evaluated and require further study.

Conclusions

The present meta-analysis indicated that ABTD is more efficacious than CSD in reducing the blood transfusion rate and the number of units transfused per patient in TKA patients. The two types of drains appear to be equivalent in terms of wound complications, deep vein thrombosis, febrile complications, post-operative hemoglobin on days 5–8, drainage volume, and length of hospital stay. The results of this meta-analysis can help TKA surgeons make clinical decisions. The development of large-volume, well-designed RCTs and clinical trials with extensive follow-up will clarify the advantages and disadvantages of ABTD.

Abbreviations

ABTD: Autologous blood transfusion drainage; B-TKA: Bilateral total knee replacement; CBM: Chinese Biomedical Literature; CIs: Confidence intervals; CNKI: China National Knowledge Infrastructure; CSD: Conventional suction drainage; ITT: Intent-to-trea; ORs: Odds ratios; SU-TKA: Selective unilateral total knee replacement; TKA: Total knee arthroplasty; WMDs: Weighted mean differences

Acknowledgements
We thank American Journal Experts for their linguistic assistance during the preparation of this manuscript.

Funding
This study was funded by National Natural Science Foundation of China (No.81473698, No.81273781), Doctoral Fund of Ministry of Education of China (No.20124425110004), TCM Standardization Projects of State Administration of Traditional Chinese Medicine of China (No. SATCM-2015-BZ115, SATCM-2015-BZ173), Science and Technology Planning Project of Guangdong Province, China (No.2011B031700027), Project of Guangdong Provincial Department of Finance (No.[2014] 157), Administration of Traditional Chinese Medicine of Guangdong Province (No.20164020), and Science and Technology Research Project of Guangdong Provincial Hospital of Chinese Medicine (No. YK2013B2N19, YN2015MS15).

Authors' contributions
Conceived and designed the SRMA: JL. Performed the SRMA: JKP, KHH, HX. Analyzed the data: JKP, KHH, HX, MHL, DG, JL. Drafted the manuscript: JKP. All authors read and approved the final manuscript.

Competing interests
The authors declare that they have no competing interests.

Consent for publication
Not applicable.

Author details
[1]Department of Orthopedics, Second Affiliated Hospital of Guangzhou University of Chinese Medicine (Guangdong Provincial Hospital of Chinese Medicine), No. 111 Dade Road, Guangzhou, Guangdong 510120, China. [2]Department of Orthopedics, Guangdong Second Traditional Chinese Medicine Hospital, No. 60 Hengfu Road, Guangzhou, Guangdong 510095, China.

References
1. Torres-Claramunt R, Hinarejos P, Perez-Prieto D, Gil-Gonzalez S, Pelfort X, Leal J, Puig L. Sealing of the intramedullar femoral canal in a TKA does not reduce postoperative blood loss: A randomized prospective study. Knee. 2014;21(4):853–857.
2. Xie H, Pan JK, Hong KH, Guo D, Fang J, Yang WY, Liu J. Postoperative autotransfusion drain after total hip arthroplasty: A meta-analysis of randomized controlled trials. Sci Rep. 2016;(6):27461.
3. Sehat KR, Evans RL, Newman JH. Hidden blood loss following hip and knee arthroplasty. Correct management of blood loss should take hidden loss into account. J Bone Joint Surg Br. 2004;86(4):561–5.
4. Keating EM, Meding JB, Faris PM, Ritter MA. Predictors of transfusion risk in elective knee surgery. Clin Orthop Relat Res. 1998;10(357):50–59.
5. Adie S, Naylor JM, Harris IA. Cryotherapy after total knee arthroplasty: a systematic review and meta-analysis of randomized controlled trials. J Arthroplasty. 2010;25(5):709–15.
6. Hong KH, Pan JK, Yang WY, et al. Comparison between autologous blood transfusion drainage and closed-suction drainage/no drainage in total knee arthroplasty: a meta-analysis. BMC Musculoskelet Disord 2016;17:142.
7. Bidolegui F, Arce G, Lugones A, Pereira S, Vindver G. Tranexamic acid reduces blood loss and transfusion in patients undergoing total knee arthroplasty without tourniquet: a prospective randomized controlled trial. Open Orthop J. 2014;7(8):250–4.
8. Tai TW, Chang CW, Yang CY. The role of drainage after total knee arthroplasty[M]. INTECH Open Access Publisher. 2012;267–74.

9. Drinkwater CJ, Neil MJ. Optimal timing of wound drain removal following total joint arthroplasty. J Arthroplasty. 1995;10(2):185–9.

10. Holt BT, Parks NL, Engh GA, Lawrence JM. Comparison of closed-suction drainage and no drainage after primary total knee arthroplasty. Orthopedics. 1997;20(12):1121–4. discussion 1124–5.

11. Martin A, Prenn M, Spiegel T, Sukopp C, von Strempel A. Relevance of wound drainage in total knee arthroplasty–a prospective comparative study. Z Orthop Ihre Grenzgeb. 2004;142(1):46–50.

12. Kim YH, Cho SH, Kim RS. Drainage versus nondrainage in simultaneous bilateral total knee arthroplasties. Clin Orthop Relat Res. 1998;2(347):188–93.

13. Gibbons CE, Solan MC, Ricketts DM, Patterson M. Cryotherapy compared with Robert Jones bandage after total knee replacement: a prospective randomized trial. Int Orthop. 2001;25(4):250–2.

14. Pavelescu D, Mirea L, Grintescu I. Combined perioperative use of tranexamic acid with a postoperative reinfusion/autotransfusion drainage system dramatically decrease the allogenic transfusion needs in total knee arthroplasty (TKA). Eur J Anaesthesiol 2014, 31((Pavelescu D.; Mirea L.; Grintescu I.) SCUB, Dept of Anaesthesiology and Intensive Care, Bucharest, Romania):103–4.

15. Kang DG, Khurana S, Baek JH, Park YS, Lee SH, Kim KI. Efficacy and safety using autotransfusion system with postoperative shed blood following total knee arthroplasty in haemophilia. Haemophilia. 2014;20(1):129–32.

16. Horstmann W, Kuipers B, Ohanis D, Slappendel R, Kollen B, Verheyen C. Autologous re-transfusion drain compared with no drain in total knee arthroplasty: a randomised controlled trial. Blood Transfus. 2014;12(Suppl 1):s176–s81.

17. Markar SR, Jones GG, Karthikesalingam A, Segaren N, Patel RV. Transfusion drains versus suction drains in total knee replacement: Meta-analysis. Knee Surg Sports Traumatol Arthrosc. 2012;20(9):1766–72.

18. Adalberth G, Byström S, Kolstad K, Mallmin H, Milbrink J. Postoperative drainage of knee arthroplasty is not necessary: a randomized study of 90 patients. Acta Orthop Scand. 1998;69(5):475–8.

19. Heddle NM, Brox WT, Klama LN, Dickson LL, Levine MN. A randomized trial on the efficacy of an autologous blood drainage and transfusion device in patients undergoing elective knee arthroplasty. Transfusion. 1992;32(8):742–6.

20. Wu XY, Tang JL, Mao C, Yuan JQ, Qin Y, Chung VC. Systematic reviews and meta-analyses of traditional chinese medicine must search chinese databases to reduce language bias. Evid Based Complement Alternat Medicine. 2013;2013:812179.

21. Egger M, Zellweger-Zahner T, Schneider M, Junker C, Lengeler C, Antes G. Language bias in randomised controlled trials published in English and German. Lancet. 1997;350(9074):326–9.

22. Thomassen BJW, Hollander PHC, Kaptijn HH, Nelissen R, Pilot P. Autologous wound drains have no effect on allogeneic blood transfusions in primary total hip and knee replacement: A three-arm randomised trial. Bone Joint J. 2014,96-B(6):765–71.

23. Cip J, Widemschek M, Benesch T, Waibel R, Martin A.Does single use of an autologous transfusion system in TKA reduce the need for allogenic blood?: A prospective randomized trial general. Clin Orthop RelatRes 2013,471(4):1319–25.

24. Dobosz B, Dutka J, Dutka L, Maleta P. Clinical and cost effectiveness-related aspects of retransfusion in total hip and knee arthroplasty. Ortop Traumatol Rehabil. 2012;14(5):421–8.

25. Liberati A, Altman DG, Tetzlaff J, Mulrow C, Gotzsche PC, Ioannidis JP, Clarke M, Devereaux PJ, Kleijnen J, Moher D. The PRISMA statement for reporting systematic reviews and meta-analyses of studies that evaluate healthcare interventions: explanation and elaboration. BMJ. 2009;339:b2700.

26. Jadad AR, Moore RA, Carroll D, Jenkinson C, Reynolds DJ, Gavaghan DJ, McQuay HJ. Assessing the quality of reports of randomized clinical trials: is blinding necessary? Control Clin Trials. 1996;17(1):1–12.

27. Huggins J, Green S. Cochrane handbook for systematic reviews of interventions. New York: Cochrane Collaboration, John Wiley and Sons; 2008.

28. Elzik ME, Dirschl DR, Dahners LE. Correlation of transfusion volume to change in hematocrit. Am J Hematol. 2006;81(2):145–6.

29. Amin A, Watson A, Mangwani J, Nawabi DH, Nawabi D, Ahluwalia R, Loeffler M.A prospective randomised controlled trial of autologous retransfusion in total knee replacement. J Bone Joint Surg. 2008;90(4):451–4.

30. Zacharopoulos A, Apostolopoulos A, Kyriakidis A. The effectiveness of reinfusion after total knee replacement. A prospective randomised controlled study. Int Orthop. 2007;31(3):303–8.

31. Abuzakuk T, Senthil Kumar V, Shenava Y, Bulstrode C, Skinner JA, Cannon SR, Briggs TW. Autotransfusion drains in total knee replacement. Are they alternatives to homologous transfusion? Int Orthop. 2007;31(2):235–9.

32. Kirkos JM, Krystallis CT, Konstantinidis PA, Papavasiliou KA, Kyrkos MJ, Ikonomidis LG. Postoperative re-perfusion of drained blood in patients undergoing total knee arthroplasty: Is it effective and cost-efficient? Acta Orthop Belg. 2006;72(1):18–23.

33. Dramis A, Plewes J. Autologous blood transfusion after primary unilateral total knee replacement surgery. Acta Orthop Belg. 2006;72(1):15–7.

34. Cheng SC, Hung TS, Tse PY. Investigation of the use of drained blood reinfusion after total knee arthroplasty: a prospective randomised controlled study. In: J Orthop Surg (Hong Kong). 2005;13(2):120–4.

35. Thomas D, Wareham K, Cohen D, Hutchings H. Autologous blood transfusion in total knee replacement surgery. Br J Anaesth. 2001;86(5):669–73.

36. Breakwell LM, Getty CJM, Dobson P. The efficacy of autologous blood transfusion in bilateral total knee arthroplasty. Knee. 2000;7(3):145–7.

37. Newman J, Bowers M, Murphy J. The clinical advantages of autologous transfusion a randomised, controlled study after knee replacement. J Bone Joint Surg Br. 1997;79(4):630–2.

38. Majkowski RS, Currie IC, Newman JH.Postoperative collection and reinfusion of autologous blood in total knee arthroplasty. Ann R Coll Surg Engl. 1991; 73(6): 381–4.

39. Sun YT, Li JY, Liu Y. The applications and effect evaluation of autologous blood transfusion device in total knee replacement postoperative. Chinese Foreign Med Res. 2014;12(9):78–9.

40. Deng YJ, Lv G, Chu LT, Fang R, Liang ZQ, Xiang WY. Observation on the effect of three different methods on blood management during perioperation of double knee replacement. HeBei Medicine (China). 2015;21(1):97–100.

41. Shen Y, Zhang MX, Liu L, Chen YX, Li H. Observation and care of wound drainage after primary total knee arthroplasty. J Nurs. 2007;14(8):43–4.

42. Jin CH. Effect of autologous blood transfusion device in primary knee arthroplasty postoperative. Med Inform. 2014;27(9):191–2.

43. Lakshmanan P, Purushothaman B, Sharma A. Impact of reinfusion drains on hemoglobin level in total knee arthroplasty. Am J Orthop. 2010;39(2):70–4.

44. Sculco TP, Gallina J. Blood management experience: relationship between autologous blood donation and transfusion in orthopedic surgery. Orthopedics. 1999;22(1 Suppl):129–34.

45. Bierbaum BE, CALLAGHAN JJ, GALANTE JO, RUBASH HE, TOOMS RE, WELCH RB. An analysis of blood management in patients having a total Hip or knee arthroplasty. J Bone Joint Surg. 1999;81(1):2–10.

46. Etchason J, Petz L, Keeler E, Calhoun L, Kleinman S, Snider C, Fink A, Brook R. The cost effectiveness of preoperative autologous blood donations. N Engl J Med. 1995;332(11):719–24.

47. Woolson ST, Wall WW. Autologous blood transfusion after total knee arthroplasty: a randomized, prospective study comparing predonated and postoperative salvage blood. J Arthroplasty. 2003;18(3):243–9.

48. Kristiansson M, Soop M, Saraste L, Sundqvist KG, Suontaka AM, Blomback M. Cytokine and coagulation characteristics of retrieved blood after arthroplasty. Intensive Care Med. 1995;21(12):989–95.

49. Peter V, Radford M, Matthews M. Re-transfusion of autologous blood from wound drains: the means for reducing tranfusion requirements in total knee arthroplasty. Knee. 2001;8(4):321–3.

50. Dalén T, Broström L-Å, Engströrn KG. Autotransfusion after total knee arthroplasty: effects on blood cells, plasma chemistry and whole blood rheology. J Arthroplasty. 1997;12(5):517–25.

51. Hand C, Henderson M, Mace P, Sherif N, Newman J, Goldie D. Methyl methacrylate levels in unwashed salvage blood following unilateral total knee arthroplasty. J Arthroplasty. 1998;13(5):576–9.

52. American Association of Blood Banks. Guidance for standards for perioperative autologous blood collection and administration. 1st ed. Bethesda, Maryland; 2002.

53. Waters JH, Dyga RM, Yazer MH. Guidelines for blood recovery and reinfusion in surgery and trauma. Bethesda, MD: American Association of Blood Banks 2010.

54. Munoz M, Kuhlmorgen B, Ariza D, Haro E, Marroqui A, Ramirez G. Which patients are more likely to benefit from postoperative shed blood salvage after unilateral total knee replacement? An analysis of 581 consecutive procedures. Vox Sang. 2007;92(2):136–41.

55. Andersson I, Tylman M, Bengtson JP, Bengtsson A. Complement split products and pro-inflammatory cytokines in salvaged blood after hip and knee arthroplasty. Can J Anaesth. 2001;48(3):251–5.

56. Innerhofer P, Klingler A, Klimmer C, Fries D, Nussbaumer W. Risk for postoperative infection after transfusion of white blood cell-filtered allogeneic or autologous blood components in orthopedic patients undergoing primary arthroplasty. Transfusion. 2005;45(1):103–10.

The efficacy and safety of autologous blood transfusion drainage in patients undergoing total knee...

35

57. Haien Z, Yong J, Baoan M, Mingjun G, Qingyu F. Post-operative auto-transfusion in total hip or knee arthroplasty: a meta-analysis of randomized controlled trials. PLoS One. 2013;8(1):e55073.
58. Diamond PT, Conaway MR, Mody SH, Bhirangi K. Influence of hemoglobin levels on inpatient rehabilitation outcomes after total knee arthroplasty. J Arthroplasty. 2006;21(5):636–41.
59. Moonen AF, Knoors NT, van Os JJ, Verburg AD, Pilot P. Retransfusion of filtered shed blood in primary total hip and knee arthroplasty: a prospective randomized clinical trial. Transfusion. 2007;47(3):379–84.
60. Strumper D, Weber EW, Gielen-Wijffels S, Van Drumpt R, Bulstra S, Slappendel R, Durieux ME, Marcus MA. Clinical efficacy of postoperative autologous transfusion of filtered shed blood in hip and knee arthroplasty. Transfusion. 2004;44(11):1567–71.

5

Patient and surgical factors affecting procedure duration and revision risk due to deep infection in primary total knee arthroplasty

Mona Badawy[1,4]*, Birgitte Espehaug[2], Anne Marie Fenstad[3], Kari Indrekvam[1,4], Håvard Dale[4], Leif I. Havelin[3,4] and Ove Furnes[3,4]

Abstract

Background: The aim of this study was to assess which patient and procedure factors affected both the risk of infection as well as procedure duration. Additionally, to assess if procedure duration affected the revision risk due to deep infection in total knee arthroplasty (TKA) patients and in a subgroup of low-risk patients.

Methods: 28,262 primary TKA with 311 revisions due to deep infection were included from the Norwegian Arthroplasty Register (NAR) and analysed from primary surgery from 2005 until 31st December 2015 with a 1 and 4 year follow up. The risk of revision due to deep infection was calculated in a multivariable Cox regression model including patient and procedure related risk factors, assessing Hazard Ratio (HR) with 95% confidence interval (CI).

Results: Multivariate analysis showed statistically significant associations with revision due to deep infection and increased procedure duration for male patients, ASA3+ (American Society of Anesthesiologists) and perioperative complications. Procedure duration ≥110 min (75 percentile) had a higher risk of deep infection compared to duration <75 min (25 percentile), in the unadjusted analysis (HR = 1.8, 95% CI 1.3-2.5, *p* = 0.001) and in the adjusted analysis (HR = 1.5, 95% CI 1.0-2.1, *p* = 0.03). For low-risk patients, procedure duration did not increase the risk of infection.

Conclusion: Male patients, ASA 3+ patients and perioperative complications were risk factors both for longer procedure duration and for deep infection revisions. Patients with a high degree of comorbidity, defined as ASA3+, are at risk of infection with longer procedure durations. The occurrence of perioperative complications potentially leading to a more complex and lengthy procedure was associated with a higher risk of infection. Long procedure duration in itself seems to have minor impact on infection since we found no association in the low-risk patient.

Keywords: Knee, Osteoarthritis, Arthroplasty, Procedure duration, Infection, Risk factors, Revision

Background

Numerous risk factors predispose patients to deep infection after total knee arthroplasty. It is critical to identify the correlation of risk factors that predispose TKA patients to deep infection, to reduce or even avoid this complication. Prolonged procedure duration has been demonstrated to increase the infection risk [1–5]. This is probably due to a combination of factors involving both the patient and the surgical environment, leading to bleeding and cautery, increased tissue damage and increased wound contamination.

Both surgeon and patient related factors can contribute to long procedure duration. Complexity of the surgery due to previous surgery to the knee or diagnoses other than primary osteoarthritis (OA) can increase procedure duration in addition to occurrence of perioperative complications. Inexperienced surgical team, low

* Correspondence: mona.badawy@helse-bergen.no
[1]Coastal Hospital in Hagavik, 5217 Hagavik, Norway
[4]Department of Clinical Medicine, Institute of Medicine and Dentistry, University of Bergen, 5021 Bergen, Norway
Full list of author information is available at the end of the article

volume hospitals/surgeons could also contribute to longer procedure duration [3, 6]. Patient related factors increasing procedure duration are male sex, comorbidities, obesity and previous fractures around the knee [7, 8]. These factors are also well known risk factors of infection [1, 9–15].

The 'Proceedings of the International Consensus Meeting on Periprosthetic Joint Infections' by Javad Parvizi and Thorsten Gehrke [16] agrees with 96% delegate votes that surgical site infection rates increase directly with the duration of surgery. Their justification is numerous studies linking increased operative time to the risk of infection after total joint arthroplasty with statistical significance [1–3, 14, 17]. A study from Naranje et al. [12] demonstrated that operative time is only one of many factors that may increase infection risk and may be influenced by numerous confounders.

There are few reports on the relationship between long procedure duration and deep infection with revision as endpoint [1, 3, 12], and few describe the factors leading to prolonged procedure duration [8, 18].

Large study populations are required to measure rare events like deep infection. We used registry data [19] to determine risk factors for both prolonged procedure duration and deep infection and if there was an association between longer procedure duration and revision risk resulting from deep infection after TKA.

Methods

TKA has been registered in the NAR since 1994. The completeness of reporting for primary procedures was 96% and 89% for revision surgery compared to data from the Norwegian Patient Registry [19]. In the present study, we included 28,262 primary TKA from 2005 to 2015. We selected the last 10 years of data to avoid outdated techniques and implants as well as less modern operating rooms. For homogeneity reasons, only cemented (with antibiotics) cruciate retaining (CR) implants (97% in the NAR) without patellar components (92% in the NAR) were included. Unicompartmental knee arthroplasty and more constrained implants were excluded (Fig. 1).

Revision was defined as complete or partial removal, exchange or addition of implant component(s). Patients with superficial wound infections treated with surgical site soft tissue debridement or with antibiotics only were

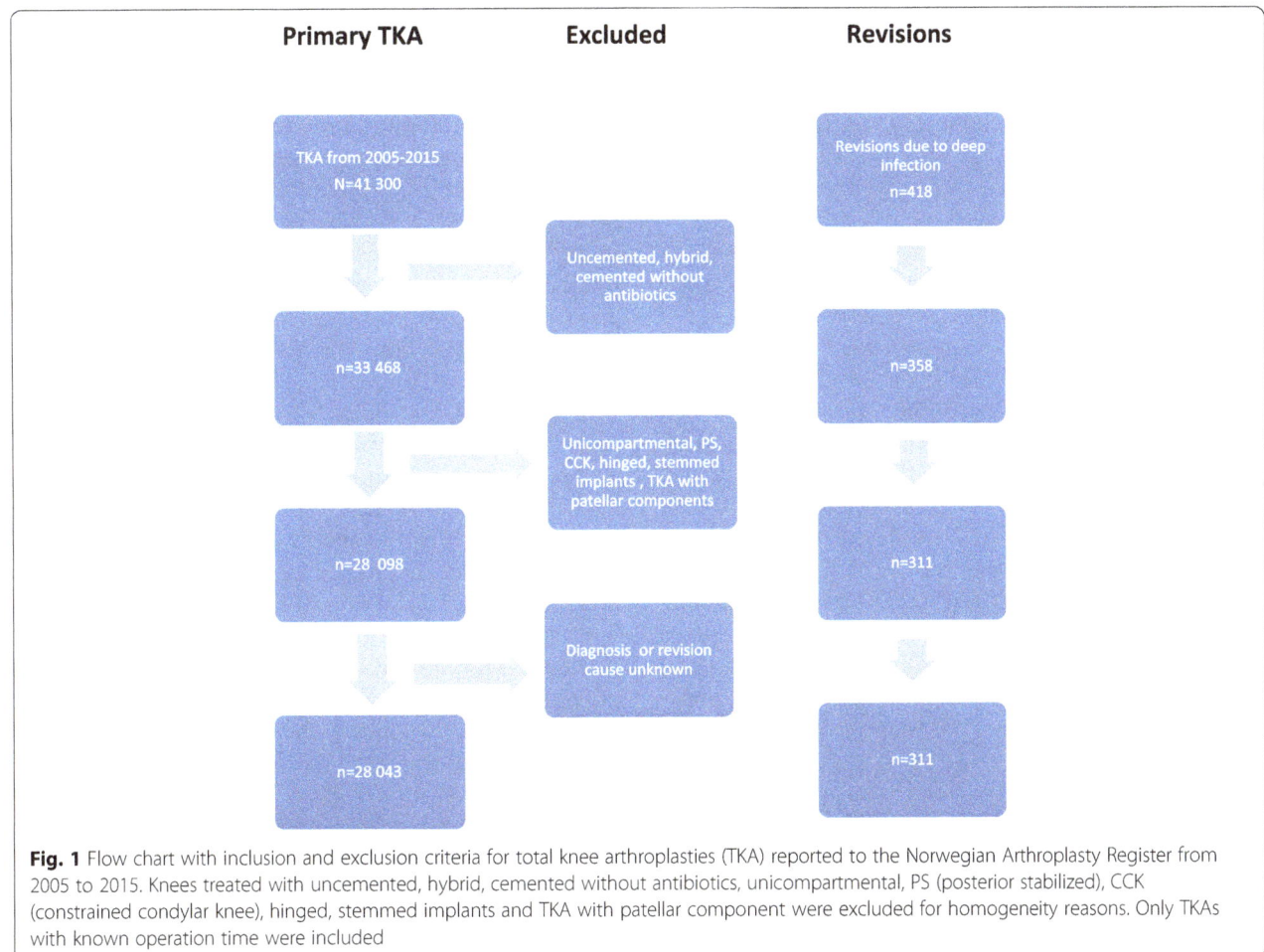

Fig. 1 Flow chart with inclusion and exclusion criteria for total knee arthroplasties (TKA) reported to the Norwegian Arthroplasty Register from 2005 to 2015. Knees treated with uncemented, hybrid, cemented without antibiotics, unicompartmental, PS (posterior stabilized), CCK (constrained condylar knee), hinged, stemmed implants and TKA with patellar component were excluded for homogeneity reasons. Only TKAs with known operation time were included

not included in this study. A suggested follow-up time of 1 year would include all post-interventional infections thought to arise during implantation. Later there may be more haematogenous spread infections [20]. 1 and 4 years Kaplan Meier revision percentages are presented in Tables 3 and 4.

Procedure duration was recorded as the time from skin incision to complete wound closure in all cases. We used four different duration categories using quartiles (<75 min, 75-89 min, 90-109 min and ≥110). Data on patient related risk factors were collected; age, sex, co-morbidity score (ASA (American Society of Anesthesiologists) classification), diagnosis and previous fractures or osteotomy to the knee. Hospital and surgery related risk factors were also collected; annual hospital volume, the occurrence of perioperative complications, the use of computer navigation (CAOS), implant brand and time period (Table 1).

The majority of reported perioperative complications were different types of fractures, various tendon and ligament ruptures and technical issues regarding instruments or cementing, all increasing the probability of prolonged procedure duration.

Finally, a low-risk patient was defined based on the least probable risk of revision TKA from the analyses of all TKA presented in Tables 2 and 3; defined as a TKA patient with primary OA, classified as ASA 1 or 2, without any previous osteotomy or fracture to the knee and without any registered occurrence of perioperative complications.

Statistics

Survival analyses were performed with first revision due to deep infection as endpoint. All cases were censored at December 31st 2015 to achieve at least 1 year follow-up for all primary TKA. Information about deaths and emigrations were obtained from the National Population Register. 1- and 4-year revision probabilities (time to revision due to deep infection) for the four procedure duration categories were calculated using the Kaplan-Meier method.

A Cox regression model was used to calculate the possible association between procedure duration and implant survival. Hazard ratios (HR) were represented with 95% confidence intervals (CI) and p-values relative to the shortest procedure duration as reference. All p-values less than 0.05 were considered statistically significant.

Both unadjusted (crude) and adjusted multivariate Cox proportional hazard models were used. Adjustment for potential confounding was performed. The model included common patient-related variables such as age, sex, diagnosis and ASA classification. The occurrence of perioperative complications were strongly associated with

prolonged procedure duration and were therefore added to the adjustment.

Similarly, unadjusted and adjusted Cox regression models were created for the low-risk patient previously described. Adjusted Cox regression curves were constructed for both models (Figs. 1 and 2).

The relative hazard assumption was tested by Schoenfeld residuals for chosen covariates and found to be valid. We found 13.3% bilateral procedures in our material and they were equally distributed in the infected and non-infected group. Death or emigration (lost to follow up) as a possible competing risk was investigated and there were no statistical significant differences in proportion of deaths within the groups, p-value equal to 0.15.

SPSS version 22 and R version 3.3.0 were used for the statistical analyses.

Results

28,262 primary TKA were included for analysis and 311 patients underwent revision surgery for deep infection after TKA (1.1%) during the 11 year study period. Revisions due to infections accounted for 46% of all revisions within 1 year, and 27% within 4 years of follow up. Patient and surgery characteristics are presented in Table 1.

The mean and median procedure duration for non-infected cases was 94 and 90 min respectively, and for infected cases 100 min in both measures. The mean difference was statistically significant ($p < 0.001$).

Risk factors for prolonged procedure duration (≥110 min) were male sex, young age, diagnosis other than OA (inflammatory arthritis, OA due to previous fracture, ligament injury or infection), ASA 3+ patients, previous surgery to the knee, low hospital volume, perioperative complications, the use of CAOS, time period from 2005 to 2009 and implant brand (Table 1).

Adjusting for the other variables, males had a two times increased risk of revision resulting from deep infection as compared to females (p < 0.001). ASA 3+ patients had a 1.8 times higher risk of revision due to deep infection compared to patients classified as ASA 1 and 2 ($p = 0.003$). The occurrence of perioperative complications resulted in a 2.1 times higher risk of revision due to deep infection ($p = 0.004$) (Table 2).

The unadjusted Cox regression analysis showed statistically significant increased risk of revision resulting from infection comparing the longest duration group ≥110 min to the shortest procedure duration of <75 min by HR = 1.8 (95% CI 1.3-2.5, $p = 0.001$). (Table 3). After adjusting the Cox model for age, sex, diagnosis, ASA classification and the occurrence of perioperative complications, the effect of procedure duration was still statistically significant showing higher risk of revision due to deep infection in the longest duration group as

Table 1 Patient and procedure characteristics at primary TKA relative to the four procedure duration groups

	Procedure Duration Groups				
	< 75 min	75 – 89	90 – 109	≥110	p-value
Number of procedures	5680	6238	8659	7685	
Year of operation 2010-2014 (n = 15,900) %	60	58	57	52	P < 0.001
Male sex (n = 10,186) %	28	31	37	44	P < 0.001
Age group %					P < 0.001
<60 (n = 4989)	15	17	17	21	
60-69 (n = 9717)	33	34	34	36	
70-79 (n = 10,009)	38	36	36	32	
≥80 (n = 3547)	14	13	13	11	
Median age (years) (range)	71 (31-96)	70 (25-94)	70 (23-101)	68 (22-93)	
Median annual hospital volume	118	113	95	86	P < 0.001
ASA %					P = 0.001
1 (n = 4167)	16	14	14	16	
2 (n = 17,918)	64	65	64	62	
3+ (n = 5621)	19	19	20	21	
Osteoarthritis (n = 25,152) %	92	90	88	87	P < 0.001
Perioperative complications (n = 640) %	0.7	1.1	1.8	4.9	P < 0.001
Previous surgery for intraarticular fracture or fracture near the joint (n = 551) %	0.8	1.3	1.7	3.6	P < 0.001
Previous high tibial osteotomy (n = 885) %	1.9	2.5	2.8	4.9	P < 0.001
Computer navigated TKA (n = 2462) %	2.5	5.6	9.0	18	P < 0.001
Systemic antibiotics (n = 28,108) %	100	100	100	100	P = 0.4
Prosthesis brand %					P < 0.01
LCS Complete (n = 8752)	26	31	31	34	
Profix (n = 6286)	23	24	23	20	
NexGen (n = 4717)	18	16	16	17	
AGC (n = 2233)	15	7.3	6.1	5.1	
Duracon (n = 2043)	5.7	6.8	6.8	9.2	
Triathlon (n = 1317)	5.2	4.0	5.2	4.1	
Vanguard (n = 741)	1.5	1.7	3.7	3.0	
PFC-Sigma (n = 697)	1.3	2.6	3.0	2.7	
LCS (n = 516)	1.3	1.2	2.0	2.5	
Other (n = 955)	3.3	5.0	2.9	2.7	

compared to the shortest duration group; HR = 1.5 (1.0-2.1, $p = 0.03$) (Table 3, Fig. 2).

Procedure duration did not influence the risk of revision due to infection in the low-risk patient (described in the methods section) neither in the crude (HR = 1.2, 95% CI 0.8-1.9, $p = 0.3$) or in the adjusted Cox regression analysis HR = 1.1, 95% CI 0.7-1.7, $p = 0.6$) (Table 4, Fig. 3).

Discussion

Males, ASA 3+ patients, diagnosis other than OA and the occurrence of perioperative complications were factors associated with long procedure duration and increased risk of deep infection in this study (Table 2). In the low-risk patient we did not find evidence that increased procedure duration increased the risk of revision due to deep infection (Table 4). It could therefore be hypothesized that healthy patients that avoid perioperative complications tolerate longer procedure durations without getting infected.

Prolonged procedure duration may be caused by the complexity of the surgery and is thought to cause prolonged exposure time to microorganisms in the operating room and from the patient, possibly

Table 2 Patient and procedure related risk factors for revision due to infection after primary TKA

Variables	No	RR (95% CI) Unadjusted p-value		RR (95% CI) Adjusted	p-value
Age					
60-69	9717	1		1	
< 60	4989	0.9 (0.7-1.3)	0.7	0.9 (0.7-1.3)	0.6
70-79	10,009	0.8 (0.6-1.0)	0.1	0.8 (0.6-1.1)	0.1
> 80	3547	0.7 (0.5-1.1)	0.1	0.7 (0.5-1.1)	0.1
Sex					
men	10,186	1		1	
women	18,076	0.5 (0.4-0.6)	<0.001	0.5 (0.4-0.6)	<0.001
Diagnosis					
OA[a]	25,152	1		1	
Other[b]	3110	1.6 (1.2-2.1)	0.004	1.4 (1.0-2.0)	0.04
ASA					
1	4167	1		1	
2	17,918	1.1 (0.8-1.5)	0.7	1.2 (0.8-1.7)	0.4
3+	5621	1.7 (1.2-2.5)	0.005	1.8 (1.2-2.7)	0.003
Hospital volume					
1-49	3953	1		1	
50-99	10,615	1.1 (0.8-1.6)	0.5	1.1(0.8-1.6)	0.5
100-149	6379	1.2 (0.8-1.7)	0.4	1.1 (0.7-1.7)	0.6
≥ 150	7315	1.2 (0.8-1.7)	0.4	1.1 (0.7-1.7)	0.6
Perioperative complications					
no	27,068	1		1	
yes	640	2.3 (1.4-3.9)	0.002	2.1 (1.3-3.6)	0.004
Computer navigation					
no	23,626	1		1	
yes	2462	1.0 (0.7-1.5)	1.0	1.0 (0.7-1.5)	1.0
Prior fracture[c]					
no	27,711	1		1	
yes	551	2.20(1.1-3.6)	0.02	1.5 (0.8-2.7)	0.2
Prior osteotomy[d]					
no	27,377	1		1	
yes	885	0.9 (0.5-1.8)	0.8	0.8 (0.4-1.5)	0.5
TKA implant brands					
LCS Complete	8752	1		1	
AGC	2233	0.8 (0.5-1.3)	0.3	0.8 (0.5-1.3)	0.3
LCS	516	1.1 (0.5-2.3)	0.9	1.3 (0.6-2.9)	0.5
Duracon	2043	1.6 (1.1-2.3)	0.02	1.5 (0.8-2.7)	0.2
NexGen	4717	1.2 (0.8-1.6)	0.4	1.0 (0.7-1.4)	1.0
Profix	6286	0.9 (0.6-1.2)	0.4	0.9 (0.6-1.2)	0.4
PFC Sigma	697	1.0 (0.4-2.3)	1.0	0.9 (0.4-2.0)	0.7
Triathlon	1317	1.0 (0.6-1.8)	1.0	0.9 (0.5-1.5)	0.6
Vanguard TM	741	0.3 (0.1-1.0)	0.06	0.2 (0.1-0.8)	0.03
Others[e]	955	0.4 (0.1-1.0)	0.05	0.4 (0.1-1.0)	0.06

Table 2 Patient and procedure related risk factors for revision due to infection after primary TKA *(Continued)*

Variables	No	RR (95% CI) Unadjusted *p*-value		RR (95% CI) Adjusted	*p*-value
Time Period					
2005-2009	12,362	1		1	
2010-2014	15,900	1.3 (1.0-1.6)	0.03	1.3 (1.0-1.6)	0.08

[a]OA = Osteoarthritis
[b]Other = other diagnosis than osteoarthritis, e.g. inflammatory diseases
[c]Intraarticular fracture or fracture in proximity to the joint with previous osteosynthesis
[d]Previous knee osteotomy for knee malalignment
[e]Implant brands used in smaller numbers than 500 during the time period from 2005 to 2014

contaminating the wound. We found that risk factors for prolonged procedure duration was male gender, probably due to more difficult exposure related to extensor muscle mass and more dense bone cuts [12]. Similarly, young age, ASA 3+, previous surgery to the knee, low hospital volume, diagnosis other than OA and the use of computer navigation increased the procedure duration (Table 1).

There are several other publications on the effect of duration of surgery on deep infection; Namba et al. [1] conducted a subanalysis regarding duration of surgery and found a 9% increased risk per 15 min increment. Additionally, they found an increased risk of infection for male sex, ASA 3+ and other diagnoses than OA comparable to our results. However, perioperative complications as a confounding factor were not included in that study. Willis-Owen et al. found that the mean duration of surgery in non-infected patients was 102 (60-315) minutes versus 125 (80-201) minutes in the infected group. They did not, however, include confounding factors of comorbidities in their analysis [21]. Perioperative complications were not included as a variable in that study. They found an increased risk of infection in the >120 min group [22]. Naranje et al. [12] concluded that there was an effect of duration of surgery, but as one of many factors.

Their conclusion was that after controlling for confounding variables, the effect of duration of surgery on risk of revision for infection was weak as an independent factor.

The strength of our study is the high number of primary TKA and the high completeness of registration in the NAR. Validation has found that 89% of all revisions after TKA were reported to the register from 2008 to 2012 [19]. However, there are some limitations to our study. The present study focuses solely on deep infection leading to revision of the knee arthroplasty either as debridement with exchange of the polyethylene bearing or as a complete 1- or 2-staged procedure. Some registry studies have shown underestimation of the incidence of reoperations due to infection [23]. A previous study on total hip arthroplasty from the Danish Hip Arthroplasty register, using multiple data sources, found nearly 40% underreporting of prosthetic joint infections [24]. The total number of deep infections in the present study is therefore probably underestimated. However, it is unlikely that the underreporting of infection cases is unevenly distributed among the duration groups.

Why males are more prone to revision for infection is probably multifactorial, but the sex difference has

Table 3 Cox regression analysis. Risk of revision due to deep infection for all TKA patients in four different procedure duration groups

Procedure duration	No of TKA	No of revisions[a]	K-M 1y %[b]	K-M 4y %[b]	Cox regression[c] Unadjusted HR (95% CI)	*p*-value	Adjusted HR (95% CI)	*p*-value
						0.01[d]		0.03[d]
<75	5680	48	0.60	0.89	1		1	
75-89	6238	54	0.58	0.85	1.1 (0.7 - 1.5)	1.0	1.0 (0.7 - 1.4)	0.9
90-109	8659	91	0.63	1.01	1.2 (0.9 – 1.7)	0.3	1.1 (0.8 – 1.6)	0.5
≥110	7685	118	0.91	1.38	1.8 (1.3 – 2.5)	0.001	1.5 (1.0 – 2.1)	0.03

[a]Number of revisions due to deep infection (*n* = 311)
[b]Kaplan-Meier estimated proportion of revisions due to deep infection at 1 and 4 years follow-up
[c]Unadjusted and adjusted Hazard ratios (HR) estimated with the Cox proportional hazards model (adjusted for sex, age, diagnosis, ASA classification and perioperative complications
[d]Overall test for group differences

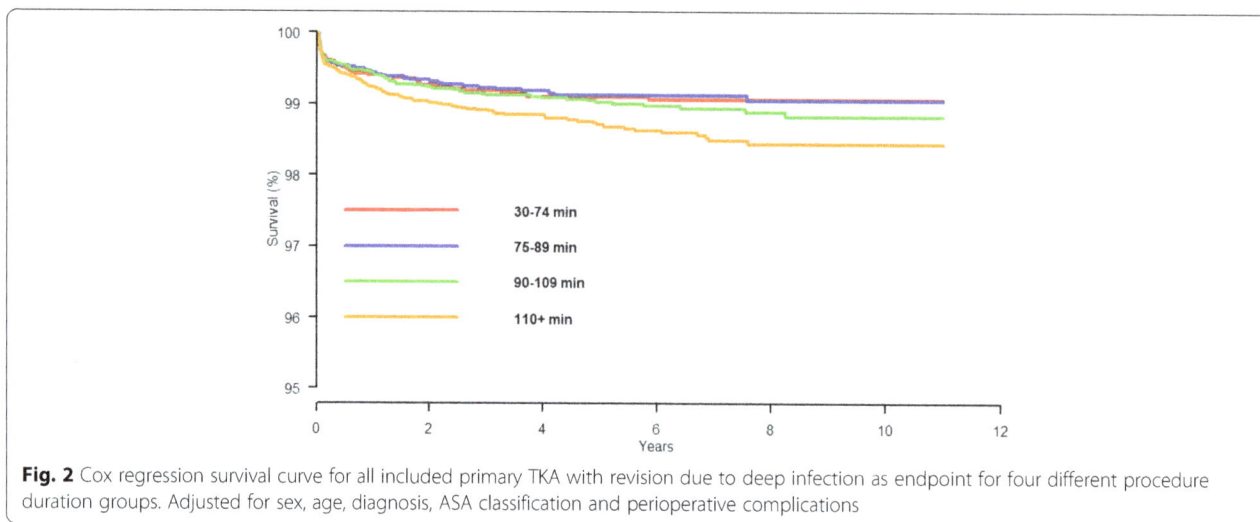

Fig. 2 Cox regression survival curve for all included primary TKA with revision due to deep infection as endpoint for four different procedure duration groups. Adjusted for sex, age, diagnosis, ASA classification and perioperative complications

been studied. Male's and female's skin differ in hormone metabolism, hair growth and sebum production [25]. There have been demonstrated sex differences in skin pH and skin thickness that are possible factors for the differences in skin colonisation [26, 27] and thereby the increased risk of infection discussed in several studies [1, 12]. Our study found evidence to support that males are at higher risk of revision due to infection after TKA.

Infection rates in orthopaedic surgery are low and therefore causal factors are difficult to determine. Endogenous transmission of for instance Staphylococci carriers has also been shown to be an important cause of surgical site infection [28, 29]. Males have a higher carrier frequency of staphylococci which may partly explain their twofold risk of revision due to infection compared to women found in several studies [13, 14].

Perioperative complications resulted in prolonged duration of surgery and also risk of revision due to deep infection after TKA in our study. The majority

of perioperative complications were different types of fractures, various tendon and ligament ruptures and technical issues regarding instruments and cementing. This highlights the importance of avoiding complications through education of surgeons and theatre staff, preoperative planning, good theatre routines and increasing volume of surgery. Perioperative complications might necessitate extended surgical approaches and added implants and devices could potentially harm the soft tissues, increasing the risk of hematomas, potentially increasing the risk of infection.

BMI (Body mass index) and other risk factors such as smoking or diabetes are not registered individually in the NAR, and is a limitation to this study. However, it is captured in the ASA classification. ASA classification has been shown to be a strong predictor of wound infection [30]. Increasing BMI is also a contributing factor to increasing duration of surgery [7] and some studies has found a correlation between increased BMI and postoperative infection after TKA

Table 4 Cox regression analysis. Risk of revision due to deep infection for the low-risk patient[a] in four different procedure duration groups

| | | | | | Cox regression[d] | | | |
| | | | | | Unadjusted | | Adjusted | |
Procedure duration	No of TKA	No of revisions[b]	K-M 1y %[c]	K-M 4y %[c]	HR (95% CI)	p-value	HR (95% CI)	p-value
<75	3232	31	0.68	1.00	1		1	
75-89	3718	30	0.57	0.84	0.8 (0.5 - 1.4)	0.5	0.8 (0.5 - 1.3)	0.4
90-109	5130	44	0.49	0.78	0.9 (0.6 – 1.4)	0.6	0.8 (0.5 – 1.3)	0.4
≥110	4177	52	0.72	1.10	1.2 (0.8 – 1.9)	0.3	1.1 (0.7 – 1.7)	0.6

[a]The low-risk TKA patient: TKA patient with primary osteoarthritis, ASA 1 or 2, without any previous surgery to the knee and no registered perioperative complications (n = 16,257)
[b]Number of revisions due to deep infection (n = 157)
[c]Kaplan-Meier estimated proportion of revisions due to deep infection at 1 and 4 years follow-up
[d]Unadjusted and adjusted Hazard ratios (HR) estimated with the Cox proportional hazards model, adjusted for sex and age

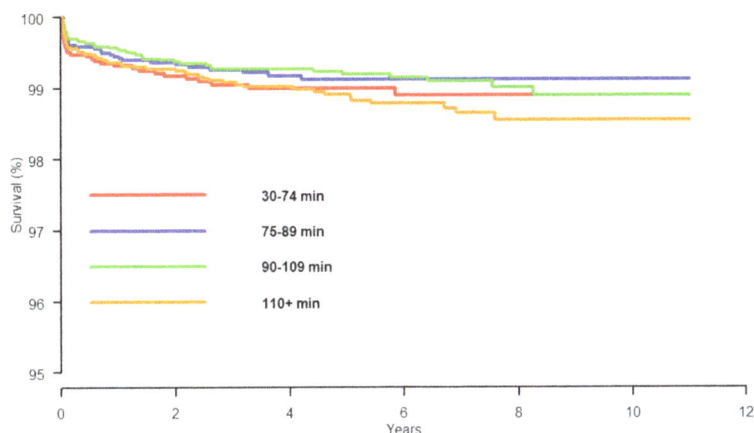

Fig. 3 Cox regression survival curve for "low-risk" primary TKA patients with revision due to deep infection as endpoint for four different procedure duration groups with adjustment for age and sex. "Low-risk" TKA patient: patient with primary osteoarthritis, with ASA 1 or 2, without any previous surgery to the knee and no registered perioperative complications

[8, 9]. Others did not find similar relationship between obesity and infection [12]. Diabetes, irradiated skin, lymphedema, history of bleeding disorder could all lead to postoperative hematomas and wound-related problems and be associated with persistent wound drainage and deep infection [31, 32]. Implant brand affected procedure duration for two different implants (Table 1). The reason for this variety could be hospital and surgeon dependent, or that some implants require more steps in the procedure itself. However, implant brand did not affect the risk of deep infection.

Conclusion

Male patients classified as ASA 3+, previous surgery to the knee and the occurrence of perioperative complications were factors requiring longer procedure duration and had a higher risk for infection after TKA in this study. Low-risk patients without perioperative complications did not have an increased risk of deep infection due to longer procedure durations. Long procedure duration in itself seems to have minor impact on infection since we found no association in the low-risk patient.

Abbreviations
ASA: American Society of Anesthesiologists; BMI: Body mass index; CAOS: Computer assisted orthopaedic surgery; CI: Confidence interval; CR: Cruciate retaining; HR: Hazard ratio; K-M: Kaplan Meier; NAR: Norwegian Arthroplasty Røegister; OA: Osteoarthritis; TKA: Total knee arthroplasty

Acknowledgements
Not applicable.

Funding
This study had no funding. The Norwegian Arthroplasty Register is financed by the Western Norway Regional Health Authority (Helse-Vest).

Author's contributions
MB, BE, AMF and OF designed the study. MB, BE, AMF, HD, KI, LIH and OF collected the data and edited the manuscript. MB wrote the manuscript and the analyses were done by AMF, BE, MB and OF. All authors have read and approved the final manuscript.

Consent for publication
Not applicable.

Competing interests
The authors declare that they have no competing interests.

Author details
[1]Coastal Hospital in Hagavik, 5217 Hagavik, Norway. [2]Center for Evidence-based Practice, Bergen University College, 5021 Bergen, Norway. [3]The Norwegian Arthroplasty Register, Department of Orthopaedic Surgery, Haukeland University Hospital, 5021 Bergen, Norway. [4]Department of Clinical Medicine, Institute of Medicine and Dentistry, University of Bergen, 5021 Bergen, Norway.

References
1. Namba RS, Inacio MC, Paxton EW. Risk factors associated with deep surgical site infections after primary total knee arthroplasty: an analysis of 56,216 knees. J Bone Joint Surg Am. 2013;95:775–82.
2. Carroll K, Dowsey M, Choong P, Peel T. Risk factors for superficial wound complications in hip and knee arthroplasty. Clin Microbiol Infect. 2014;20:130–5.
3. Peersman G, Laskin R, Davis J, Peterson MG, Richart T. Prolonged operative time correlates with increased infection rate after total knee arthroplasty. HSS journal: the musculoskeletal journal of Hospital for Special Surgery. 2006;2:70–2.
4. Smabrekke A, Espehaug B, Havelin LI, Furnes O. Operating time and survival of primary total hip replacements: an analysis of 31,745 primary cemented and uncemented total hip replacements from local hospitals reported to the Norwegian Arthroplasty register 1987-2001. Acta Orthop Scand. 2004;75:524–32.
5. Campbell DA, Jr., Henderson WG, Englesbe MJ, Hall BL, O'Reilly M, Bratzler D, et al. Surgical site infection prevention: the importance of operative duration and blood transfusion–results of the first American College of Surgeons-National Surgical Quality Improvement Program Best Practices Initiative. J Am Coll Surg 2008;207: 810-820.

6.   Strum DP, Sampson AR, May JH, Vargas LG. Surgeon and type of anesthesia predict variability in surgical procedure times. Anesthesiology. 2000;92:1454–66.

7.   Raphael IJ, Parmar M, Mehrganpour N, Sharkey PF, Parvizi J. Obesity and operative time in primary total joint arthroplasty. The journal of knee surgery. 2013;26:95–9.

8.   Liabaud B, Patrick DA, Jr., Geller JA. Higher body mass index leads to longer operative time in total knee arthroplasty. J Arthroplast 2013;28: 563-565.

9.   Maoz G, Phillips M, Bosco J, Slover J, Stachel A, Inneh I, et al. The Otto Aufranc award: modifiable versus nonmodifiable risk factors for infection after hip arthroplasty. Clin Orthop Relat Res. 2015;473:453–9.

10. Baker P, Petheram T, Jameson S, Reed M, Gregg P, Deehan D. The association between body mass index and the outcomes of total knee arthroplasty. The Journal of bone and joint surgery American. 2012;94:1501–8.

11. Dale H, Skramm I, Lower HL, Eriksen HM, Espehaug B, Furnes O, et al. Infection after primary hip arthroplasty: a comparison of 3 Norwegian health registers. Acta Orthop. 2011;82:646–54.

12. Naranje S, Lendway L, Mehle S, Gioe TJ. Does operative time affect infection rate in primary total knee arthroplasty? Clin Orthop Relat Res. 2015;473:64–9.

13. Kurtz SM, Ong KL, Lau E, Bozic KJ, Berry D, Parvizi J. Prosthetic joint infection risk after TKA in the Medicare population. Clin Orthop Relat Res. 2010;468:52–6.

14. Pedersen AB, Svendsson JE, Johnsen SP, Riis A, Overgaard S. Risk factors for revision due to infection after primary total hip arthroplasty. A population-based study of 80,756 primary procedures in the Danish hip Arthroplasty registry. Acta Orthop. 2010;81:542–7.

15. Dale H, Fenstad AM, Hallan G, Havelin LI, Furnes O, Overgaard S, et al. Increasing risk of prosthetic joint infection after total hip arthroplasty. Acta Orthop. 2012;83:449–58.

16. Parvizi J, Gehrke T, Chen AF. Proceedings of the international consensus on Periprosthetic joint infection. The bone & joint journal. 2013;95-b:1450–2.

17. Skramm I, Saltyte Benth J, Bukholm G. Decreasing time trend in SSI incidence for orthopaedic procedures: surveillance matters. The Journal of hospital infection. 2012;82:243–7.

18. Lozano LM, Nunez M, Segur JM, Macule F, Sastre S, Nunez E, et al. Relationship between knee anthropometry and surgical time in total knee arthroplasty in severely and morbidly obese patients: a new prognostic index of surgical difficulty. Obes Surg. 2008;18:1149–53.

19. NorwegianArthroplastyRegister. Norwegian Arthroplasty register annual report 2015. Rapport2015.pdf.

20. Kapadia BH, Berg RA, Daley JA, Fritz J, Bhave A, Mont MA. Periprosthetic joint infection. Lancet. 387:386–94.

21. Willis-Owen CA, Konyves A, Martin DK. Factors affecting the incidence of infection in hip and knee replacement: an analysis of 5277 cases. The Journal of bone and joint surgery British volume. 2010;92:1128–33.

22. Ridgeway S, Wilson J, Charlet A, Kafatos G, Pearson A, Coello R. Infection of the surgical site after arthroplasty of the hip. The Journal of bone and joint surgery British volume. 2005;87:844–50.

23. Jamsen E, Huotari K, Huhtala H, Nevalainen J, Konttinen YT. Low rate of infected knee replacements in a nationwide series–is it an underestimate? Acta Orthop. 2009;80:205–12.

24. Gundtoft PH, Overgaard S, Schonheyder HC, Moller JK, Kjaersgaard-Andersen P, Pedersen AB. The "true" incidence of surgically treated deep prosthetic joint infection after 32,896 primary total hip arthroplasties. Acta Orthop. 2015:1–9.

25. Giacomoni PU, Mammone T, Teri M. Gender-linked differences in human skin. J Dermatol Sci. 2009;55:144–9.

26. Fierer N, Hamady M, Lauber CL, Knight R. The influence of sex, handedness, and washing on the diversity of hand surface bacteria. Proc Natl Acad Sci U S A. 2008;105:17994–9.

27. Dao H Jr, Kazin RA. Gender differences in skin: a review of the literature. Gender medicine. 2007;4:308–28.

28. Mansson E, Hellmark B, Sundqvist M, Soderquist B. Sequence types of Staphylococcus Epidermidis associated with prosthetic joint infections are not present in the laminar airflow during prosthetic joint surgery. APMIS. 2015;123:589–95.

29. Skramm I, Fossum Moen AE, Aroen A, Bukholm G. Surgical site infections in Orthopaedic surgery demonstrate clones similar to those in Orthopaedic Staphylococcus Aureus nasal carriers. J Bone Joint Surg Am. 2014;96:882–8.

30. Woodfield JC, Beshay NM, Pettigrew RA, Plank LD, van Rij AM. American Society of Anesthesiologists classification of physical status as a predictor of wound infection. ANZ J Surg. 2007;77:738–41.

31. Simons MJ, Amin NH, Scuderi GR. Acute wound complications after Total knee Arthroplasty: prevention and management. The Journal of the American Academy of Orthopaedic Surgeons. 2017;25:547–55.

32. Galat DD, McGovern SC, Larson DR, Harrington JR, Hanssen AD, Clarke HD. Surgical treatment of early wound complications following primary total knee arthroplasty. J Bone Joint Surg Am. 2009;91:48–54.

6

Risk factors and outcomes in asymmetrical femoral component size for posterior referencing bilateral total knee arthroplasty

Piya Pinsornsak[1]* (iD), Adisai Chaiwuttisak[1] and Krit Boontanapibul[2]

Abstract

Background: Theoretically, potential errors in femoral component (FC) sizing can affect postoperative functional outcomes after total knee arthroplasty (TKA), including range of motion (ROM), anterior knee pain, and flexion stability. Incidences of asymmetrical femoral components (AFC) in bilateral TKA have been reported; however; there is a lack of data on exactly why AFC size selection may differ in patients who have had posterior referencing system bilateral TKA. Therefore, this study was conducted to determine risk factors of AFC size selection in patients specifically undergoing posterior referencing bilateral TKA and to compare clinical outcomes between those with AFC or symmetrical femoral component (SFC) sizes.

Methods: We conducted a retrospective matched-pair study comparing thirty-four patients who had undergone simultaneous and staged bilateral TKA using AFC size (Group I) and thirty-five patients with SFC size (Group II). Patients were matched according to gender, body mass index, prosthesis type, and operative technique. Preoperative radiographic morphology of both distal femurs including anteroposterior/mediolateral diameters, anterior-posterior femoral offset, and postoperative radiographic data of FC comprising flexion and valgus angle were recorded. The postoperative functional outcomes including ROM, anterior knee pain, knee society score, and functional score at 6 weeks, 3, 6, 12 and 24 months were compared.

Results: There were no differences in morphology between left and right distal femurs from preoperative radiographic data in both groups. The postoperative radiograph showed a significantly greater FC flexion angle difference in Group I vs. Group II (2.18° ± 1.29° and 1.36° ± 1.08° $P = 0.007$), while the other parameters were the same. The postoperative clinical outcomes displayed no distinction between groups.

Conclusion: The factor primarily associated with AFC size selection in bilateral TKAs is the difference in FC flexion angle but not the morphological diversity between sides. The postoperative functional outcomes were not inferior in AFC patients in comparison with SFC patients.

Keywords: Bilateral total knee arthroplasty, Femoral component, Asymmetrical femoral component size, Anterior femoral offset, Posterior femoral offset, Femoral component flexion

* Correspondence: pinpiya2003@yahoo.com
[1]Department of Orthopaedics, Faculty of Medicine, Thammasat University, 99 Moo 18, Khlong Nueng, Khlong Luang, Pathum Thani 12120, Thailand
Full list of author information is available at the end of the article

Background

The number of patients undergoing Total Knee Arthroplasty (TKA) has mirrored the growth in aging populations; some 20 % of elderly patients need bilateral TKA [1]. The proper choice of component size is thought to be essential for a good clinical outcome [2].

Theoretically, the femoral component size affects the flexion gap, stability, range of motion (ROM) and functional outcome after surgery. If the selected component is too small, the result could be flexion instability and pain, recurrent effusion, cam jump and dislocation in a posterior-stabilised prosthesis, and premature loosening of the component itself [3]. Conversely, too large of a femoral component can limit the ROM, create a painful and stiff knee, lead to anterior knee pain with patellar over-stuff, and result in a poor functional outcome [4, 5]. In the mediolateral (ML) plane, too small of a component creates an under hang which may result in subsiding of the component, increased bleeding from the raw surface, and, finally, osteolysis [6] whilst too large of a femoral component enhances component overhang and may increase knee pain [5, 7].

An overview of previously published work shows that 7–9.2%of patients who had undergone a bilateral TKA had an asymmetrical femoral component (AFC) [8–10]. Asymmetrical incidences for anterior referenced femoral component were significantly higher than those using the posterior referencing system. This may be because of the irreproducibility of the flexion gap which will possibly create variability in femoral component sizing [9]. Many factors can influence AFC size selection, including asymmetrical patient anatomy between the left and right knees, the ligament laxity or tightness, the thickness of distal femoral cut which affects the extension gap, errors in distal femoral cutting angle, and the potential variability of the different anatomical landmarks used to measure (between surgeons) over the anterior surface of distal femur [11]. Overall, though, we consider that there is a lack of data on exactly why specific AFC sizes are chosen for patients using posterior referencing bilateral TKA. Therefore, the primary objective of this study was to determine the risk factors affecting AFC size selection for patients undergoing posterior referencing bilateral TKA, including the preoperative patient's anatomy on both sides of the knee and the position of prosthesis component placement in sagittal and coronal plane. The secondary objective was to compare the clinical outcomes of patients who underwent posterior referencing bilateral TKA between AFC or SFC.

Methods

Study design and participants

For our retrospective review, we had 374 cases of bilateral TKA that were operated on, between March 2012 and June 2015, by a single surgeon (PP). We included all varus gonarthrosis patients classified with Kellgren-Lawrence Grade 3 to 4 who underwent either simultaneous bilateral (operation on both sides with the same anaesthesia) or staged bilateral (each side operated on independently with separate anaesthesia and admission) TKA. We excluded patients with previous knee injuries, deformed bone anatomy, post-traumatic knee arthritis, extra-articular knee deformity, inflammatory arthritis, and other deformities classified as severe (preoperative varus deformity $> 20°$, limited knee flexion $< 90°$, and flexion contracture $> 20°$). Inadequate preoperative and postoperative radiographs, including improper exposure, position and techniques affecting radiographic measurement, were also excluded. Therefore, we finally enrolled 319 patients from the original total of 374 bilateral TKA patients.

Among these cases, we identified thirty-five patients with AFC (Group I), and all had cemented posterior-stabilized total knee prosthesis (Vanguard® Knee System, Zimmer Biomet, Warsaw, Indiana, USA) using the posterior referencing system. SFC patients (Group II) were then place into matched pair in a 1:1 fashion. To do this, we selected 35 SFC from the total of 284 SFC bilateral TKA patients; this was based on gender, age at bilateral TKA (performed within a range of 5 years), body mass index [BMI (within 5 kg/m^2)], prosthesis type, and operative technique. This study was approved by our institutional ethics committee.

Sample size

We calculated sample size based on our pilot study. We estimated that a sample size of at least 33 patients in each treatment group would have 80% power to detect a mean femoral component size difference of at least 0.8 mm for the asymmetrical size group compared with the symmetrical size group, assuming an SD of 0.21, with a 5% one-sided type I error. We rounded this up to 35 patients in each group.

Operative procedure

A standard medial parapatellar approach was used on all patients. Femoral preparation was performed first by drilling the insertion point of the femoral step reamer 1 cm above the posterior cruciate ligament insertion. After the intramedullary drill guide diameter 9 mm was inserted, the distal femoral cut was carried out with the valgus angle perpendicular to the mechanical axis, measured from the whole leg standing posteroanterior weight-bearing radiograph. Anterior cruciate and posterior cruciate ligaments were removed. The tibial extramedullary guide system was applied, and proximal tibial cut was made with a posterior slope aiming for 3 degrees and perpendicular to the mechanical axis. Ligament balancing to create a rectangular extension gap was performed and checked with a spacer block.

Lower extremity alignment was measured, and the valgus-varus stability of knee was tested in full extension. The posterior referencing system for the AP cut was chosen. The femoral anteroposterior (AP) cut using the AP cutting guide was inserted with a 3-degree external rotation from the posterior condyle. The AP sizing was measured using an anterior boom position at the highest point of the anterolateral femoral cortex. In-between femoral component size was determined by using the closest size of the component. After finishing the AP cut, the flexion gap was balanced and checked with the spacer block in 90-degree knee flexion. The cemented posterior-stabilized total knee prosthesis (Vanguard® Knee System, Zimmer Biomet, Warsaw, Indiana, USA) was inserted, and the patella was resurfaced by restoring of natural patella thickness. Standard postoperative pain control and rehabilitation protocols were employed in all cases.

Outcome measures

The primary outcome measure was the preoperative evaluation of patient's anatomy on both sides of distal femurs including the AP and ML diameters of the femoral condyle, the AP diameter of femoral canal, and the anterior and posterior femoral offset (Fig. 1). We also examined the postoperative radiographs to evaluate the femoral component flexion angle, femoral component valgus angle, the anterior and posterior femoral offset of the component, AP diameter of femoral canal, and AP and ML diameters of the femoral component (Fig. 2). Only good quality radiographs were selected for pre and postoperative evaluation, including AP and lateral views with good exposure: having a uniform controlled distance of beam to the cassette was essential. Measurements were analysed by the Picture Archiving and Communication System (PACS), also known as Synapse (FUJIFILM Medical Systems Inc., Hanover Park, Illinois). All the radiographs were blinded from assessors by computerized random selection. Two independent orthopaedists were assigned to evaluate inter-observer and intra-observer reliability in radiographic measurement.

Our secondary outcome was the postoperative clinical results of patients who had AFC or SFC, including knee society score (KSS), functional score, knee ROM, and anterior knee pain at 6 weeks, 3 months, 6 months, 12 months and 24 months. We excluded staged bilateral TKA from clinical outcome evaluations to reduce the confounding effects of differing recovery protocols and operating intervals between sides. The outcome assessors were blinded to treatment groups during the study period.

Statistical analysis

The measurements collected from radiographs and clinical results were analysed by descriptive statistics as means and standard deviations. The difference between sides in

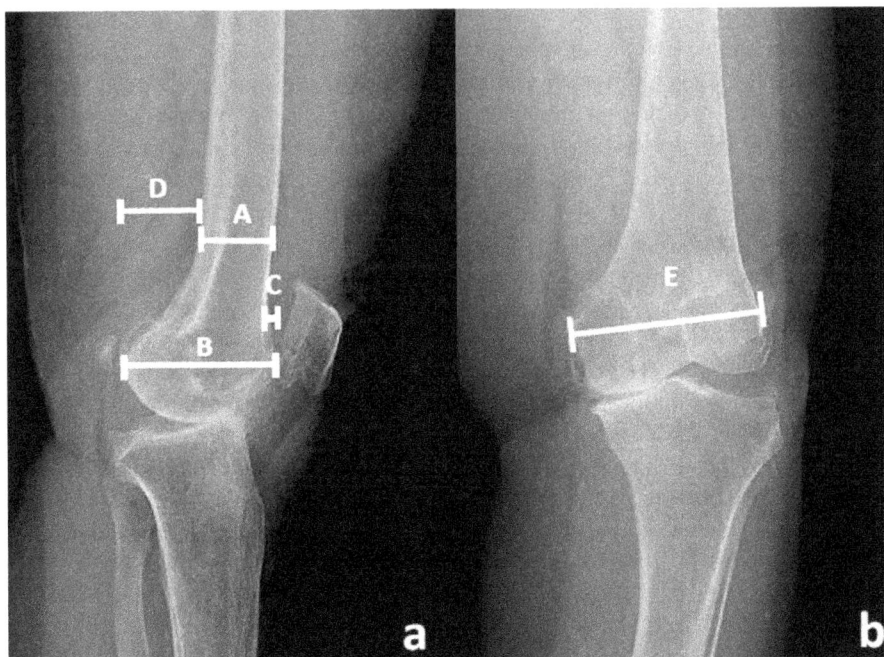

Fig. 1 Preoperative radiographic measurements of distal femoral morphology. **a**: Measurement technique of diameter of AP femoral canal (A), diameter of AP femoral condyle (B), anterior femoral offset (C) and posterior femoral offset (D) in lateral view. **b**: Measurement technique of ML diameter of femoral condyle in AP view (E)

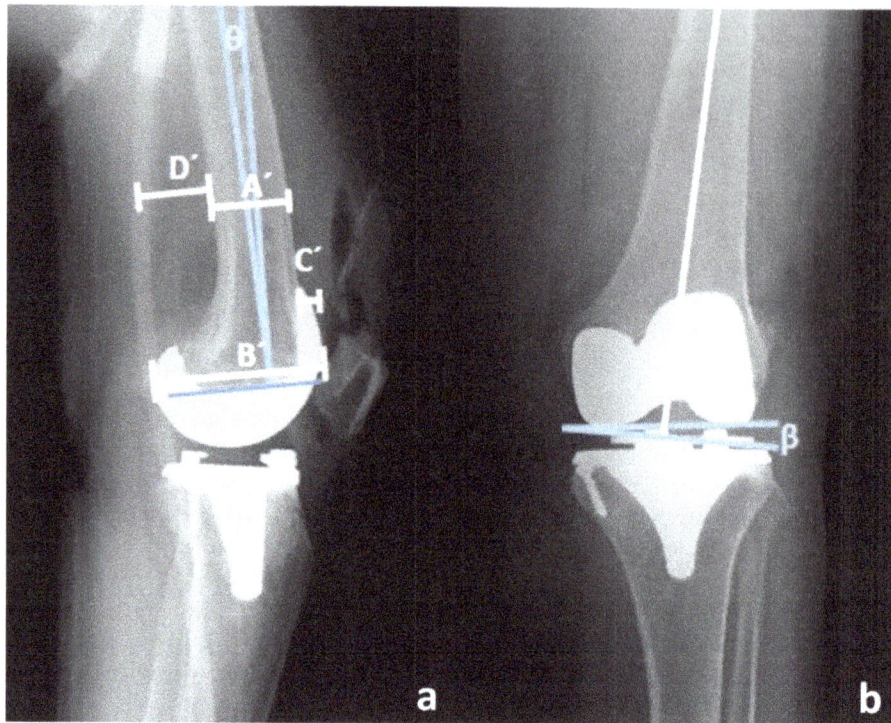

Fig. 2 Postoperative radiographic measurements of femoral component. **a**: Measurement technique of diameter of AP femoral canal (A'), diameter of AP femoral condyle (B'), anterior femoral offset (C'), posterior femoral offset (D') and femoral component flexion angle (θ) in lateral view. **b**: Measurement technique of femoral valgus angle (β)

individual patients was evaluated by using independent simple t-test and proportional data were analysed by Fisher's exact test.

Both inter-observer reliability and intra-observer reproducibility for pre and postoperative radiograph measurements among evaluators were calculated by using an intra-class correlation coefficient (ICC). For the inter-observer reliability, measurements were performed by two adult reconstruction fellows (AC, KB). For intra-observer reproducibility, measurements were performed twice with an interval of three weeks between.

Results

A total of 374 patient notes were evaluated for entry (STROBE profile, Fig. 3). Fifty-five patients were excluded: 29 did not meet the ineligibility criteria and 26 had inadequate radiographs. We enrolled 319 patients and grouped them according to individual size of femoral components. Then, a retrospective matched pair (1:1) study of 70 patients who underwent bilateral TKA by a single surgeon; thirty-five patients with AFC size (Group I) and 35 patients with SFC size (Group II) were included. Only sixty-nine patients were analysed due to incomplete data collection for one patient who did not have a recorded KSS at 6 months after surgery in Group I. There were 20

patients of simultaneous bilateral TKA in each group. The incidence of AFC size in our study was 9.89% (37/374).

Preoperative demographic data are shown in Table 1. In Group I, 28 were female, and 6 were male, with an average age of 67.57 ± 8.9 years old; of the 35 patients in Group II, 27 were female, and 8 were male with an average age of 68.14 ± 6.8 years old. Patient demographics were not significantly different between the two groups. Preoperative radiographic data (Table 2) comparing the anatomy of both knees between Group I and Group II showed no outstanding discrepancies in AP femoral condyle diameters, AP femoral canal diameters, anterior and posterior femoral offsets, and ML diameter of femoral condyles.

The postoperative radiograph (Table 3) noted a statistically significant ($p = 0.007$) imbalance in femoral component flexion of 2.18° ± 1.29° in Group I and 1.37° ± 1.08° in Group II. As the femoral component size was asymmetrical in Group I, the AP and ML femoral component diameters were significantly greater than those in Group II ($p = 0.015$ and $p = 0.000$, respectively). Group II had a slightly greater femoral valgus angle difference of the femoral component but was not statistically significant (1.64° ± 1.67°, and 1.41° ± 1.13°, $p = 0.524$). No statistically significant deviations in the other parameters (AP femoral canal

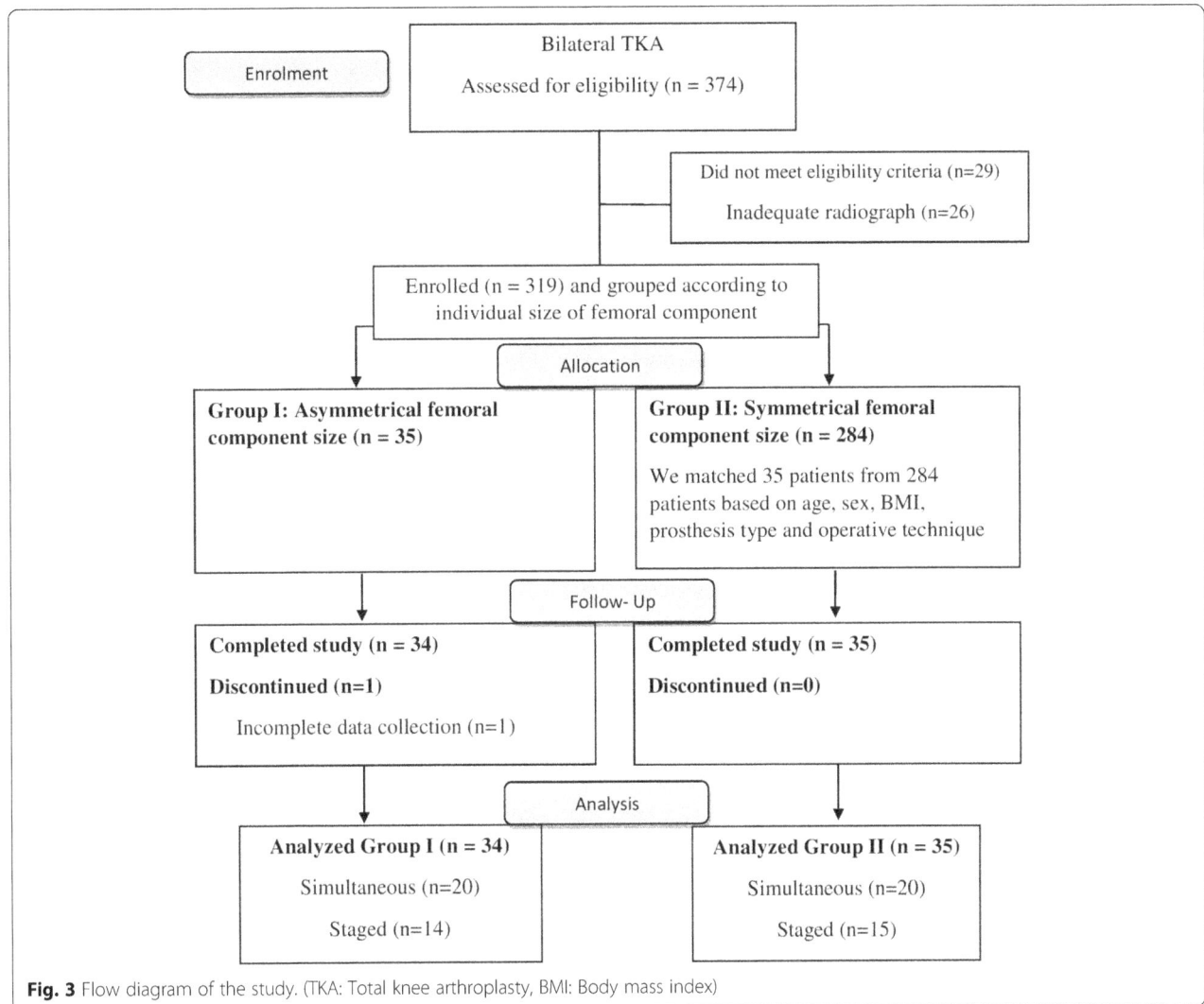

Fig. 3 Flow diagram of the study. (TKA: Total knee arthroplasty, BMI: Body mass index)

diameter, anterior and posterior femoral component offset) were seen.

For preoperative radiographs, the intra- and inter-observer kappa values (κ) were 0.69 and 0.63, respectively. For postoperative radiographs intra and inter observer kappa values (κ) were 0.72 and 0.64, respectively. Therefore, the reliability of the radiographic measurements was acceptable.

Table 1 Demographic data for patients in the study

Characteristics	Group I	Group II	P-value
	Asymmetrical femoral component	Symmetrical femoral component group	
	(n = 34)	(n = 35)	
Gender (F/M)	28/6	27/8	0.76*
Age (years)	67.57 ± 8.9	68.14 ± 6.8	0.85†
BMI (kg/m²)	28.51 ± 3.4	28.04 ± 2.7	0.69†

*data analyses were performed with exact probability
†data analyses were performed with Student's t-test

The postoperative clinical outcomes were measured only in the simultaneous bilateral TKA patients in each group to reduce the effect of confounding factors. No significant differences in postoperative clinical outcomes between the two groups were seen in the pre- and postoperative KSS, functional score, and knee ROM at 3 months, 6 months, 12 months and 24 months (Table 4). Of interest, both groups had the same incidence of anterior knee pain in each time period (Table 5).

Discussion

Asymmetrical component sizes in bilateral TKA have been studied extensively [8, 9]. However, clinical data have not been incorporated in determining the causes of bilateral asymmetry. In the study of Brown et al....., of the 268 bilateral TKAs studied, there was a 6.7% size gap in femoral components between left and right knees, a 1.1% difference in tibial components, and a 0.3% distinction in patellar components [8]. Capeci et al evaluated 253

Table 2 Measured preoperative radiographic parameters for the left and right knees and their mean differences for Groups I and II

Parameter	Group I Asymmetrical femoral component (n = 34)			Group II Symmetrical femoral component (n = 35)			P value[†]
	Rt (mm)	Lt (mm)	Difference (Each patient)	Rt (mm)	Lt (mm)	Difference (Each patient)	
AP femoral canal diameter (A)	28.69 ± 2.55	28.57 ± 2.62	0.50 ± 0.46	28.65 ± 2.35	28.74 ± 2.41	0.53 ± 0.41	0.78
AP femoral condyle diameter (B)	64.34 ± 5.11	64.52 ± 4.62	2.11 ± 1.99	64.79 ± 4.67	65.06 ± 3.01	2.19 ± 1.69	0.87
Anterior femoral offset (C)	7.05 ± 1.75	7.37 ± 1.71	1.21 ± 0.95	6.67 ± 1.77	6.90 ± 1.86	1.16 ± 1.19	0.84
Posterior femoral offset (D)	27.19 ± 3.97	27.36 ± 4.14	2.14 ± 2.08	27.93 ± 4.30	27.57 ± 4.45	2.17 ± 2.31	0.95
ML femoral condyle diameter	74.88 ± 6.66	74.82 ± 6.00	1.03 ± 1.58	75.42 ± 5.41	75.45 ± 5.53	0.75 ± 0.94	0.38

[†]data analyses were performed with Student's t-test

patients with simultaneous bilateral TKA and found 8.7%, 6.7% and 5.1% had femoral, tibial and patellar component asymmetry, respectively [9]. Reddy et al also reported 9.2% and 8.7% disparities in femoral and tibial component asymmetry within a total of 289 bilateral TKAs, respectively [10].

In our study, we noted just under 10% of our patients had AFC sizes following bilateral TKA that was performed by the same surgeon with the same surgical technique and prosthesis. Theoretically, asymmetry of bony anatomy and geometry could determine femoral component size selection, but this phenomenon has not yet been recorded in bilateral TKA patients. Yet, we observed no great variation in preoperative knee anatomy between the two groups. This implies that femoral bone geometry did not affect femoral component size selection for our patients (including AP and ML distal femoral bone geometry, anterior and posterior offset of distal femoral bone geometry). The imbalance between flexion and extension gap is one of the key factors that affected the femoral component size choice especially in the anterior refencing system where a bigger initial extension gap has typically resulted in surgeons selecting smaller femoral component size while a smaller initial extension gap has forced surgeons to choose the bigger femoral components to compensate for these gaps. However, in our

study, we have particularly chosen femoral component size by using the "measure-resection bone cutting technique with posterior referencing system"; this creates the same amount of posterior femoral bone cut and flexion gap in all patients. Thus, any possible differences in femoral component size selection would not be affected by ligament laxity in our study.

Our study ascertained that the selection of the femoral component size was related to its angle of flexion and its coronal plane deviation. The difference in femoral component flexion could have resulted from different points of entry on the distal femur when the distal femoral cutting guide was inserted, bone cutting errors due to flexure of the thin cutting saw blade, forceful misdirection of the cutting saw blade, or movement of the cutting guide during osteotomy [12, 13]. A drill hole placement that is positioned too anteriorly generally leads to extension of the femoral component, whereas an excessive posterior drill hole placement might lead to flexion of the femoral component. An entry point deviation of just 5 mm anteriorly or posteriorly brought about a significant degree of flexion or extension (ranging from 2.2° of extension to 8.7° of flexion) [14]. Sagittal malalignment could create a 1-size-up or 1-size-down error in femoral sizing in TKA.

A computer simulation of TKA found that a femoral component flexion from 0° to 6° significantly resulted

Table 3 Measured postoperative radiographic parameters in Groups I and II

Parameter	Group I Asymmetrical femoral component (Different each patient)	Group II Symmetrical femoral component (Different each patient)	P value[†]
AP femoral canal diameter (A') (mm)	0.48 ± 0.44	0.60 ± 0.56	0.312
AP prosthesis diameter (B') (mm)	2.33 ± 1.74	1.46 ± 1.05	0.015
Anterior femoral offset (C') (mm)	1.13 ± 0.93	1.29 ± 0.99	0.500
Posterior femoral offset (D') (mm)	2.23 ± 1.73	1.56 ± 1.12	0.066
ML prosthesis diameter (mm)	2.23 ± 1.41	0.72 ± 0.61	0.000
Femoral component flexion angle (β) (degrees)	2.18° ± 1.29°	1.36° ± 1.08°	0.007
Femoral component valgus angle (α) (degrees)	1.41° ± 1.13°	1.64° ± 1.67°	0.524

[†]data analyses were performed with Student's t-test

Table 4 Postoperative clinical outcomes of bilateral simultaneous TKA between Groups I and II

Parameter	Group I	Group II	P value†
	Asymmetrical femoral component (n = 20)	Symmetrical femoral component (n = 20)	
Mean Knee Society Score			
Pre-op	53.32 ± 11.63	50.30 ± 13.84	0.29
6 weeks Post-op	78.55 ± 5.14	79.22 ± 4.55	0.53
3 months Post-op	86.82 ± 5.69	87.50 ± 5.15	0.57
6 months Post-op	91.95 ± 4.26	92.45 ± 4.16	0.59
12 months Post-op	92.10 ± 4.25	92.52 ± 4.08	0.65
24 months Post-op	92.17 ± 4.22	92.65 ± 4.02	0.60
Mean Functional Score			
Pre-op	45.5 ± 12.59	46.75 ± 10.03	0.62
6 weeks Post-op	60.75 ± 12.38	61.25 ± 8.71	0.88
3 months Post-op	73.25 ± 10.42	75.50 ± 8.25	0.45
6 months Post-op	84.50 ± 6.67	85.25 ± 6.78	0.72
12 months Post-op	84.25 ± 7.12	85.50 ± 6.47	0.56
24 months Post-op	84.75 ± 7.15	85.75 ± 7.12	0.66
Mean Maximum Knee Flexion Difference (Each patient)			
Pre-op	5.50° ± 4.68°	4.70° ± 4.49°	0.58
6 weeks Post-op	4.65° ± 3.76°	3.40° ± 3.59°	0.29
3 months Post-op	3.15° ± 2.85°	2.80° ± 2.67°	0.69
6 months Post-op	3.35° ± 4.04°	2.45° ± 2.82°	0.42
12 months Post-op	2.70° ± 3.23°	2.25° ± 2.17°	0.62
24 months Post-op	2.55° ± 3.02°	2.15° ± 1.93°	0.61

†data analyses were performed with Student's t-test

in smaller femoral size without changing flexion gap [15, 16]. Three dimensional imaging with prosthesis template software found that a 3° and a 5° extension of the distal femoral cut increased the AP femoral diameters by 2 and 3 mm, respectively, while a 3° and a 5° flexion decreased the AP femoral diameter by 2 and 3 mm, respectively [17]. Therefore, surgeons should carefully focus on the best distal femoral cutting angle to ensure an appropriate size selection of femoral component.

Theoretically, the component size would affect the functionality of the knee, but this was not borne out by our results. We found that the KSS, functional score and postoperative ROM were similar between AFC size and SFC size for patients; moreover, these findings are in agreement with previous studies [9, 10]. The similar postoperative ROM in both groups from our study could be due to the referencing system we used for femoral AP cuts. We used the posterior referencing system, which typically has the same posterior femoral bone thickness cut and does not affect the flexion gap. We had also anticipated differences in possible anterior knee pain which might have been due to the use of larger femoral component sizes. Larger components normally associated with increasing anterior offset, anterior overstuff, and

Table 5 Incidence of anterior knee pain of bilateral simultaneous TKA between groups

Parameter	Asymmetrical femoral component size (yes/no)	Symmetrical femoral component size (yes/no)	P-value*
Preoperation	23 (13 patients)/17	15 (8 patients)/25	0.12
6 weeks postoperation	3 (2 patients)/37	5 (3 patients)/35	0.71
3 months postoperation	0/40	1 (1 patients)/39	1.00
6 months postoperation	0/40	1 (1 patients)/39	1.00
12 months postoperation	0/40	0/39	1.00
24 months postoperation	0/40	0/39	1.00

*data analyses were performed with exact probability

patellofemoral contact force. Nonetheless, we did not see any of these outcomes in our study [5].

Different recovery of knee function (i.e. active ROM, quadriceps strength, and visual analogue scale pain score) between sides in simultaneous bilateral TKA has previously been examined and shown to be associated with risk factors such as female gender, old age, high BMI, high levels of anxiety, diagnostic differences, and different component sizes. We did not analyse these variables in our study; rather we focused on femoral component sizes [18].

Other limitations of our study were its retrospective design and small sample size which may not have completely represented the bilateral TKA population. We did not evaluate anterior bowing of femur from lateral radiographic view which may be a factor that influences femoral component size choice. All operations were performed by one surgeon with a specific type of prosthesis; therefore, decision making for component size choice will only reflect this particular surgeon's experience, and the results are only generalizable to the same type of prosthesis. For the postoperative clinical outcome measures, our study utilized self-reported questionnaires which only represented the patients' impression of their physical function. Performance-based tests such as the 2-min walking test and timed up and go tests may address other more objective aspects and complement these types of subjective questionnaires [19]. Furthermore, postoperative functional scores were included only in simultaneous bilateral TKA but not staged bilateral TKA because of the difficulty in interpreting data based on differing recovery protocols and confounding effects of different interval recovery times between the two sides.

Conclusions

Our study showed that flexion of the femoral component and not preoperative bone anatomy determined the size of the AFC in patients undergoing bilateral TKA. Surgeons may want to be very careful to use a uniform cutting technique when performing distal femoral cutting during bilateral replacements as this affects the femoral component flexion and femoral size selection. The true lateral view of distal femur radiographs may assist surgeons in centralizing intramedullary drill guide into femoral canal and reduce the incidence of error in femoral flexion angle. In our study, AFC selection in bilateral TKA did not appear to greatly affect the outcome. Size selection remained independent of favourable clinical outcomes, including KSS, functional score, ROM in both asymmetrical and SFC size groups. Nonetheless, surgeons should still carefully and uniformly perform the distal femoral cutting as long-term studies need to be done on different

prosthesis design and the outcomes of AFC size selection in bilateral TKA.

Abbreviations
AFC: Asymmetrical femoral component; AP: Anteroposterior; BMI: Body mass index; ICC: Intra-class correlation coefficient; KSS: Knee society score; ML: Mediolateral; PACS: Picture archiving and communication system; ROM: Range of motion; SFC: Symmetrical femoral component; TKA: Total knee arthroplasty

Acknowledgements
We thank Prof. J. Patumanond, MD, for help with the statistical analysis and Dr. Bob Taylor, MD, and D. Kim Liwiski for reviewing the manuscript. We also thank all study participants.

Funding
The study has not received any external funding.

Authors' contributions
PP participated in the design, performed the surgeries, drafting the article, critical revision of the article and final approval of the version to be published. AC participated in gathered data of patients and analysis. KB participated in the analysis and interpretation of the data and manuscript writing or revising. All authors read and approved the final manuscript.

Consent for publication
Not applicable.

Competing interests
We declare that none of the authors have any competing interests.

Author details
[1]Department of Orthopaedics, Faculty of Medicine, Thammasat University, 99 Moo 18, Khlong Nueng, Khlong Luang, Pathum Thani 12120, Thailand. [2]Department of Orthopaedics, Chulabhorn International College of Medicine, Thammasat University, 99 Moo 18, Khlong Nueng, Khlong Luang, Pathum Thani 12120, Thailand.

References
1. Ritter M, Mamlin LA, Melfi CA, Katz BP, Freund DA, Arthur DS. Outcome implications for the timing of bilateral total knee arthroplasties. Clin Orthop Relat Res. 1997;345:99–105.
2. Daluga D, Lombardi AV Jr, Mallory TH, Vaughn BK. Knee manipulation following total knee arthroplasty. Analysis of prognostic variables. J Arthroplasty. 1991;6(2):119–28.
3. Baldini A, Scuderi GR, Aglietti P, Chalnick D, Insall JN. Flexion-extension gap changes during total knee arthroplasty: effect of posterior cruciate ligament and posterior osteophytes removal. J Knee Surg. 2004;17(2):69–72.
4. Mihalko W, Fishkin Z, Krackow K. Patellofemoral overstuff and its relationship to flexion after total knee arthroplasty. Clin Orthop Relat Res. 2006;449:283–7.
5. Kawahara S, Matsuda S, Fukagawa S, Mitsuyasu H, Nakahara H, Higaki H, et al. Upsizing the femoral component increases patellofemoral contact force in total knee replacement. J Bone Joint Surg Br. 2012;94(1):56–61.

Risk factors and outcomes in asymmetrical femoral component size for posterior referencing bilateral...

53

6. Hitt K, Shurman JR 2nd, Greene K, McCarthy J, Moskal J, Hoeman T, et al. Anthropometric measurements of the human knee: correlation to the sizing of current knee arthroplasty systems. J Bone Joint Surg Am. 2003;85-A(Suppl 4):115–22.

7. Mahoney OM, Kinsey T. Overhang of the femoral component in total knee arthroplasty: risk factors and clinical consequences. J Bone Joint Surg Am. 2010;92(5):1115–21.

8. Brown TE, Diduch DR, Moskal JT. Component size asymmetry in bilateral total knee arthroplasty. Am J Knee Surg. 2001;14(2):81–4.

9. Capeci CM, Brown EC 3rd, Scuderi GR, Scott WN. Component asymmetry in simultaneous bilateral total knee arthroplasty. J Arthroplast. 2006;21(5):749–53.

10. Reddy VG, Mootha AK, Thayi C, Kantesaria P, Kumar RV, Reddy D. Are both the knees of the same size? Analysis of component asymmetry in 289 bilateral knee arthroplasties. Indian J Orthop. 2011;45(3):251–4.

11. Ng FY, Jiang XF, Zhou WZ, Chiu KY, Yan CH, Fok MW. The accuracy of sizing of the femoral component in total knee replacement. Knee Surg Sports Traumatol Arthrosc. 2013;21(10):2309–13.

12. Otani T, Whiteside LA, White SE. Cutting errors in preparation of femoral components in total knee arthroplasty. J Arthroplasty. 1993;8(5):503–10.

13. Plaskos C, Hodgson AJ, Inkpen K, McGraw RW. Bone cutting errors in total knee arthroplasty. J Arthroplast. 2002;17(6):698–705.

14. Mihalko WM, Boyle J, Clark LD, Krackow KA. The variability of intramedullary alignment of the femoral component during total knee arthroplasty. J Arthroplast. 2005;20(1):25–8.

15. Chen S, Zeng Y, Yan M, Yue B, Zhang J, Wang Y. Morphological evaluation of the sagittal plane femoral load-bearing surface in computer-simulated virtual total knee arthroplasty implantation at different flexion angles. Knee Surg Sports Traumatol Arthrosc. 2017;25(9):2880–6.

16. Tsukeoka T, Lee TH. Sagittal flexion of the femoral component affects flexion gap and sizing in total knee arthroplasty. J Arthroplast. 2012;27(6):1094–9.

17. Nakahara H, Matsuda S, Okazaki K, Tashiro Y, Iwamoto Y. Sagittal cutting error changes femoral anteroposterior sizing in total knee arthroplasty. Clin Orthop Relat Res. 2012;470(12):3560–5.

18. Yang Y, Long G, Zhenhu W. Analysis of Interlimb asymmetry in patients undergoing simultaneous bilateral Total knee Arthroplasty. PLoS One. 2015;10(6):e0129783.

19. Unnanuntana A, Mait JE, Shaffer AD, Lane JM, Mancuso CA. Performance-based tests and self-reported questionnaires provide distinct information for the preoperative evaluation of Total hip Arthroplasty patients. J Arthroplast. 2012;27(5):770–5.

7

No difference in the functional improvements between unilateral and bilateral total knee replacements

Yu-Hao Huang[10], Chin Lin[1], Jia-Hwa Yang[2], Leou-Chyr Lin[3], Chih-Yuan Mou[4], Kwo-Tsao Chiang[1], Man-Gang Lee[5], Hsien-Feng Chang[1], Hsueh-Lu Chang[1], Wen Su[6], Shih-Jen Yeh[7], Hung Chang[8,9], Chih-Chien Wang[3*†] and Sui-Lung Su[1,10*†]

Abstract

Background: Differences between staged bilateral total knee replacement (TKR) and simultaneous bilateral TKR have been investigated, but few studies have investigated differences in the functional improvements resulting from these methods. Therefore, this study investigates the different functional improvements between staged bilateral total knee TKR and simultaneous bilateral TKR.

Methods: Among 144 potential bilateral TKR patients who were included in this study, 93 (64.6%) patients selected unilateral TKR and 51 (35.4%) selected bilateral TKR. Functional improvements were assessed using the Western Ontario and McMaster University osteoarthritis index (WOMAC) and the Medical Outcomes Trust Short Form-36 (SF-36), and patients were interviewed pre-operatively and after 6 months. A generalized equation was used to test for differences in functional improvements.

Results: After TKR, pain, stiffness, function and total WOMAC scores were significantly reduced in both groups, with mean changes from − 26.6 to − 41.4 and from − 27.5 to − 42.2.The mean health change of SF-36 scores, physical component and mental component scores changed to 45.2 ± 18.2, 74.0 ± 15.4 and 77.0 ± 9.6, respectively, in Group 1 and 47.1 ± 17.1, 74.0 ± 15.2 and 75.5 ± 12.1, respectively, in Group 2.
Unilateral and simultaneous bilateral TKR produce similar functional improvements, although current work status may be a novel impact factor.

Conclusion: No differences in functional improvements were identified between patients who selected unilateral versus bilateral TKR, indicating no recommendation for one procedure over the other.

Keywords: Total knee replacement, Bilateral TKR, Unilateral TKR, Functional improvement, WOMAC, SF-36

Background

Total knee replacement (TKR) is mainly offered to patients with end-stage osteoarthritis (OA) and has become more prevalent in recent years [1]. TKR is an effective intervention that improves quality of life, reduces pain and increases functional capability [2].

Many diagnoses of osteoarthritis (OA) are caused by aging, and the prevalence of bilateral symptomatic knees in these patients is 63.3% [3]. Patients with bilateral symptoms frequently require bilateral TKR, which can be performed as a one-stage simultaneous operation, or as a two-stage unilateral operation [4, 5]. Although patients are free to select the mode of TKR, it remains controversial which mode is better.

Previous studies have investigated differences in responses to staged bilateral and simultaneous bilateral TKR in terms of short-term discomfort [6], morbidity and mortality [7–10] and cost-effectiveness [11]. However, few studies have investigated differences in

---

* Correspondence: tsghcc@yahoo.com.tw; a131419@gmail.com
†Equal contributors
[3]Department of Orthopedics, Tri-Service General Hospital and National Defense Medical Center, No.325, Sec.2, Chenggong Rd., Neihu District, Taipei 114, Taiwan, Republic of China
[1]School of Public Health, National Defense Medical Center, No.161, Min-Chun E. Rd., Sec. 6, Neihu, Taipei 114, Taiwan, Republic of China
Full list of author information is available at the end of the article

functional improvements. An Indian study described changes in functional improvements using the Western Ontario and McMaster University Osteoarthritis Index (WOMAC) in patients receiving simultaneous bilateral TKR [12], and another study from the United Kingdom reported changes in WOMAC scores in patients who received staged bilateral TKR [13]. However, these studies lacked suitable controls, precluding group comparisons between studies.

An Australian study compared the functional improvements between simultaneous bilateral and unilateral TKR [14], and this study reported that bilateral replacement patients reported better physical function and general health. However, the patients receiving bilateral and unilateral TKR in the above study had significant differences in the source of their health insurance [14], and this difference might cause a false result. The bilateral TKR group was younger and less likely to receive a pension. Instead, the group was more likely to have private health insurance, and most of them lived with others. Either of these situations may influence the patient's costs over the post-operative year [14]. Taiwan had National Health Insurance (NHI), which almost covered the entire cost of TKR. This advantage might have reduced the economic inequalities and increased the homogeneity between patients receiving bilateral or unilateral TKR.

In summary, the available evidence is insufficient to explain with certainty the benefit of simultaneous bilateral TKR in functional outcomes. Thus, to inform clinical decisions, we investigated differences in functional improvements and assessed the potential impact factors between patients receiving unilateral and bilateral TKR.

Methods

Ethics statement and subject recruitment
The study was reviewed and approved by the institutional ethics committee. Written informed consent was obtained from all participants after thorough explanation of the study. Inclusion criteria were defined previously [15] and included (1) TKR surgery patients for the first time, (2) patients with bilateral knee OA and (3) patients with bilateral symptomatic knees. All patients were expected to eventually require bilateral TKR, and all TKRs were performed by a single surgeon. Moreover, patients choosing staged procedures needed more than 6 months of waiting time for the second surgery, and they followed the same post-operative recovery protocol. The waiting time included approximately 3 months for recovery and approximately 3 months for rehabilitation. Patients with serious co-morbidities (cancer, renal failure and infection) were excluded because of influences on functional measurements [16]. The above included criteria improved the homogeneity in the study population and might help to reduce potential confounding factors.

The patients who met the above criteria would attend an approximately half-hour explanation. The following information about the two TKR methods would be provided: (1) the waiting time in two-stage unilateral TKR, (2) higher anesthesia risks in simultaneous TKR [17], and (3) the short term discomfort in simultaneous TKR may be higher than in unilateral TKR [6]. In addition, physicians informed patients of the surgical options but did not influence patient decisions. Thus, modes of TKR were based on patient selection.

During the study period (from July 2009 to April 2010), a total of 169 TKR patients consented to participate in the study. Although 25 patients (16 patients who selected unilateral TKR and 9 patients who selected bilateral TKR) were lost to follow-up, no differences in the investigated characteristics were found in the missing patients (detailed data is shown in Additional file 1: Table S1). Finally, a total of 144 (85.2%) potential bilateral TKR patients were included. Among these, 93 (64.6%) patients selected unilateral TKR (Group 1), and 51 (35.4%) patients selected bilateral TKR (Group 2).

Data source and definition
Data analyses were performed as a comparative cohort study, and data were collected prospectively from a single center. Demographic details including age, gender, medical history, height and weight were retrieved from hospital records. In addition, self-reported education, income and current work status before TKR surgery were recorded. The functional improvements were based on patient reported outcomes and assessed according to the WOMAC [18] and Medical Outcomes Trust Short Form-36 (SF-36) [19]. Questionnaires pertaining to socio-economic factors and patient reported outcomes were conducted during face-to-face interviews with each participant by well-trained investigators before TKR.

The WOMAC index included 24 questions divided into 3 sub-scales: pain, stiffness and function. These sub-scales were combined to produce a total measure of knee health. Each question had a visual analogue scale (VAS) for assessing functional scores (0–100-point scale; 0 best). Scores of questions in each subscale were averaged to calculate pain, stiffness, function and total scores. The SF-36 index included 36 questions, divided into 9 sub-scales: health change, physical function, role of function/physical, pain, general health, role of function/emotion, energy/fatigue, emotional well-being and social function. These sub-scales were combined as a measure of general health. Scores were transformed to produce a 0–100-point scale (100 best), and scores from each sub-scale were calculated according to a previous study [19]. Scores for physical function, role of function/physical, pain and general health were averaged to give a physical component score, and scores for role of function/emotion, energy/fatigue, and emotional well-being while social were averaged to give the mental component score. Health changes were assessed as an independent subscale.

Potential impact factors included gender, age, BMI (body mass index), education, income, current work, other bone disease, low back pain and history of disease. BMI was calculated from self-reported height and weight. Education was divided into two groups ($\leq$ 6 years and > 6 years) because compulsory education was previously 6 years in Taiwan. To maintain privacy, income was assessed as enough or lacking. Because some patients > 65 years of age had not yet retired, we asked for current work status (without or with employment). Other bone diseases and low back pain were self-reported as with or without. History of disease was assessed using the open-ended question "Has a doctor ever diagnosed you as having any disease?" However, most diseases were rare in the present patient cohort. Only histories of cardiovascular disease (CVD), diabetes mellitus (DM) and hypertension (HTN) were analyzed because their prevalence was > 10%.

In the primary analysis, the three primary outcomes were as follows: (1) patient reported outcomes before TKR in each group, (2) patient reported outcomes after 6 months in each group and (3) changes in patient reported outcomes in each group. The first and second primary analyses used independent sample t-tests to compare the means of patient reported outcomes before and after TKR. The third primary analysis used paired t-tests to compare the means of the changes in functional outcomes in each group. It is noteworthy that assessing for change of functional outcomes after TKR within 6 months is a short follow up compared with related studies [14, 22]. However, the patients receiving unilateral TKR will continue with the second stage surgery after 6 months, so follow up after more than 6 months would be impacted by second stage surgery in patients receiving unilateral TKR. This might reduce the comparability between two groups, so this study only followed up within 6 months.

Sample size calculation

Prior to the study, we used G*Power to perform a t-test of the difference between two independent means to calculate the required sample size [20], and effects were detected in a two-sided test with a power of $(1 - \beta) = 80\%$ at a significance level of 0.05. Other calculation settings were as follows: (1) the hypothetical proportion of patients selecting bilateral TKR was 40% based on clinical experience, (2) minimally clinically important differences (MCID) were at least 15 points for the WOMAC and 10 points for the SF-36 [21], and (3) the standard deviations of functional changes were approximately 20, as shown in a previous study [22]. Based on these settings, the required sample size for calculation was at least 60 subjects for the WOMAC and 133 subjects for the SF-36.

Statistical method

All data were analyzed using the R statistical program (version 3.1.1) with the geepack package, and graphs were drawn using bear, ggplot2 and metafor packages.

Association analysis

Categorical and continuous variables were presented as numbers (proportions) and means $\pm$ standard deviations. Differences between variables of patients in each group were tested using the Student's t-test or the χ^2 test where appropriate. The significance level was set at $0.05/11 = 0.0045$ based on Bonferroni correction to avoid errors of multiple testing.

Impact factor analysis

To infer the progression of a primary parameter and then apply parameter ranking to investigate which behavioral data had the highest 'impact' on patient reported outcomes, we used a generalized estimating equation to analyze the association between possible impact factors and changes in patient reported outcomes. Significance levels were again set at $0.05/11 = 0.0045$. Accordingly, the results were presented using forest plots with 99.54% confidence intervals. Significantly associated factors in both association analyses and impact factor analyses were considered confounders and were adjusted in subsequent analyses. However, no factors met these criteria.

Patient reported outcomes before and after TKR in each group were presented as the means $\pm$ standard deviations, and changes in patient reported outcomes in each group were presented as the means with 95% confidence intervals. To investigate the association between surgery type and changes in patient reported outcomes and adjust the confounders, the generalized estimating equation was used to analyze repeated data. GEE models were adjusted by all factors (gender, age, BMI, education, income, current work, other bone disease, low back pain, history of CVD, history of DM and history of HTN). The significance level was set at 0.05. Although no potential confounders were present, fully adjusted changes in patient reported outcomes were presented for each group.

Results
Association analysis

Table 1 shows differences in characteristics between Groups 1 (unilateral TKR) and 2 (bilateral TKR). Group 1 comprised 75.3% females aged 70.4 $\pm$ 7.2 years old, and Group 2 comprised 90.2% females aged 70.0 $\pm$ 6.2 years old. The p-value for the association between gender and

Table 1 Demographics and patient characteristics

		Group 1 (n = 93)	Group 2 (n = 51)	p-value
Gender	Male	23 (24.7%)	5 (9.8%)	0.030
	Female	70 (75.3%)	46 (90.2%)	
Age (years)		70.4 ± 7.2	70.0 ± 6.2	0.707
BMI (kg/m^2)		27.1 ± 3.5	27.4 ± 3.4	0.615
Education (years)	≤ 6	69 (74.2%)	44 (86.3%)	0.092
	> 6	24 (25.8%)	7 (13.7%)	
Income	Enough	86 (92.5%)	49 (96.1%)	0.393
	Lacking	7 (7.5%)	2 (3.9%)	
Current work status	Without	70 (75.3%)	39 (76.5%)	0.872
	With	23 (24.7%)	12 (23.5%)	
Other bone disease	Without	69 (74.2%)	37 (72.5%)	0.860
	With	24 (25.8%)	14 (27.5%)	
Low back pain	Without	44 (47.3%)	27 (52.9%)	0.518
	With	49 (52.7%)	24 (47.1%)	
CVD	Without	71 (76.3%)	45 (88.2%)	0.085
	With	22 (23.7%)	6 (11.8%)	
DM	Without	73 (78.5%)	40 (78.4%)	0.993
	With	20 (21.5%)	11 (21.6%)	
HTN	Without	41 (44.1%)	16 (31.4%)	0.136
	With	52 (55.9%)	35 (68.6%)	

Group 1, unilateral TKR; Group 2, bilateral TKR; CVD, history of cardiovascular disease; DM, history of diabetes mellitus; HTN, history of hypertension
Statistical significance was set at $p < 0.0045$, as described in the statistical analysis section

group was < 0.05 ($p = 0.030$) but was not significant after Bonferroni correction (significance level = 0.0045). Other factors such as age, BMI, education, income, current work, other bone disease, low back pain, history of CVD, history of DM and history of HTN were not associated with treatment selections.

Impact factor analysis

Associations of potential impact factors with WOMAC and SF-36 scores (Figs. 1 and 2) indicated that patients with current work may benefit from TKR more than patients without current work (slope difference, – 11.1; 99.42% CI, from – 18.7 to – 3.5) and predominantly reflected function scores (slope difference, – 12.1; 99.42% CI, from – 19.5 to – 4.8). No other factors were associated with changes in total WOMAC scores in either univariate or multivariate models (data not shown). According to the stiffness scores, patients with a history of HTN may receive less benefit from TKR than those without a history of HTN (slope difference, 12.2; 99.42% CI, 0.9–23.5). However, history of HTN was not a significant impact factor after adjusting for current work status (p-value before adjustment, 0.002; p-value after adjustment, 0.010).

No significant impact factors were found among SF-36 scores, including in changes in health, physical components and mental component scores. However, current work status ($p = 0.0047$) and history of HTN ($p = 0.0052$) were almost significantly associated with physical component and mental component scores, respectively.

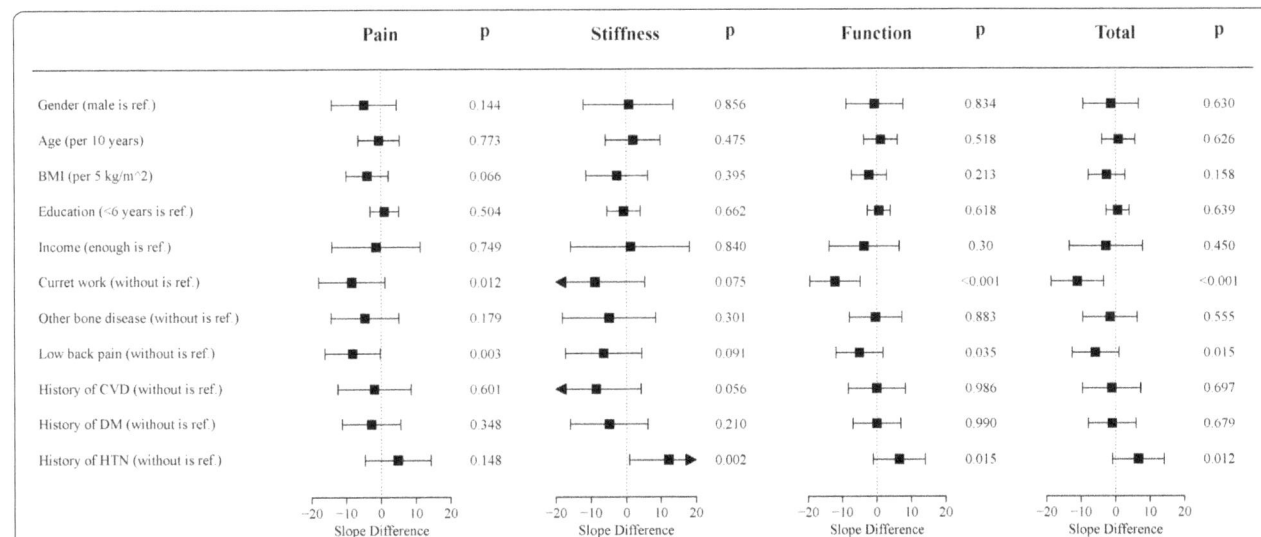

Fig. 1 Impact and 99.54% conference interval of potential impact factors on WOMAC score. CVD: cardiovascular disease; DM: diabetes mellitus; HTN: hypertension. This forest plot included 11 potential impact factors on WOMAC score: Gender (female versus male); Age (10 years is a unit); BMI (5 kg/m^2 is a unit); Education (> 6 versus ≤6 years); Income (lacking versus enough); Current work (with versus without); Other bone disease (with versus without); Lower back pain (with versus without); CVD (with versus without); DM (with versus without); HTN (with versus without). For each potential impact factor, generalized estimating equation analysis was used to interaction between time and impact factor

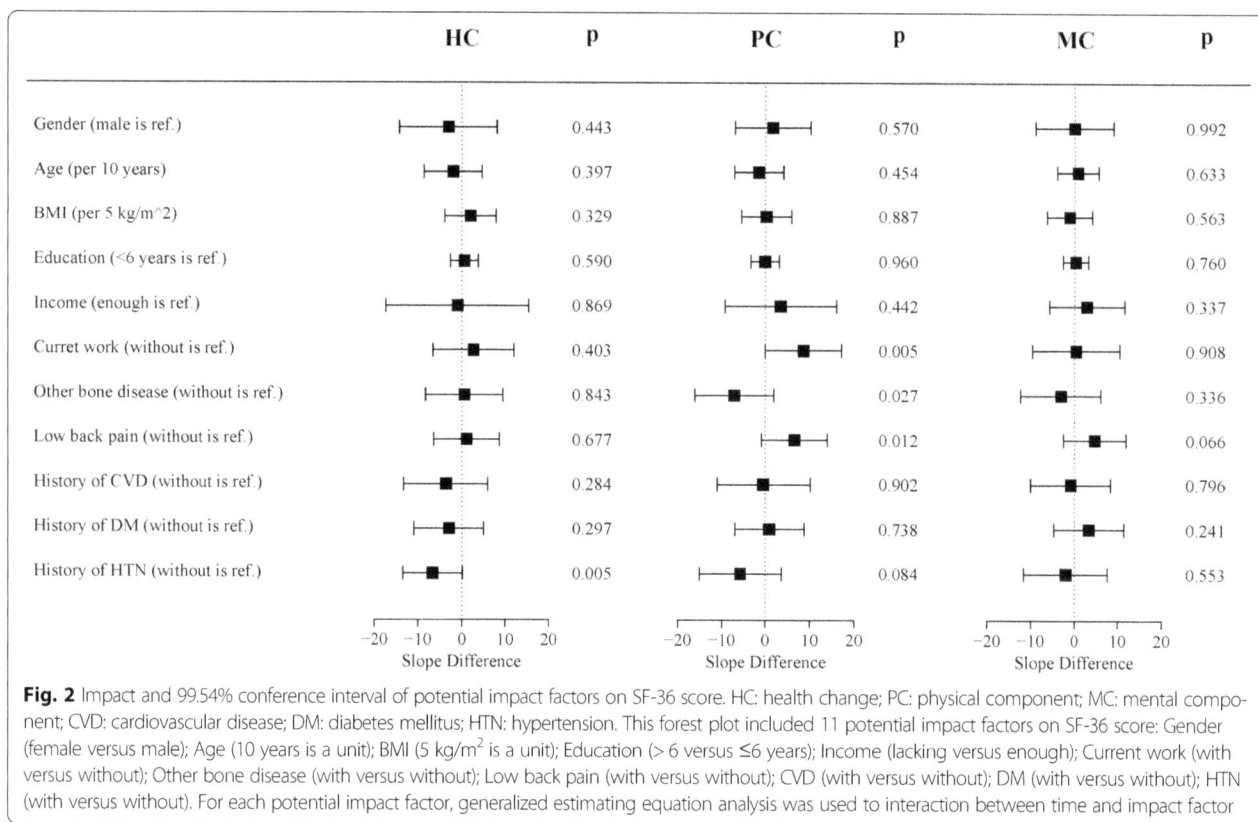

	HC	**p**		**PC**	**p**		**MC**	**p**
Gender (male is ref.)		0.443			0.570			0.992
Age (per 10 years)		0.397			0.454			0.633
BMI (per 5 kg/m^2)		0.329			0.887			0.563
Education (<6 years is ref.)		0.590			0.960			0.760
Income (enough is ref.)		0.869			0.442			0.337
Curret work (without is ref.)		0.403			0.005			0.908
Other bone disease (without is ref.)		0.843			0.027			0.336
Low back pain (without is ref.)		0.677			0.012			0.066
History of CVD (without is ref.)		0.284			0.902			0.796
History of DM (without is ref.)		0.297			0.738			0.241
History of HTN (without is ref.)		0.005			0.084			0.553

−20 −10 0 10 20 Slope Difference −20 −10 0 10 20 Slope Difference −20 −10 0 10 20 Slope Difference

Fig. 2 Impact and 99.54% conference interval of potential impact factors on SF-36 score. HC: health change; PC: physical component; MC: mental component; CVD: cardiovascular disease; DM: diabetes mellitus; HTN: hypertension. This forest plot included 11 potential impact factors on SF-36 score: Gender (female versus male); Age (10 years is a unit); BMI (5 kg/m^2 is a unit); Education (> 6 versus ≤6 years); Income (lacking versus enough); Current work (with versus without); Other bone disease (with versus without); Low back pain (with versus without); CVD (with versus without); DM (with versus without); HTN (with versus without). For each potential impact factor, generalized estimating equation analysis was used to interaction between time and impact factor

Primary analysis
WOMAC

A breakdown of WOMAC scores for the 2 groups is shown in Table 2 and Fig. 3. Among Group 1 patients, mean pre-operative and 6-months total WOMAC scores were 56.8 ± 11.3 and 20.4 ± 14.2, respectively, and those among Group 2 patients were 57.1 ± 10.3 and 19.8 ± 13.8, respectively. Changes in total WOMAC scores following TKR were -36.3 (95% CI, from -39.3 to -33.4) and -37.3 (from -41.4 to -33.1) in Groups 1 and 2, respectively. After TKR, pain, stiffness, function and total WOMAC scores were significantly reduced in both groups, with mean changes from -26.6 to -41.4 and from -27.5 to -42.2, respectively. Both groups showed similar trends in the various sub-scales, and no significant differences in any sub-scale were observed between treatment groups before and after adjustment. The most improved sub-scale was pain, whereas only minimal improvements were observed in the stiffness sub-scale.

SF-36

Table 2 and Fig. 4 show the breakdown of SF-36 scores among patients of the two groups. Before TKR, the mean health change, physical component and mental component scores were 36.3 ± 17.9, 28.6 ± 11.3 and 46.4 ± 15.0, respectively, in Group 1 and 34.8 ± 17.9, 28.2 ± 10.8 and 48.8 ± 15.6, respectively, in Group 2. After TKR, the mean

health change, physical component and mental component scores changed to 45.2 ± 18.2, 74.0 ± 15.4 and 77.0 ± 9.6, respectively, in Group 1 and 47.1 ± 17.1, 74.0 ± 15.2 and 75.5 ± 12.1, respectively, in Group 2.

Health change, physical component and mental component SF-36 scores were significantly increased after TKR by 8.9 (95% CI, 5.7–12.0), 45.3 (95% CI, 42.2–48.5) and 30.6 (95% CI, 27.6–33.7), respectively, among Group 1 patients and 12.3 (95% CI, 7.6–16.9), 45.7 (95% CI, 41.0–50.4) and 26.7 (95% CI, 22.2–31.2), respectively, among Group 2 patients. In agreement with the WOMAC scores, trends in sub-scales of SF-36 scores were similar in the two treatment groups, and no significant differences were identified before or after adjustment. Moreover, the greatest improvement following TKR was in the physical component sub-scale.

Discussion

In the present study, no differences in investigated characteristics were found between patients receiving unilateral and bilateral TKR. In addition, all patients had substantial functional improvements following surgery. Although no differences in functional improvement sub-scales were found between treatment groups, current work status influenced the perceived benefits of the interventions.

This study population had similar characteristics to those of other studies [12–14, 22], with a mean age of

Table 2 Comparison of the WOMAC and SF-36 scores for the 2 groups

		Group 1 (n = 93)	Group 2 (n = 51)	95%CI	p-value#	p-value$
WOMAC						
Pain	Pre-op	61.1 ± 14.7	60.6 ± 13.5	−4.38~ 5.43	0.833	0.464
	Post-op	19.7 ± 14.6	18.3 ± 12.7	−3.43~ 6.19	0.572	0.397
	Change	−41.4 (from − 44.9 to −37.9)	− 42.2 (from − 47.2 to −37.3)	−5.14~ 6.85	0.779	0.931
Stiffness	Pre-op	48.6 ± 26.9	52.0 ± 26.8	−12.56~ 5.93	0.876	0.608
	Post-op	22.0 ± 21.2	24.5 ± 21.6	−9.87~ 4.86	0.503	0.757
	Change	−26.6 (from −31.2 to −22.0)	−27.5 (−34.1 to −20.8)	−7.19~ 8.81	0.841	0.741
Function	Pre-op	56.5 ± 11.5	56.6 ± 10.9	−4.07~ 3.71	0.926	0.821
	Post-op	20.5 ± 14.5	19.7 ± 14.1	−4.19~ 5.70	0.764	0.517
	Change	−36.0 (from − 39.0 to − 33.1)	−36.9 (from −41.1 to − 32.8)	− 4.13~ 6.01	0.716	0.631
Total	Pre-op	56.8 ± 11.3	57.1 ± 10.3	−4.06~ 3.46	0.876	0.795
	Post-op	20.4 ± 14.2	19.8 ± 13.8	−4.22~ 5.44	0.803	0.541
	Change	−36.3 (from − 39.3 to −33.4)	−37.3 (from −41.4 to − 33.1)	− 4.17~ 5.99	0.724	0.684
SF-36						
Health change	Pre-op	36.3 ± 17.9	34.8 ± 16.6	−4.52~ 7.49	0.626	0.899
	Post-op	45.2 ± 18.2	47.1 ± 17.1	−8.02~ 4.22	0.541	0.254
	Change	8.9 (5.7–12.0)	12.3 (7.6–16.9)	−8.88~ 2.12	0.226	0.166
Physical	Pre-op	28.6 ± 11.3	28.2 ± 10.8	−3.45~ 4.22	0.842	0.887
	Post-op	74.0 ± 15.4	74.0 ± 15.2	−5.25~ 5.28	0.996	0.680
	Change	45.3 (42.2–48.5)	45.7 (41.0–50.4)	−5.94~ 5.19	0.895	0.774
Mental	Pre-op	46.4 ± 15.0	48.8 ± 15.6	−7.67~ 2.78	0.357	0.254
	Post-op	77.0 ± 9.6	75.5 ± 12.1	−2.17~ 5.09	0.429	0.585
	Change	30.6 (27.6–33.7)	26.7 (22.2–31.2)	−1.41~ 9.21	0.149	0.124

Group 1, unilateral TKR; Group 2, bilateral TKR; Pre-op, pre-operative; Post-op, 6 months after surgery
#, The p-value
$, adjusted p-value; Models were adjusted by all factors (gender, age, BMI, education, income, current work, other bone disease, low back pain, history of CVD, history of DM and history of HTN)

approximately 70 years and more females than males. The proportion of patients who selected bilateral TKR was 36.6% in a previous study [14] and 35.4% in the present study. In addition, the range of mean WOMAC scores at baseline was 50–60 in both studies, and the ranges of mean physical component and mental component SF-36 scores at baseline were 20–30 and 40–50, respectively, indicating that the present cohort is representative.

It is widely recognized that TKR improves quality of life for OA patients [2]. In agreement, the present functional improvements in patients receiving unilateral and bilateral TKR were both statistically and clinically significant and were greater than MCID [21].

Previous studies also report significant differences in functional improvements between patients receiving unilateral and bilateral TKR, and the present patient groups had differences in health insurance because of the high rate of private health insurance [14]. In particular, patients receiving bilateral TKR suffered from increased

discomfort in the short-term compared with those receiving unilateral TKR [6], but this might not impact the functional outcome after rehabilitation. Nonetheless, other factors in addition to functional improvements may require consideration during decision making for bilateral or unilateral TKR. Functional outcomes might not be the only factor to decide the modes of TKR: safety and financial matters are also variables to consider when deciding between bilateral TKA and staged procedures. Although it might be disputed, some evidence exists that the risk of complications following simultaneous bilateral TKR is not increased compared with that following unilateral TKR [10, 23, 24]. In addition, simultaneous bilateral TKR is reportedly more cost effective than staged bilateral TKR, although the ensuing functional improvements do not differ [11]. The above evidence needs to be considered in the decision surrounding the method of TKR, and the functional outcomes are also a critical factor in decision making.

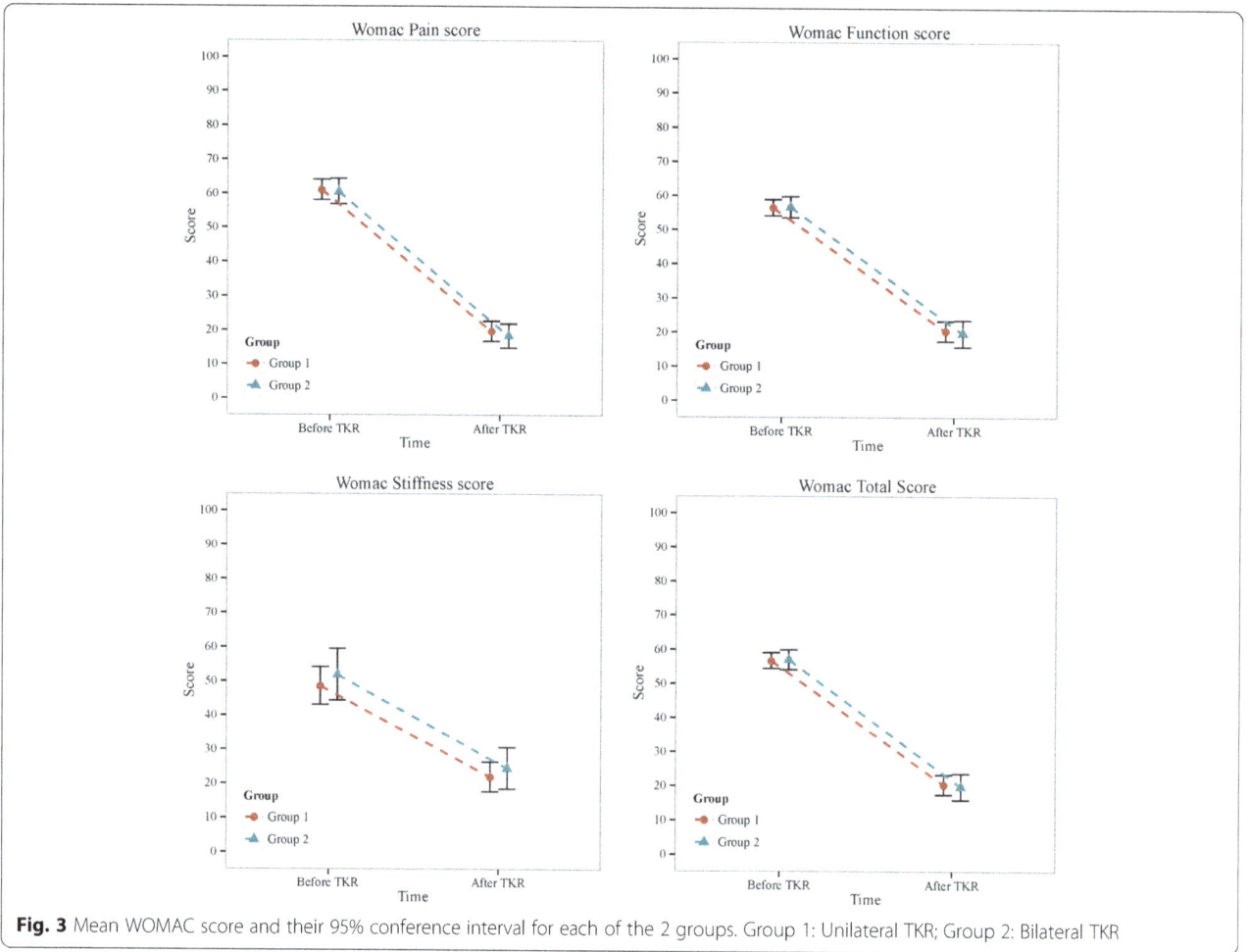

Fig. 3 Mean WOMAC score and their 95% conference interval for each of the 2 groups. Group 1: Unilateral TKR; Group 2: Bilateral TKR

Among the present patients, current work status was a significant impact factor, with greater improvements in WOMAC function scores following TKR in working patients. This observation may reflect greater perceptions of functional improvement among working patients who use their knees more often than non-working patients. Moreover, working patients may benefit because they will miss less work. Accordingly, current work status can be considered a novel impact factor for functional improvement following TKR. Moreover, history of HTN was significantly predictive of functional improvements following TKR but was not

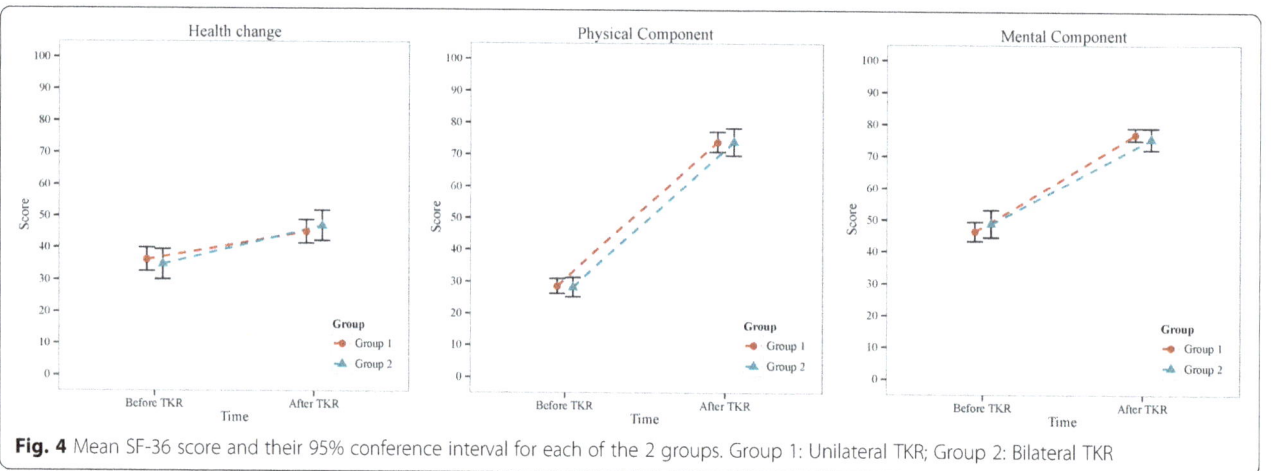

Fig. 4 Mean SF-36 score and their 95% conference interval for each of the 2 groups. Group 1: Unilateral TKR; Group 2: Bilateral TKR

an independent risk factor after adjusting for work status, reflecting the prevalence of hypertension among retired patients. In agreement with the present study, a previous Saudi Arabian study of potential impact factors for the effect of TKR showed no association between gender and functional improvement [25]. Moreover, a study from the United Kingdom showed no association of BMI with functional improvements following TKR [22].

This study had 3 limitations. First, although the present study was not an authentic randomized controlled trial, it had an important advantage in the homogeneity between patients receiving bilateral or unilateral TKR. Previous studies of this issue encountered some challenges, namely, patients who selected bilateral TKR had a higher proportion of private health insurance [14]. The differences in financial capability might be a potential confounder of this issue. Thus, the absence of economic influences, because the cost of TKR was covered by NHI, on patient selections of surgical procedures adds credibility. Moreover, Hooper and his co-workers noted some differences between patients receiving unilateral and bilateral TKR in the New Zealand National Joint Registry [24]. This real-world observation showed that age, pain, and activities of daily living might impact the selection of surgery. However, this study attempted to reduce the potential confounders, such as to exclude patients with a high risk of complications. These efforts allowed some patients who selected to carry out unilateral TKR to be excluded and reduced the potential confounders in our result. Finally, we also observed significant baseline differences between the two groups. Thus, we considered the homogeneity between two groups in our study to be acceptable. Second, assessments of outcome were based on a structured questionnaire, and self-reporting may have led to misclassification. Therefore, highly trained interviewers regularly re-standardized analyses. In addition, patients were well informed prior to interviews. Third, this was not long-term research, so there was not much time to follow the patients. We cannot completely evaluate the functional difference between the 12 month follow-up of the one-stage, simultaneous operation group and the 6 month follow-up of the second operation of the two-stage operation group.

Conclusions

In conclusion, no differences in functional improvements were identified between patients who selected unilateral or bilateral TKR, resulting in no recommendation for one or the other procedure. It was noteworthy that we excluded the patients with serious co-morbidities, so this conclusion might be not extrapolated to them. Nonetheless, it remains critical that physicians inform patients of the differences in short-term discomfort, cost effectiveness, morbidity and mortality between the procedures.

Elderly patients, or those with serious co-morbidities, might be not appropriate for bilateral TKR because they might be at increased risk for perioperative complications. Finally, the present analyses identified current work status as a novel impact factor, as those patients might be more sensitive and miss less time from work. Future studies are required to confirm this observation.

Abbreviations
BMI: Body mass index; CVD: Cardiovascular disease; DM: Diabetes mellitus; HTN: Hypertension; MCID: Minimally clinically important differences; NHI: National Health Insurance; OA: Osteoarthritis; SF-36: Medical Outcomes Trust Short Form-36; TKR: Total knee replacement; VAS: Visual analogue scale; WOMAC: Western Ontario and McMaster University osteoarthritis index

Acknowledgements
Not applicable.

Funding
Not applicable.

Authors' contributions
YHH, CCW, SLS: Conception and design. YHH, SLS: Acquisition of data. YHH, CL: Data analysis. YHH, CL, SLS: Drafting the article. YHH, CL, JHY, LCL, CYM, KTC, MGL, HFC, HLC, WS, SJY, HC, CCW and SLS have made substantial contributions in the interpretation of data, revising the article critically, and all approved of the final version for submission.

Consent for publication
Not applicable.

Competing interests
The authors declare that they have no competing interests.

Author details
[1]School of Public Health, National Defense Medical Center, No.161, Min-Chun E. Rd., Sec. 6, Neihu, Taipei 114, Taiwan, Republic of China. [2]Graduate Institute of Life Sciences, National Defense Medical Center, No.161, Min-Chun E. Rd., Sec. 6, Neihu, Taipei 114, Taiwan, Republic of China. [3]Department of Orthopedics, Tri-Service General Hospital and National Defense Medical Center, No.325, Sec.2, Chenggong Rd., Neihu District, Taipei 114, Taiwan, Republic of China. [4]Department of Aviation Medicine and Physical examination, National Defense Medical Center and Tri-Service General Hospital Songshan Branch, No.131, Jiankang Rd., Songshan District, Taipei 10581, Taiwan, Republic of China. [5]Department of Surgery, Zuoying Branch of Kaohsiung Armed Forces General Hospital, No.553, Junxiao Rd., Zuoying Dist., Kaohsiung City 813, Taiwan, Republic of China. [6]Department of Nursing, Tri-Service General Hospital, No.]61, Min-Chun E. Rd., Sec. 6, Neihu, Taipei 114, Taiwan, Republic of China. [7]Department of Research and Development, Da-Yeh University, No. 168, Xuefu Road, Dacun Township, Changhua County 515, Taiwan, Republic of China. [8]Department of Physiology and Biophysics, National Defense Medical Center, No.325, Sec. 2, Chenggong Rd., Neihu District, Taipei City 114, Taiwan, Republic of China. [9]Division of Thoracic Surgery, Tri-Service General Hospital, National Defense Medical Center, No.325, Sec. 2, Chenggong Rd., Neihu District, Taipei City 114, Taiwan, Republic of China. [10]Graduate Institute of Medical Sciences, National Defense Medical Center, No.161, Min-Chun E. Rd., Sec. 6, Neihu, Taipei 114, Taiwan, Republic of China.

References

1. Kurtz S, Mowat F, Ong K, Chan N, Lau E, Halpern M. Prevalence of primary and revision total hip and knee arthroplasty in the United States from 1990 through 2002. J Bone Joint Surg Am. 2005;87(7):1487.
2. Waimann CA, Fernandez-Mazarambroz RJ, Cantor SB, Lopez-Olivo MA, Zhang H, Landon GC, Siff SJ, Suarez-Almazor ME. Cost-effectiveness of total knee replacement: a prospective cohort study. Arthritis Care Res. 2014;66(4):592.
3. White DK, Zhang Y, Felson DT, Niu J, Keysor JJ, Nevitt MC, Lewis CE, Torner JC, Neogi T. The independent effect of pain in one versus two knees on the presence of low physical function in a multicenter knee osteoarthritis study. Arthritis Care Res. 2010;62(7):938.
4. Mangaleshkar SR, Prasad PS, Chugh S, Thomas AP. Staged bilateral total knee replacement–a safer approach in older patients. Knee. 2001;8(3):207.
5. Jankiewicz JJ, Sculco TP, Ranawat CS, Behr C, Tarrentino S. One-stage versus 2-stage bilateral total knee arthroplasty. Clin Orthop Relat Res. 1994;(309):94–101.
6. Wang YC, Teng WN, Kuo IT, Chang KY, Chang WK, Tsou MY, Chan KH, Ting CK. Patient-machine interactions of intravenous patient-controlled analgesia in bilateral versus unilateral total knee arthroplasty: a retrospective study. J Chin Med Assoc. 2013;76(6):330.
7. Restrepo C, Parvizi J, Dietrich T, Einhorn TA. Safety of simultaneous bilateral total knee arthroplasty. A meta-analysis. J Bone Joint Surg Am. 2007;89(6):1220.
8. Courtney PM, Melnic CM, Alosh H, Shah RP, Nelson CL, Israelite CL. Is bilateral total knee arthroplasty staged at a one-week interval safe? A matched case control study. J Arthroplast. 1946;29(10):2014.
9. Cahill CW, Schwarzkopf R, Sinha S, Scott RD. Simultaneous bilateral knee arthroplasty in octogenarians: can it be safe and effective? J Arthroplast. 2014;29(5):998.
10. Ritter MA, Harty LD, Davis KE, Meding JB, Berend M. Simultaneous bilateral, staged bilateral, and unilateral total knee arthroplasty. A survival analysis. J Bone Joint Surg Am. 2003;85-a(8):1532.
11. Lin A, Chao E, Yang CM, Wen HC, Ma HL, Lu TC. Costs of staged versus simultaneous bilateral total knee arthroplasty: a population-based study of the Taiwanese National Health Insurance Database. J Orthop Surg Res. 2014;9(1):59.
12. Jain S, Wasnik S, Mittal A, Sohoni S, Kasture S. Simultaneous bilateral total knee replacement: a prospective study of 150 patients. J Orthop Surg (Hong Kong). 2013;21(1):19.
13. Gabr A, Withers D, Pope J, Santini A. Functional outcome of staged bilateral knee replacements. Ann R Coll Surg Engl. 2011;93(7):537.
14. March LM, Cross M, Tribe KL, Lapsley HM, Courtenay BG, Cross MJ, Brooks PM, Cass C, Coolican M, Neil M, Pinczewski L, Quain S, Robertson F, Ruff S, Walter W, Zicat B. Two knees or not two knees? Patient costs and outcomes following bilateral and unilateral total knee joint replacement surgery for OA. Osteoarthr Cartil. 2004;12(5):400.
15. Minter JE, Dorr LD. Indications for bilateral total knee replacement. Contemp Orthop. 1995;31(2):108.
16. Vulcano E, Memtsoudis S, Della Valle AG. Bilateral total knee arthroplasty guidelines: are we there yet? J Knee Surg. 2013;26(4):273.
17. Oakes DA, Hanssen AD. Bilateral total knee replacement using the same anesthetic is not justified by assessment of the risks. Clin Orthop Relat Res. 2004;(428):87–91.
18. Bellamy N, Buchanan WW, Goldsmith CH, Campbell J, Stitt LW. Validation study of WOMAC: a health status instrument for measuring clinically important patient relevant outcomes to antirheumatic drug therapy in patients with osteoarthritis of the hip or knee. J Rheumatol. 1833;15(12):1988.
19. Ware JE Jr, Sherbourne CD. The MOS 36-item short-form health survey (SF-36). I. Conceptual framework and item selection. Med Care. 1992;30(6):473.
20. Faul F, Erdfelder E, Lang AG, Buchner A. G*power 3: a flexible statistical power analysis program for the social, behavioral, and biomedical sciences. Behav Res Methods. 2007;39(2):175.
21. Escobar A, Quintana JM, Bilbao A, Arostegui I, Lafuente I, Vidaurreta I. Responsiveness and clinically important differences for the WOMAC and SF-36 after total knee replacement. Osteoarthritis and cartilage / OARS. Osteoarthritis Res Soc. 2007;15(3):273.
22. Baker P, Muthumayandi K, Gerrand C, Kleim B, Bettinson K, Deehan D. Influence of body mass index (BMI) on functional improvements at 3 years following total knee replacement: a retrospective cohort study. PLoS One. 2013;8(3):e59079.
23. Jenny JY, Trojani C, Prudhon JL, Vielpeau C, Saragaglia D, Houillon C, Ameline T, Steffan F, Bugnas B, Arndt J. Simultaneous bilateral total knee arthroplasty. A multicenter feasibility study. Orthop Traumatol Surg Res. 2013;99(2):191.
24. Hooper GJ, Hooper NM, Rothwell AG, Hobbs T. Bilateral total joint arthroplasty: the early results from the New Zealand National Joint Registry. J Arthroplast. 2009;24(8):1174.
25. Al-Omran AS. The quality of life (QOL) after Total knee arthroplasties among Saudi Arabians: a pilot study. Int J Biomed Sci. 2014;10(3):196.

8

Comparison of intravenous and topical tranexamic acid in total knee arthroplasty

Wenbo Wei[1,2], Shajie Dang[2,3], Dapeng Duan[1] and Ling Wei[4*]

Abstract

Background: To investigate the clinical effectiveness of intravenous (IV) and topical tranexamic acid (TXA) in patients undergoing total knee arthroplasty (TKA) by comparing safety, efficacy and patient-reported outcomes.

Methods: In this prospective single-blind clinical trial, 64 patients were randomized into two groups ($n = 32$ each). The Intravenous Group was administered TXA 10 mg/kg IV (Reyong, Shandong, China) 10 min prior to tourniquet deflation. In the Topical Group, 1.0 g TXA diluted in 50 ml of normal saline was injected into the surgical site, which was bathed in the solution for at least 5 min prior to tourniquet deflation. Outcomes included changes in hemoglobin levels, intra-operative, post-operative, and total blood loss, number of transfusions and number of transfused units, patient-reported postoperative Visual Analog Scale (VAS) score for knee pain, and complications.

Results: There were no significant differences in intra-operative blood loss, post-operative blood loss, total blood loss, or post-operative decrease in hemoglobin in the Intravenous Group versus the Topical Group. The number of transfused red blood cell units was significantly greater and-post-operative VAS score was significantly lower in the Intravenous Group. There were no differences in post-operative thromboembolic complications between groups.

Conclusions: Topical TXA is not inferior to IV administration in reducing perioperative blood loss in primary TKA. However, the influence of injection volume of locally applied TXA on post-operative knee pain warrants further investigation.

Keywords: Total knee arthroplasty, Tranexamic acid, Hemoglobin drop, Intravenous injection, Topical injection

Background

Since the 1960s, total knee arthroplasty (TKA) has become one of the most commonly performed orthopedic operations for the treatment of end-stage knee arthritis. Although TKA provides substantial pain relief and greatly improves orthopedic patients' quality of life, the surgery is associated with complications; in particular, patients undergoing TKA are at risk for bleeding and may require transfusion. As transfusions extend patients' rehabilitation time, prolong length of hospital stay, and represent a considerable cost [1–5], control of bleeding using antifibrinolytic agents such as tranexamic acid (TXA) is a primary focus in TKA [6–10].

TXA exerts its antifibrinolytic effects by inhibiting plasminogen, which prevents plasminogen activation and the binding of plasmin to fibrin. This leads to clot stabilization and decreases blood loss in surgical patients [11].

Previous publications have reported on the safety and efficacy of intravenous (IV) TXA for TKA. IV TXA is associated with decreased intra-operative blood loss, transfusion rates, and drop in post-operative hemoglobin concentrations, with no increase in the incidence of post-operative infections or thromboembolic events compared to placebo in patients undergoing orthopedic surgery [12–16]. However, patients with medical conditions such as renal insufficiency, history of previous deep vein thrombosis (DVT), and cerebrovascular and cardiac disease [17] may not tolerate intraoperative IV TXA; topical administration of TXA maybe more appropriate for these patients. Evidence suggests that topical and IV

* Correspondence: wwb560@163.com
[4]Department of Pain, YangLing Demonstration Zone Hospital, No.15 Kangle street, Yang ling, Xi'an 712100, China
Full list of author information is available at the end of the article

TXA have similar safety and efficacy in TKA; however, there is no consensus regarding the most clinically effective regimen for TXA administration. Clinical effectiveness is determined by the therapeutic benefit and adverse effects of a therapeutic approach, as evaluated by patients and clinicians. To the authors' knowledge, no studies comparing different regimens of TXA administration in TKA include patient-reported outcomes, such as patient-reported knee pain, which may have a substantial impact on length of hospital stay and delay rehabilitation, resulting in increased cost associated with surgery. Therefore, the purpose of this study was to investigate the clinical effectiveness of IV and topical TXA in patients undergoing TKA by comparing safety, efficacy, and patient reported outcomes represented by the postoperative Visual Analog Scale (VAS) score for knee pain.

Methods

This prospective single-blind randomized controlled trial included patients with knee osteoarthritis undergoing unilateral primary TKA performed by senior surgeons at the Department of Orthopedic Surgery, Shannxi Provincial People's Hospital between March, 2010 and October, 2013. The study protocol was approved by the institutional review board (Clinical ethics committee of Shaanxi People's Hospital, Shaanxi, China), and all study participants provided written informed consent.

Inclusion criteria were 1) ≥18 years old; 2) American Society of Anesthesiologists (ASA) score ≤ 3; and 3) planned TKA due to degenerative arthritis of the knee. Exclusion criteria were 1) cardiovascular problems (e.g., myocardial infarction, atrial fibrillation, angina); 2) cerebrovascular conditions (e.g., previous stroke or previous vascular surgery); 3) thromboembolic disorders; and 4) renal insufficiency.

On the day of surgery, included patients were randomized 1:1 into two groups using a random number table and closed envelopes (n = 32 each group). The Intravenous Group was administered TXA 10 mg/kg IV (Reyong, Shandong, China) 10 min after placement of a loose tourniquet. In the topical group, 1 g of TXA was diluted in 50 ml of normal saline, injected into the surgical site (posterior and anterior capsule, medial and lateral retinaculum), and the surgical site was soaked in the solution for 5 min before deflation of the tourniquet. Treatment dose was determined from previous reports that indicate TXA 10–20 mg/kg IV and 1.0–3.0 g applied topically is effective for reducing blood loss in primary TKA [18–22]. Patients and investigators responsible for evaluating the results were blind to the treatment allocation, while two authors of the study were unblinded on the day of surgery.

All operations were carried out by the same surgeon. Patients' limbs were elevated, bleeding was controlled with an Esmarch bandage, and the tourniquet was inflated to 350 mmHg. Operative techniques included a median skin incision followed by a joint incision. Gentamicin cement was used for prosthetic fixation. A polyethylene liner was inserted and wounds were closed. An intra-articular drain was used until post-operative day 2. All patients were given low-molecular-weight heparin to prevent DVT unless they took another cardiovascular medication before surgery.

Indications for blood transfusion were hemoglobin < 8.0 g/dl or hemoglobin < 10.0 g/dl with concomitant symptoms of anemia (tachycardia, tachypnea, decreased exercise tolerance) or anemia-related organ dysfunction.

All subjects underwent the same postoperative recovery and rehabilitation program. Routine follow-up was performed at postoperative 2, 6, and 12 weeks, and imaging analysis was performed at postoperative 6 weeks.

Outcomes

The primary outcome measure was the difference in pre-operative and postoperative hemoglobin levels. Secondary outcome measures include intra-operative, post-operative, and total blood loss, number of transfusions and number of transfused units, post-operative VAS score for knee pain, and complications.

Hemoglobin was measured before the operation and at 24 h, 48 h, and 96 h post-operatively. The difference in pre-operative and postoperative hemoglobin levels was calculated. The postoperative hemoglobin level was defined as the lowest level of hemoglobin among three levels measured postoperatively. The amount of postoperative bleeding was estimated from the drainage volume. The VAS score for knee pain was measured using a 10 cm visual analog scale.

Statistical analyses

Statistical analyses were conducted using IBM SPSS 12.0 for Windows (Microsoft Corporation, Redmond WA). Data are expressed as mean ± standard deviations (SDs). Continuous variables are presented as means and standard deviations. Categorical variables are summarized as the number and percentage of the total study population. Normally distributed continuous variables were compared with a two-sided independent t-test. Categorical variables were combined with Chi-square. Statistical significance was defined as $P < 0.05$.

Results

This prospective randomized clinical trial included 64 patients undergoing TKA due to degenerative arthritis of the knee. Patients' baseline demographic and clinical characteristics are shown in Table 1. Mean age of patients in the Intravenous Group was 66.47 years (range, 56–79 years); mean age of patients in the Topical Group was 66.43 years (range, 54–78 years). There were no significant differences in age, gender, height, weight, body

Table 1 Patient baseline demographic and clinical characteristics

	IV group	Topical group	P value
Age (year)	66.47 ± 8.28	66.43 ± 7.69	0.984
Male: Female	14:18	16:16	0.25
Body mass index (kg/m2)	32.39 ± 3.73	34.15 ± 5.02	0.084
American Society of Anesthesiologists classification	2.03 ± 0.14	1.79 ± 0.26	0.153
hemoglobin (g/l)	11.26 ± 1.60	10.97 ± 1.19	0.21
Red blood cell(10^{12}/l)	3.72 ± 0.75	4.05 ± 1.04	0.35
prothrombin time(s)	11.51 ± 3.51	11.85 ± 4.62	0.16

mass index, prothrombin time, hemoglobin, American Society of Anesthesiologists score, or comorbidities between the two groups.

There were no significant differences in intra-operative blood loss (intravenous: 122.81 ± 41.60 mL [range 60–200 mL] vs. topical: 109.06 ± 33.38 mL [range 70–200 mL]), post-operative blood loss (intravenous: 125.31 ± 35.649 mL [range 80–240 mL] vs. topical: 110.00 ± 30.900 mL [range 20–180 mL]), or total blood loss (intravenous: 254.38 ± 52.544 mL [range 140–420 mL] vs. topical: 210.00 ± 41.426 mL [range 100–400 mL]) in the Intravenous Group versus the Topical Group.

There were no significant differences in post-operative drop in hemoglobin (intravenous: 2.84 ± 0.68 [range 1.95–4.36] vs. topical: 2.66 ± 0.60 [range 1.73–3.84]). However, the number of transfused red blood cell units was significantly greater in the Intravenous Group (42 units red cell suspension; 1.28 units/patient) compared to the Topical Group (20 units red cell suspension; 0.63 units/patient) (P < 0.05) (Table 2).

Post-operative VAS score was significantly lower in the Intravenous Group compared to the Topical Group at 12 and 24 h after surgery. In the Intravenous Group, the VAS score was 5.41 ± 0.875 at post-operative 12 h and 3.88 ± 0.976 at post-operative 24 h. In the Topical Group, the VAS score was 6.69 ± 0.998 at post-operative 12 h and 5.50 ± 0.842 at post-operative 24 h. At 48 h after surgery,

there was no significant difference in VAS score (intravenous: 2.75 ± 0.568 vs. topical: 2.97 ± 0.647).

There were no differences in post-operative thromboembolic complications between the Intravenous Group and Topical Group. No infusion-related complications related to TXA dosing, no allergic reactions, and no deaths were reported.

Discussion

This study sought to compare the clinical effectiveness of IV and topical TXA in primary TKA using a prospective randomized controlled trial. Our results indicate that topical TXA and IV-TXA have similar safety and efficacy for reducing perioperative blood loss in TKA. There was no significant difference in the change in hemoglobin levels or therapeutic effect between topical TXA and IV administration. However, patients reported a significantly higher VAS score for knee pain in the Topical Group compared to the Intravenous Group at 12 and 24 h after surgery; there was no significant difference at 48 h. The higher VAS score at 12–24 h after the surgery may result from increased pressure in the knee joint due to the topical administration of TXA. A previous study [22] found that topical administration of TXA via a drain tube significantly increased joint swelling following TKA; rehabilitation in these patients took longer because of the pain. Further studies are warranted to elucidate the

Table 2 Outcomes

	IV group	Topical group	P value
Post-Operative Transfusion (Units)	1.28	0.63	0.016
Intra-operative blood loss (ml)	122.81 ± 41.60 mL	109.06 ± 33.38 ml	0.150
Post-operative blood loss(ml)	125.31 ± 35.649 mL	110.00 ± 30.900 mL	0.071
Total blood loss	254.38 ± 52.544 mL	210.00 ± 41.426 mL	0.143
Hb Fall (mg/dl)	2.84 ± 0.68	2.66 ± 0.60	0.261
VAS			
12 h	5.41 ± 0.875	6.69 ± 0.998	0.001
24 h	3.88 ± 0.976	5.50 ± 0.842	0.008
48 h	2.75 ± 0.568	2.97 ± 0.647	0.157
comorbidities	no	no	

clinical and economic implications of the increased VAS score in patients receiving topical administration of TXA in primary TKA.

The current study confirmed the results of previous studies showing that IV and topical TXA have similar safety and efficacy profiles in TKA [12–16]. However, to the authors' knowledge, this is the first study to include patient-reported outcomes in a study investigating the effectiveness of different regimens of TXA administration. Results showed that IV TXA administration may be the optimal approach as patients reported less pain during the initial 24 h after surgery, suggesting this regimen is associated with the potential for faster rehabilitation and shorter length of hospital stay.

TKA has good outcomes for the treatment of end-stage knee arthritis; however, blood loss may vary from 800 ml to 1800 ml [1–5], and the incidence of transfusion may range from 11 to 67% [6, 7]. Allogeneic blood transfusions are an economic burden and may result in the transmission of bloodborne pathogens, an immunomodulatory response, and periprosthetic joint infection [23]. Control of perioperative blood loss is associated with lower transfusion rates and shorter length of hospital stay [24, 25]. Currently, perioperative blood loss is controlled by the use of a tourniquet, hypotension, re-infusion drains, bipolar radiofrequency ablation, and antifibrinolytic drugs such as TXA.

TXA is an anti fibrinolytic drug that is used to reduce hemorrhage. TXA enhances microvascular hemostasis by preventing the dissolution of fibrin clots [26]. TXA is rapidly distributed to the synovial fluid and synovial membranes. The biological half-life of TXA in synovial fluid is estimated at 3 h [27]. TXA is eliminated through glomerular filtration; excretion of an Intravenous infusion of 10 mg / kg may reach 30% at 1 h, 55% at 3 h, and 90% at 24 h [27]. Methods of TXA administration include intravenous or Intramuscular injection or oral, [28], which result in maximal plasma levels of TXA at 5 to 15 min, 30 min, or2 hours, respectively [29, 30]. TXA may also be administered by intra-articular injection.

Renal insufficiency, previous history of DVT, and cerebrovascular and heart disease are contraindications to the use of IV TXA. In these patients, topical application of TXA to the knee joint is considered the safest route of administration as drug activity is delivered directly to the site of action and systemic sequelae are limited [31]. To target the bleeding, TXA is applied locally before wound closure. This reduces the significant increase in local fibrinolysis associated with tourniquet release [32]. Akizuki first described the use of topical TXA in orthopedic surgery [33]. They found that intra-articular application of 250 mg TXA in 50 ml saline effectively reduced bleeding in patients with cementless TKA. Since then, other studies have demonstrated similar outcomes.

A prospective, double-blind, placebo-controlled randomized trial of 124 patients who received 1.5 g or 3 g of TXA or placebo in 100 ml of saline in the joint after surgery showed that TXA administration resulted in a significantly lower drop in hemoglobin loss and blood loss with no differences in thromboembolic complications. In accordance with our findings, a prospective randomized study involving 89 patients showed no significant difference in lowest post-operative hemoglobin level or total drain output following topical administration of 2.0 g TXA or 10 mg/kg TXA IV [34].

The authors acknowledge that the current study has several limitations. First, the study was conducted in a small sample of patients. Second, the clinical characteristics of thromboembolic complications were not documented. A longer follow-up period is required to adequately compare the safety profile and functional outcome differences between the two groups.

Conclusion

This study showed that topical TXA is not inferior to IV administration in reducing perioperative blood loss in primary TKA. However, the VAS score in the Topical Group was significantly higher than the Intravenous Group at 12 and 24 h after surgery. The influence of the injection volume of locally applied TXA on post-operative pain in surgical patients warrants further investigation.

Abbreviations
DVT: Deep vein thrombosis; IV: Intravenous; TKA: Total knee arthroplasty; TXA: Tranexamic acid; VAS: Visual Analog Scale

Acknowledgements
We greatly appreciate the assistance of the company Medjaden Bioscience Limited., which provided English language editing.

Authors' contributions
WBW was in charge and contributed to all stages of the present study.; DPD was responsible for participated in the design of the study, made revisions of the manuscript and approved the final version. WBW and SJD contributed to interpreting the data and writing the final manuscript; LW was a contributor in writing and editing the manuscript. All authors read and approved the final manuscript.

Competing interests
The authors declare that they have no competing interests.

Author details
[1]Department of Orthopedics, Shaanxi Province People Hospital, Xi'an 710004, China. [2]Xi'an JiaoTong University, Xi'an 710004, China. [3]Department of Anesthesiology, Shaanxi Provincial Cancer Hospital, Xi'an 710001, China. [4]Department of Pain, YangLing Demonstration Zone Hospital, No.15 Kangle street, Yang ling, Xi'an 712100, China.

References

1. Benoni G, Fredin H. Fibrinolytic inhibition with tranexamic acid reduces blood loss and blood transfusion after knee arthroplasty: a prospective, randomized, double-blind study of 86 patients. J Bone Joint Surg (Br). 1996;78:434.
2. Cushner FD, Friedman RJ. Blood loss in total knee arthroplasty. Clin Orthop Relat Res. 1991;269:98.
3. Hiippala S, Strid L, Wennerstrand M, et al. Tranexamic acid (Cyklokapron) reduces perioperative blood loss associated with total knee arthroplasty. Br J Anaesth. 1995;74:534.
4. Lotke PA, Faralli VJ, Orenstein EM, et al. Blood loss after total knee replacement: effects of tourniquet release and continuous passivemotion. J Bone Joint Surg Am. 1991;73:1037.
5. Sehat KR, Evans R, Newman JH. How much blood is really lost in total knee arthroplasty? Correct blood loss management should take hidden loss into account. Knee. 2000;7:151.
6. Bierbaum BE, Callaghan JJ, Galante JO, et al. An analysis of blood management in patients having a total hip or knee arthroplasty. J Bone Joint Surg Am. 1999;81(1):2.
7. Noticewala MS, Nyce JD, Wang W, et al. Predicting need for allogeneic transfusion after total knee arthroplasty. J Arthroplast. 2012;27(6):961.
8. Sharrock NE, Go G, Williams-Russo P, et al. Comparison of extradural and general anaesthesia on the fibrinolytic response to total knee arthroplasty. Br J Anaesth. 1997;79(1):29.
9. Sculco TP. Global blood management in orthopaedic surgery. Clin Orthop Relat Res. 1998;357:43.
10. Bezwada HR, Nazarian DG, Henry DH, et al. Blood management in total joint arthroplasty. Am J Orthop. 2006;35(10):458.
11. Jansen J, Andreica S, Claeys M, et al. Use of tranexamic acid for an effective blood conservation strategy after total knee arthroplasty. Br J Anaesth. 1999;83:596.
12. Yang ZG, Chen WP, Wu LD. Effectiveness and safety of tranexamic acid in reducing blood loss in total knee arthroplasty: a meta-analysis. J Bone Joint Surg Am. 2012;94(13):1153.
13. Zhang H, Chen J, Chen F, et al. The effect of tranexamic acid on blood loss and use of blood products in total knee arthroplasty: a meta-analysis. Knee Surg Sports Traumatol Arthrosc. 2012;20(9):1742.
14. Dahuja A, Dahuja G, Jaswal V, et al. A prospective study on role of tranexamic acid in reducing postoperative blood loss in total knee arthroplasty and its effect on coagulation profile. J Arthroplast. 2013;29:733.
15. Karam JA, Bloomfield MR, Diiorio TM, et al. Evaluation of the efficacy and safety of tranexamic acid for reducing blood loss in bilateral total knee arthroplasty. J Arthroplast. 2014;29(3):501.
16. Tan J, Chen H, Liu Q, et al. A meta-analysis of the effectiveness and safety of using tranexamic acid in primary unilateral total knee arthroplasty. J Surg Res. 2013;184(2):880.
17. McCormack PL. Tranexamic acid: a review of its use in the treatment of hyperfibrinolysis. Drugs. 2012;72:585–617.
18. Kagoma YK, Crowther MA, Douketis J, et al. Use of antifibrinolytic therapy to reduce transfusion in patients undergoing orthopedic surgery: a systematic review of randomized trials. Thromb Res. 2009;123(5):687.
19. Patel JN, Spanyer JM, Smith LS, Huang J, Yakkanti MR, Malkani AL. Comparison of intravenous versus topical tranexamic acid in total knee arthroplasty: a prospective randomized study. J Arthroplasty. 2014;29(8):1528–31.
20. Alshryda S, Sarda P, Sukeik M, et al. Tranexamic acid in total knee replacement: a systematic review and meta-analysis. J Bone Joint Surg Br. 2011;93(12):1577.
21. Soni A, Saini R, Gulati A, Paul R, Bhatty S, Rajoli SR. Comparison between intravenous and intra-articular regimens of tranexamic acid in reducing blood loss during total knee arthroplasty. J Arthroplasty. 2014;29(8):1525.
22. Sarzaeem MM, Razi M, Kazemian G, Moghaddam ME, et al. Comparing efficacy of three methods of tranexamic acid administration in reducing hemoglobin drop following total knee arthroplasty. J Arthroplast. 2014;29(8):1521–4.
23. Alter HJ, Klein HG. The hazards of blood transfusion in historical perspective. Blood. 2008;112(7):2617–26.
24. Raut S, Mertes SC, Muniz-Terrera G, et al. Factors associated with prolonged length of stay following a total knee replacement in patients aged over 75. Int Orthod. 2012;36(8):1601.
25. Diamond PT, Conaway MR, Mody SH, et al. Influence of hemoglobin levels on inpatient rehabilitation outcomes after total knee arthroplasty. J Arthroplast. 2006;21(5):636.
26. Katsumata S, Nagashima M, Kato K, et al. Changes in coagulation-fibrinolysis marker and neutrophil elastase following the use of tourniquet during total knee arthroplasty and the influence of neutrophil elastase on thromboembolism. Acta Anaesthesiol Scand. 2005;49(4):510.
27. Ahlberg A, Eriksson O, Kjellman H. Diffusion of tranexamic acid to the joint. Acta Orthop Scand. 1976;47(5):486.
28. TanakaN SH, Sato E, et al. Timing of the administration of tranexamic acidfor maximum reduction in blood loss in arthroplasty of the knee. J Bone Joint Surg (Br). 2001;83:p:702.
29. Sano M, Hakusui H, Kojima C, et al. Absorption and excretion of tranexamic acid following intravenous, intramuscular and oral administrations in healthy volunteers. Jpn J Clin Pharmacol Ther. 1976;7:375.
30. Benoni G, Bjorkman S, Fredin H. Application of pharmacokinetic data from healthy volunteers for the prediction of plasma concentrations of tranexamic acid in surgical patients. Clin Drug Investig. 1995;10:280.
31. Seo JG, Moon YW, Park SH, et al. The comparative efficacies of intraarticular and IV tranexamic acid for reducing blood loss during total knee arthroplasty. Knee Surg Sports Traumatol Arthrosc. 2013;21:1869.
32. Aglietti P, Baldini A, Vena LM, et al. Effect of tourniquet use on activation of coagulation in total knee replacement. Clin Orthop Relat Res. 2000;371:169.
33. Akizuki S, Yasukawa Y, Takizawan T. A new method of hemostasis for cementless total knee arthroplasty. Bull Hosp Jt Dis. 1997;56:222.
34. Patel JN, Spanyer JM, Smith LS, Huang J, et al. Comparison of intravenous versus topical tranexamic acid in total knee arthroplasty: a prospective randomized study. The Journal of Arthroplasty. 2014;29:1528–31.

9

A comparative study of flat surface design and medial pivot design in posterior cruciate-retaining total knee arthroplasty: a matched pair cohort study of two years

Junichi Nakamura*[ID], Takaki Inoue, Toru Suguro, Masahiko Suzuki, Takahisa Sasho, Shigeo Hagiwara, Ryuichiro Akagi, Sumihisa Orita, Kazuhide Inage, Tsutomu Akazawa and Seiji Ohtori

Abstract

Background: Component design is one of the contributory factors affecting the postoperative flexion angle. The purpose of this study was to compare short-term outcomes of flat surface and medial pivot designs in posterior cruciate-retaining (CR) total knee arthroplasty (TKA).

Methods: A retrospective, case-control, and observational cohort study consisted of matched-pairs of the flat surface design (Hi-Tech Knee II) and the medial pivot design (FINE Knee) in CR-TKA with a two-year follow-up period.

Results: Hi-Tech Knee II and FINE knee groups each included 7 males and 38 females. Surgical time was significantly shorter in the FINE Knee group than in the Hi-Tech Knee II group (104.8 min versus 154.9 min, $p = 0.001$). Estimated total blood loss was significantly lower in the FINE Knee group than in the Hi-Tech Knee II group (654 ml versus 1158 ml, $p = 0.001$). The postoperative flexion angle was significantly better in the FINE Knee group than in the Hi-Tech Knee II group (119.3 degrees versus 112.5 degrees), and was positively correlated with the preoperative flexion angle. Postoperative Knee Society scores were significantly better in the FINE Knee group than in the Hi-Tech Knee II group (93.0 points versus 85.0 points, $p = 0.001$), especially for postoperative pain relief (46.0 points versus 39.0 points out of 50, $p = 0.001$). Complications were not observed in either group over a two-year follow-up period.

Conclusion: The short-term outcome of the medial pivot design used in CR-TKA was more favorable than the flat surface design, especially for surgical time, estimated total blood loss, postoperative flexion angle, and knee pain.

Keywords: Total knee arthroplasty, Comparative study, Posterior cruciate-retaining, Flat surface, Medial pivot

Background

Total knee arthroplasty (TKA) is associated with pain relief and improvement in activities of daily living. The decisions regarding whether the posterior cruciate ligament (PCL) should be replaced or retained and whether the prosthesis should be fixed using cement or not are made at the surgeon's discretion. Studies of cruciate-retaining (CR) TKA without cement fixation of the prosthesis in patients with rheumatoid arthritis (RA) indicated prosthesis survival rates of over 90% after 10 years [1].

Hi-Tech Knee II CR-type cementless TKA (Teijin Nakashima Medical, Okayama, Japan) was developed in 1994 at Chiba University in Japan [2] and has been used for 1918 cases at 73 hospitals until 2016. This prosthesis was designed for the Japanese knee, with 6 fins at the anterior of the femoral component with the same radii in the sagittal plane, with aspect ratios (anteroposterior/mediolateral) of 0.86, PCL retention, flat-on-flat surface component geometry with 5 degrees of posterior tilt, all-polyethylene patella fixed without cement, strong initial fixation by the center screw of the tibial base plate, 10 layers of titanium alloy fiber mesh, and direct compression molded ultra-high molecular weight polyethylene (UHMWPE) [3]. The

* Correspondence: njonedr@chiba-u.j
Department of Orthopedic Surgery, Graduate School of Medicine, Chiba University, 1-8-1 Inohana, Chuo-ku, Chiba 260-8677, Japan

mid-term (5–12 year) results of Hi-Tech Knee II CR-type cementless TKA in 31 RA patients were satisfactory [4].

The FINE knee (Teijin Nakashima Medical, Okayama, Japan) was subsequently developed by Professor Suguro in 2001 [5]. Up to 2016, the FINE knee has been one of the most popular implants in Japan, used in 14,266 cases at 293 hospitals. The FINE knee was designed based on morphological study of Japanese normal knees to allow deeper flexion matching the Japanese lifestyle. The FINE knee has a design concept to guide tibial internal movements by medial pivot motion. The femoral component was designed to reproduce the physiologic joint line at an oblique angle of 3 degrees on the posterior condyle by osteotomy in parallel with the surgical epicondylar axis. The articular surface of the tibial medial condyle was designed to show high conformity with the femoral component and thereby enhance tibial internal rotation and secure stability during the early phase of flexion. The articular surface of the tibial lateral condyle was designed flat to allow femoral rollback, thereby allowing tibial internal rotation by medial pivot motion.

The purpose of this study was to compare short-term clinical outcomes of these two different implants with the flat surface design and the medial pivot design in CR TKA.

Methods

The protocol for this retrospective, case-control, and observational cohort study was approved by the institutional review board. Written informed consent was obtained from all patients before surgery.

From January 2005 to December 2014, a matched-pair study was conducted for TKA. Two types of implants were compared the Hi-Tech Knee II and the FINE Knee. Inclusion criteria were a diagnosis of osteoarthritis or rheumatoid arthritis, primary TKA without previous knee surgery, CR-type component, and a minimum follow-up period of two years. Cementless fixation was applied in the Hi-Tech Knee II group and cemented fixation was used in the FINE Knee group. Osteotomy of the femur and the tibia were performed with an intramedullary guide and the proximal tibia was cut perpendicular to the axis of the tibial shaft. A posterior slope of 5 degrees was built in the tibial plates of both groups. Pairs were matched by gender and age categories (younger than 60 years, 60–64, 65–69, 70–74, 75–79, and older than 80 years). Patient condition preoperatively was documented by age, diagnosis, height, weight, body mass index (BMI, [weight]/[height]^2), surgical approach, Knee Society score (KSS) [6], range of motion (ROM), femoro-tibial angle (FTA), joint line, and posterior condylar offset. Perioperative factors were recorded such as surgical time time and estimated total blood loss by following Gross's formula [7]; Estimated total blood loss =

estimated blood volume × (preoperative hemoglobin concentration [Hb] - postoperative day-one Hb)/(preoperative Hb + postoperative day-one Hb) × 2 + autologous blood transfusion + allogeneic blood transfusion. Estimated blood volume was calculated by 70 × body weight in men and 65 × body weight in women. Two years postoperatively, KSS, ROM, FTA, level of joint line, posterior condylar offset, α angle, β angle, γ angle, δ angle [8], and complications were compared between the Hi-Tech Knee II and FINE Knee groups.

Statistical analysis

The Fisher's exact probability test was calculated for differences of gender, diagnosis, and surgical approach. The Wilcoxon signed rank test was calculated for age, height, weight, BMI, KSS, ROM, and X-ray measurements with 95% confidence interval [CI]. Inter-observer and intra-observer reliability of X-ray measurements was calculated with intraclass correlation coefficients (ICC) and measurement error by minimal detectable change with Bland-Altman plot. Simple regression analysis was calculated for some correlations followed by step-wise multiple regression analysis. A p value less than 0.05 was considered significant (JMP Pro 12.0, SAS, North Carolina).

Results

Hi-tech Knee II for 383 cases and FINE knee group for only 49 cases were registered. Firstly, 4 cases of FINE knee were excluded because posterior stabilizing type of knee prosthesis was applied. The remaining 45 FINE knee cases were matched to the historical cohort of Hi-tech Knee II group by gender and age categories. Patients were similar in age, BMI, and preoperative ROM in the Hi-Tech Knee II and FINE Knee groups, although height and weight were greater in the Hi-Tech Knee II group (Table 1). This study involved three consultant surgeons; A performed 53 operations, B performed 20 operations, and C performed 17 operations. All the surgeons preferred PCL retaining TKA. The mid-vastus approach was used more frequently in the FINE Knee group than in the Hi-Tech Knee II group (91% versus 64%, $p = 0.005$). The preoperative KSS indicated more severe pathology in the FINE Knee group than in the Hi-Tech Knee II group (knee score 55.1 points [95%CI, 50.9 to 59.3] versus 64.6 points [95%CI, 61.1 to 68.1], $p = 0.005$; functional score 33.3 points [95%CI, 27.2 to 39.5] versus 43.5 points [95%CI, 38.6 to 48.5], $p = 0.013$). Preoperative pain was more severe in the FINE Knee group than in the Hi-Tech Knee II group (16.9 points [95%CI, 14.1 to 19.7] versus 24.6 points [95%CI, 22.1 to 27.0] out of 50, $p = 0.001$).

Surgical time was significantly shorter in the FINE Knee group than in the Hi-Tech Knee II group (104.8 min [95%CI, 97.9 to 111.7] versus 154.9 min

Table 1 Patient characteristics in the Hi-Tech Knee II and FINE Knee groups

	Hi-Tech Knee II (n = 45)	FINE Knee (n = 45)	p values
Gender (male:female)	7:38	7:38	1.000[a]
Age, years	74.1 (8.1)	74.3 (10.3)	0.351[b]
Diagnosis (OA:RA)	38:7	30:15	0.846[a]
Height, cm	149.5 (8.6)	147.8(7.2)	0.015[b]
Weight, kg	60.3 (9.5)	55.7(8.4)	0.035[b]
BMI	25.8 (3.1)	25.6 (3.7)	0.566[b]
Surgical approach (Mid-vastus: Medial parapatellar)	29:16	41:4	0.005[a]
Preoperative knee score[c]	64.6 (12.0)	55.1 (14.3)	0.006[b]
Preoperative functional score[c]	45.6 (16.9)	33.3 (21.1)	0.013[b]
Preoperative total ROM, degrees	104 (23)	104 (23)	0.961[b]
Preoperative maximum flexion, degrees	114 (17)	116 (19)	0.436[b]
Preoperative flexion contracture, degrees	11 (10)	13 (10)	0.226[b]
Preoperative FTA, degrees	183.7 (6.8)	181.3 (5.2)	0.069[b]

Mean (standard deviation)
[a]Fisher's exact probability test
[b]Wilcoxon signed rank test, [c]Knee Society score
OA osteoarthritis, RA rheumatoid arthritis, BMI body mass index, ROM range of motion, FTA femoro-tibial angle

[95%CI, 145.2 to 164.6], Fig. 1). Estimated total blood loss was significantly lower in the FINE Knee group than in the Hi-Tech Knee II group (654 ml [95%CI, 550 to 758] versus 1158 ml [95%CI, 1031 to 1439], $p = 0.001$). Estimated total blood loss increased with body weight (Fig. 2).

Postoperative ROM was improved in both groups, but it was significantly better in the FINE Knee group than in the Hi-Tech Knee II group (119.3 degrees [95%CI, 113.9 to 123.0] versus 112.5 degrees [95%CI, 108.1 to 117.0], $p = 0.036$). Postoperative ROM was better in patients with greater preoperative ROM (Fig. 3). FINE knee group showed a significant improvement of ROM from

less than 125 degrees before to 125 degrees and more after the surgery (16 of 36 patients [44%] in FINE group versus 5 of 37 patients [14%] in Hi-tech Knee II group, $p = 0.005$, Fisher's exact probability test, Tables 2 and 3). Postoperative knee scores of KSS were improved in both groups, but the values were significantly better in the FINE Knee group than in the Hi-Tech Knee II group (92.2 points [95%CI, 89.4 to 95.1] versus 85.0 points [95%CI, 82.7 to 87.4], $p = 0.001$). There was less postoperative pain in the FINE Knee group than in the Hi-Tech Knee II group (45.9 points [95%CI, 44.1 to

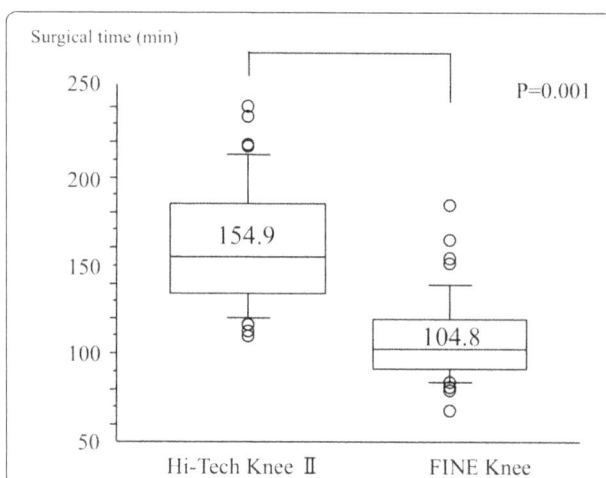

Fig. 1 Surgical time for Hi-Tech Knee II and FINE Knee groups. Box-and-whisker plot shows the mean surgical time and standard deviation. Wilcoxon signed rank test

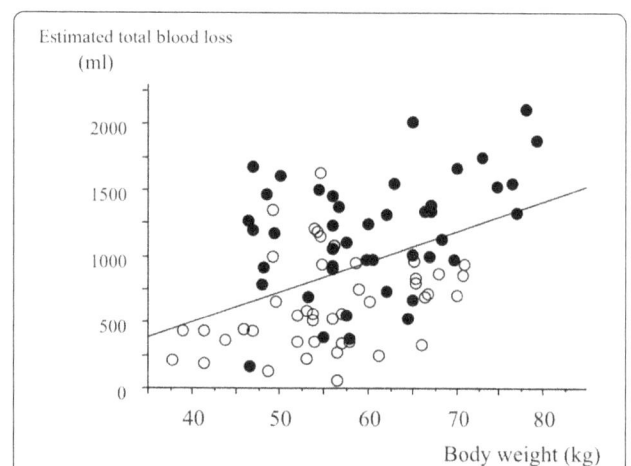

Fig. 2 Relationship of estimated total blood loss and body weight. (Estimated total blood loss) =22 × (body weight) − 401, R = 0.441, $p = 0.001$, simple regression analysis. White dots: FINE Knee group and black dots: Hi-Tech Knee II group

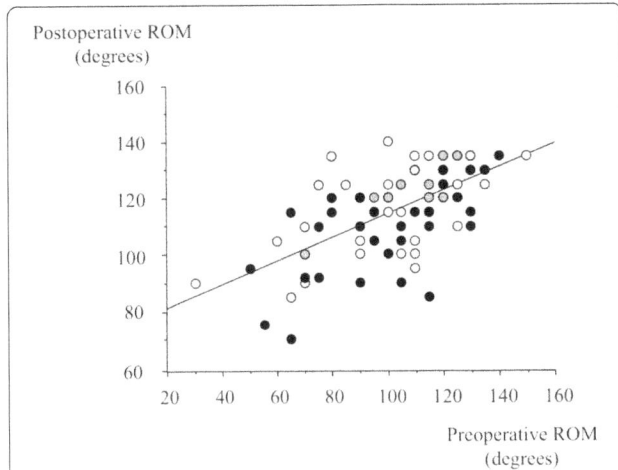

Fig. 3 Relationship of preoperative and postoperative ROM. (Postoperative ROM) = 73 + 0.4× (preoperative ROM), R = 0.622, p = 0.001, simple regression analysis. White dots: FINE Knee group, black dots: Hi-Tech Knee II group, and gray dots: overlapping of FINE Knee and Hi-Tech Knee II groups

Table 3 Number of patients with 125 degrees of total ROM in Fine Knee group

		Preoperative total ROM (degrees)	
		< 125	125≤
Postoperative total ROM (degrees)	< 125	20	2
	125≤	16	7

$P = 0.135$, Fisher's exact probability test

47.7] versus 39.3 points [95%CI, 37.5 to 41.2] out of 50, p = 0.001).

As for X-ray measurement, Inter-observer ICCs were 0.754 (95%CI, 0.639 to 0.835) in α angle, 0.544 (95%CI, 0.365 to 0.681) in β angle, 0.440 (95%CI, 0.258 to 0.592) in γ angle, and 0.460 (95%CI, 0.282 to 0.608) in δ angle. Intra-observer ICCs were 0.836 (95%CI, 0.760 to 0.889) in α angle, 0.827 (95%CI, 0.748 to 0.883) in β angle, 0.753 (95%CI, 0.646 to 0.831) in γ angle, and 0.602 (95%CI, 0.451 to 0.720) in δ angle. Therefore, α angle was substantial to perfect, β angle was moderate to perfect, γ angle was moderate to substantial, and δ angle was moderate to substantial. The measurement errors were 3.5 degrees in α angle, 2.9 degrees in β angle, 3.7 degrees in γ angle, and 3.9 degrees in δ angle. Postoperative X-ray findings showed that postoperative FTA was closer to normal both in the Hi-Tech Knee II and FINE Knee groups (174.8 degrees versus 174.2 degrees, p = 0.339). The joint line became 0.7 mm lower in the Hi-Tech Knee II group [95%CI, – 1.5 to 0.0] and 0.9 mm higher in the FINE Knee group (95%CI, 0.3 to 1.3, p = 0.001). Posterior condylar offset became smaller by 0.8 mm in the Hi-Tech Knee II group and 0.3 mm in the FINE Knee group (p = 0.802). The α angle was

Table 2 Number of patients with 125 degrees of total ROM in Hi-tech Knee II group

		Preoperative total ROM (degrees)	
		< 125	125≤
Postoperative total ROM (degrees)	< 125	32	4
	125≤	5	4

$P = 0.039$, Fisher's exact probability test

significantly larger in the FINE Knee group than in the Hi-Tech Knee II group (100.0 degrees [95%CI, 99.5 to 100.6] versus 95.4 degrees [95%CI, 94.9 to 95.9], p = 0.001). The β angle and γ angle were similar in the Hi-Tech Knee II and FINE Knee groups (89.1 degrees versus 88.1 degrees and 5.9 degrees versus 6.2 degrees). The δ angle was significantly smaller in the FINE Knee group than in the Hi-Tech Knee II group (87.8 degrees [95%CI, 87.0 to 88.5] versus 89.0 degrees [95%CI, 88.0 to 89.9], $p = 0.0365$).

The effect of prosthesis type and surgical approach on the duration of the surgery can be estimated by:

(Surgical time) = 168–45 × (group: 0 for Hi-Tech Knee II and 1 for FINE Knee) – 21× (approach: 0 for parapatellar and 1 for mid-vastus), $R^2 = 0.481$, $p = 0.001$.

The effect of body weight and prosthesis type on total blood loss can be estimated by:

(Estimated total blood loss) =22–498 × (group: 0 for Hi-Tech Knee II and 1 for FINE Knee) + 20 × (body weight), $R^2 = 0.301$, $p = 0.001$.

The effect of prosthesis type and preoperative ROM on postoperative ROM can be estimated by: (Postoperative ROM) = 69.8 + 6.5 × (group: 0 for Hi-Tech Knee II and 1 for FINE Knee) + 0.42× (preoperative ROM), $R^2 = 0.432$, p = 0.001.

Complications were not observed in either group at a two-year follow-up (Additional file 1).

Discussion

The two-year clinical outcome was better with the medial pivot design (FINE knee) than with the flat surface design (Hi-Tech Knee II) following CR-TKA, resulting in a 6.8 degree greater ROM. The ideal TKA would guarantee restoration of ROM. At present, 125 degrees may be enough to satisfy the patients because the much more deep flexion may lead to implant failure due to the impingement or subluxation (Fig. 4). Component design contributes to the postoperative flexion angle. Kaneyama et al. [2] performed three-dimensional kinematic analysis of the flat surface design with CR-TKA (Hi-Tech Knee II) and reported that the lateral contact point moved only slightly, but the medial contact point showed both roll-back and anterior sliding movements, with lateral pivot motions. The ten-year follow-up of the Hi-Tech Knee II shows an average flexion angle of 113.3 degrees

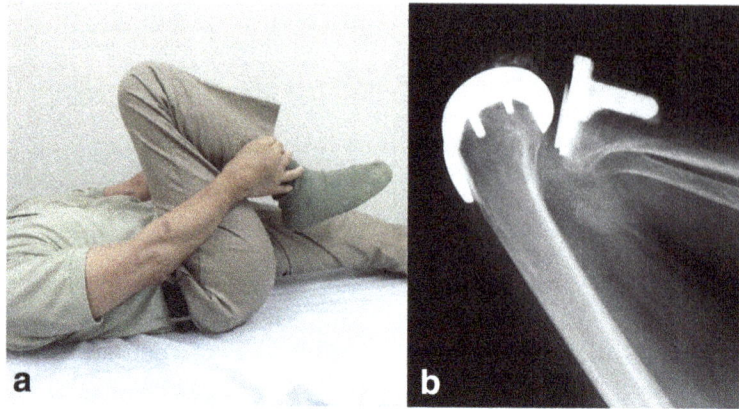

Fig. 4 Clinical appearance (**a**) and X-ray (**b**) in a patient of FINE knee group with 140 degrees of flexion. You can see enough roll back but bone-implant impingement between the posterior femoral condyle and the posterior part of tibial plate and the polyethylene, indicating the limit of deep flexion

in the medial pivot motion and 108.8 degrees in the lateral pivot motion without loosening or polyethylene wear [9]. Stiehl et al. [10] reported paradoxical movement, condylar lift-odd, and erratic screw home motion as risk factors related to abnormal wear characteristics when using a flat surface design for CR-TKA. On the other hand, rotation of the healthy knee occurs around an axis medial to the midline, and the lateral femoral condyle moves posteriorly an average of 22 mm on knee flexion to 120 degrees [11]. Magnetic resonance studies showed medial pivot motion in healthy knees and emphasized the importance of medial pivot motion in deep flexion [12]. The FINE Knee has a medially-constrained conformation to induce medial pivot motion with a postoperative flexion angle of 130.6 degrees [5]. The FINE Knee was designed to allow tibial internal rotation of 25 degrees to approximately 30 degrees, and to allow high conformity of the inside and rollback of the outside. Furthermore, the largerα angle might help the medial pivot motion and the smaller δ angle might lead the roll-back movement in the FINE knee group. We conclude that the medial pivot characteristics allow deeper flexion than the flat surface design.

Soft tissue balance plays a role in stabilizing the knee, and the choice of CR- or PS-TKA might affect the postoperative flexion angle [13]. CR-TKA can reproduce tibial rotation during flexion-extension more physiologically. The PCL kept the knee stable against distal traction force in flexion, and sacrifice of this ligament caused joint laxity [14]. Moreover, the slackness of the lateral collateral ligament makes the medial pivot motion possible [15].

The preoperative flexion angle is known to be the principal predictive factor of the postoperative angle [16]. In the current study, the postoperative ROM was better in patients with greater preoperative ROM. Other contributory factors affecting the postoperative flexion angle include both patient factors (age, comorbidity, gender, and BMI) [16, 17], and surgically modifiable factors (surgical approach, level of the joint line, tibial slope, and posterior condylar offset) [13, 17]. To equalize the patient factors, this study matched pairs by gender and age. The surgical approach did not affect postoperative flexion angle, but surgical time using the mid-vastus approach was 21 min faster than for the parapatellar approach. X-ray findings of the joint line, α angle, and δ angle were significantly different between the FINE Knee and the Hi-Tech Knee II group, although they were not predictive of the postoperative flexion angle.

The fixation method (cementless or cemented TKA) is still controversial [18]. In the Japanese registry, 83% of TKAs were cemented and 11% were cementless in 2017 [19]. Kim et al. [20] observed bone ingrowth at the surface of the titanium fiber mesh of 50.8% at 3 weeks and 62.7% at 8 weeks. Hydroxyapatite powder enhanced osteointegration to the titanium fiber [21]. Fricka et al. [22] reported equivalent survivorship at two-years in a prospective, randomized study comparing cemented versus cementless TKA. In our study, the cementless Hi-Tech Knee II group did not have any complications or revisions, but showed more estimated total blood loss than the cemented FINE knee group.

There are several limitations to this study. First, this was a short-term comparative study and long-term outcomes are unclear. However, Tamai et al. [9] reported that after 10 years, the KSS was 85.8 points in the medial pivot group and 82.9 points in the lateral pivot group when using the Hi-Tech Knee II. Yamanaka et al. [4] reported that prosthetic survival was 96.9% at 12 years postoperatively in RA patients. Long-term results of the FINE knee have not been reported. Second, because of the study's retrospective nature, patient characteristics were heterogeneous, even though gender and age were matched. It is true that a comparative study should combine factors (disease category, surgeon, possible measurement error, pre-operative range of motion, and tilt) to match the pairs. However, it was too strict for small sample size to match the complete characteristics. Third, this study involved three consultant surgeons and permitted the surgeon's preference. Multiple regression analysis was used to try to control confounding factors. Forth, measurement error should be taken into account. Unfortunately, the measurement error for range of motion could not be provided because of the retrospective nature in this study. As for X-ray measurement, inter-observer and intra-observer reliability was acceptable, because Brazier et al. showed radiographic measurement of the tibial psterior slope with measurement error of error of 3 degrees or more in 39.3% [23].

Conclusion

The two-year results of the medial pivot design for CR TKA was more favorable than the flat surface design, especially for surgical time, estimated total blood loss, postoperative flexion angle, and knee pain.

Abbreviations
BMI: body mass index; CR: cruciate-retaining; FTA: femoro-tibial angle; Hb: hemoglobin concentration; KSS: Knee Society score; PCL: posterior cruciate ligament; RA: rheumatoid arthritis; ROM: range of motion; TKA: total knee arthroplasty

Acknowledgements
The authors appreciate Yasunori Sato, Ph.D., Associate Professor, Department of Global Clinical Research / Biostatistics, Graduate School of Medicine, Chiba University, for his statistical assistance.

Funding
The corresponding author, Junichi Nakamura, receive JSPS KAKENHI Grant Number 17 K10954.

Authors' contributions
JN, TI, TS, MS, and TS analyzed and interpreted the patient data regarding the clinical outcome. JN, TI, SO1, KI, and TA measured the X-rays. JN and SO2 planed the study design. KI and TA made substantial contributions to conception. SH and RA performed the patient matching. JN wrote the manuscript. SH and RA revised it critically for important intellectual content. JN and TI equally contributed the article as the first author. All authors read and approved the final manuscript.

Consent for publication
Not applicable.

Competing interests
The authors declare that they have no competing interests.

References
1. Gill GS, Joshi AB. Long-term results of retention of the posterior cruciate ligament in total knee replacement in rheumatoid arthritis. J Bone Joint Surg Br. 2001;83:510–2.
2. Kaneyama R, Suzuki M, Moriya H, Banks SA, Hodge WA. Fluoroscopic analysis of knee kinematics after total knee arthroplasty in osteoarthritis and rheumatoid arthritis. Chiba Med J. 2002;78:193–201.
3. Watanabe E, Suzuki M, Nagata K, Kaneeda T, Harada Y, Utsumi M, Mori A, Moriya H. Oxidation-induced dynamic changes in morphology reflected on freeze-fractured surface of gamma-irradiated ultra-high molecular weight polyethylene components. J Biomed Mater Res. 2002;62:540–9.
4. Yamanaka H, Goto K, Suzuki M. Clinical results of hi-tech knee II total knee arthroplasty in patients with rheumatoid athritis: 5- to 12-year follow-up. J Orthop Surg Res. 2012;7:9.
5. Miyazaki Y, Nakamura T, Kogame K, Saito M, Yamamoto K, Suguro T. Analysis of the kinematics of total knee prostheses with a medial pivot design. J Arthroplast. 2011;26:1038–44.
6. Insall JN, Dorr LD, Scott RD, Scott WN. Rationale of the knee society clinical rating system. Clin Orthop Relat Res. 1989;248:13–4.
7. Gross JB. Estimating allowable blood loss: corrected for dilution. Anesthesiology. 1985;58:277–80.
8. Ewald FC. The knee society total knee arthroplasty roentgenographic evaluation and scoring system. Clin Orthop Relat Res. 1989;248:9–12.
9. Tamai H, Suzuki M, Tsuneizumi Y, Tsukeoka T, Banks SA, Moriya H, Takahashi K. Knee kinematics do not influence the long-term results in posterior cruciate-retaining total knee arthroplasties. Chiba Med J. 2008;84:269–76.
10. Stiehl JB, Komistek RD, Dennis DA. Detrimental kinematics of a flat on flat total condylar knee arthroplasty. Clin Orthop Relat Res. 1999;365:139–48.
11. Johal P, Williams A, Wragg P, Hunt D, Gedroyc W. Tibio-femoral movement in the living knee. A study of weight bearing and non-weight bearing knee kinematics using 'interventional' MRI. J Biomech. 2005;38:269–76.
12. Nakagawa S, Kadoya Y, Todo S, Kobayashi A, Sakamoto H, Freeman MA, Yamano Y. Tibiofemoral movement 3: full flexion in the living knee studied by MRI. J Bone Joint Surg Br. 2000;82(8):1199–200.
13. Maruyama S, Yoshiya S, Matsui N, Kuroda R, Kurosaka M. Functional comparison of posterior cruciate-retaining versus posterior stabilized total knee arthroplasty. J Arthroplast. 2004;19:349–53.
14. Tsuneizumi Y, Suzuki M, Miyagi J, Tamai H, Tsukeoka T, Moriya H, Takahashi K. Evaluation of joint laxity against distal traction force upon flexion in cruciate-retaining and posterior-stabilized total knee arthroplasty. J Orthop Sci. 2008;13:504–9.
15. Kobayashi T, Suzuki M, Sasho T, Nakagawa K, Tsuneizumi Y, Takahashi K. Lateral laxity in flexion increases the postoperative flexion angle in cruciate-retaining total knee arthroplasty. J Arthroplast. 2012;27:260–5.
16. Lizaur A, Marco L, Cebrian R. Preoperative factors influencing the range of movement after total knee arthroplasty for severe osteoarthritis. J Bone Joint Surg Br. 1997;79:626–9.
17. Arabori M, Matsui N, Kuroda R, Mizuno K, Doita M, Kurosaka M, Yoshiya S. Posterior condylar offset and flexion in posterior cruciate-retaining and posterior stabilized TKA. J Orthop Sci. 2008;13:46–50.
18. Dalury DF. Cementless total knee arthroplasty: current concepts review. Bone Joint J. 2016;98-B:867–73.
19. The Japanese Society for Replacement Arthroplasty http://jsra.info/pdf/TKA20170331.pdf (accessed 2017/7/28).
20. Kim T, Suzuki M, Ohtsuki C, Masuda K, Tamai H, Watanabe E, Osaka A, Moriya H. Enhancement of bone growth in titanium fiber mesh by surface modification with hydrogen peroxide solution containing tantalum chloride. J Biomed Mater Res B Appl Biomater. 2003;64:19–26.
21. Tsukeoka T, Suzuki M, Ohtsuki C, Tsuneizumi Y, Miyagi J, Sugino A, Inoue T, Michihiro R, Moriya H. Enhanced fixation of implants by bone ingrowth to titanium fiber mesh: effect of incorporation of hydroxyapatite powder. J Biomed Mater Res B Appl Biomater. 2005;75:168–76.
22. Fricka KB, Sritulanondha S, McAsey CJ. To cement or not? Two-year results of a prospective, randomized study comparing cemented vs. Cementless Total knee arthroplasty (TKA). J Arthroplast. 2015;30(9 Suppl):55–8.
23. Brazier J, Migaud H, Gougeon F, Cotten A, Fontaine C, Duquennoy A. Evaluation of methods for radiographic measurement of the tibial slope. A study of 83 healthy knees. Rev Chir Orthop Reparatrice Appar Mot. 1996; 82(3):195–200. French

10

A prospective evaluation of a largely cementless total knee arthroplasty cohort without patellar resurfacing: 10-year outcomes and survivorship

Richard J. Napier[1][*], Christopher O'Neill[1], Seamus O'Brien[1], Emer Doran[1], Brian Mockford[1], Jens Boldt[2] and David E. Beverland[1]

Abstract

Background: The theoretical benefits of a mobile bearing design in Total Knee Arthroplasty (TKA) include increased articular surface conformity with a reduction in both polyethylene wear and implant interface shear. However, to date these theoretical advantages have not been translated into published evidence of superior survivorship. This paper presents the results of a prospective, non-comparative study evaluating the performance of the mobile bearing Low Contact Stress LCS Complete Rotating Platform TKA in a largely cementless cohort without patellar resurfacing.

Methods: 237 consecutive patients (240 knees) undergoing primary TKA were prospectively recruited. All received the LCS Complete Rotating Platform TKA (DePuy International, Leeds, UK). Clinical and radiographic assessments were performed at 3, 12, 60 and 120 months post-operatively. Radiographic evaluation was performed by an independent external surgeon.

Results: The mean age was 70.3 years. 77.5% of cases were cementless. Radiographic assessment suggested excellent femoral component fixation. 22 tibial radiolucent lines (RLLs) > 1 mm were observed in 12 knees. No RLLs were progressive. There have been two revisions; one for late infection and one for aseptic loosening. No patients underwent secondary patellar resurfacing. The cumulative implant survivorship, using component revision for any reason as the endpoint, was 98.9% (95% CI, 95.6 to 99.7%) at 10 years.

Conclusions: The excellent survivorship at a minimum 10-year follow-up supports the use of uncemented porous coated fixation without patellar resurfacing with the non-posterior stabilized LCS Complete Rotating Platform TKA.

Keywords: Cementless TKA, LCS total knee, Cementless knee survivorship, Knee replacement

Background

The theoretical benefits of a rotating platform design in Total Knee Arthroplasty (TKA) are well-documented [1, 2]. The concept of increasing the congruity of the articular surface to reduce polyethylene wear rates, coupled with the use of a mobile bearing (MB) to minimize constraint forces associated with mechanical loosening should theoretically be associated with greater long-term survivorship [3]. However to date

such advantages have not been demonstrated in the literature [4–9].

Although cemented fixation for TKA is supported within the literature as offering excellent long-term survivorship [10], cementless fixation has many benefits including shorter surgical time, which may reduce infection rates [11], preservation of bone stock for revision procedures [12], and prevention of third body cement wear. The most common cause of late failure in TKA remains aseptic loosening particularly the tibial component [13–16]. A recent Cochrane review suggested if good early fixation is achieved the potential for later

* Correspondence: rjnapier@doctors.org.uk
[1]Orthopaedic Outcomes Assessment Unit, Musgrave Park Hospital, Stockman's Lane, Belfast BT9 7JB, Northern Ireland
Full list of author information is available at the end of the article

aseptic loosening is reduced by up to half compared to cemented TKA [17].

Patellar resurfacing also creates significant debate among knee surgeons with numerous studies both for [18–21] and against [22, 23]. Due to the wide variety of trochlear geometry between TKA designs, it may be more appropriate to refer to specific designs when debating patellar resurfacing [24–26]. Additional factors such as surgical technique and the primary indication for knee arthroplasty also contribute to reducing anterior knee pain post-operatively [27, 28]. This prospective, non-comparative study aimed to evaluating the performance of a rotating platform TKA using predominantly cementless fixation and without patellar resurfacing at a minimum 10-year follow-up.

Methods

Between March 2002–January 2003, 237 consecutive patients (240 knees) scheduled for primary TKA at a regional orthopaedic centre were prospectively recruited. Exclusion criteria included: previous knee surgery (except for open or arthroscopic meniscectomy) and/or an inability to give informed consent. Institutional Review Board (IRB) approval was obtained from the regional research and ethics committee. (Study reference ORECNI-335-01) and written consent was obtained from all patients.

All patients received a LCS Complete Rotating Platform TKA (DePuy International, Leeds, UK), without patellar resurfacing. Surgery was performed under the care of the senior author. The philosophy for alignment was to achieve a balanced knee through bone cuts rather than soft tissue releases, and not to aim for a neutral mechanical axis [29, 30]. At the beginning of the study hybrid fixation with a cemented tibia was used in female patients with valgus deformities due to concern regarding early post-operative tibial insufficiency fractures [31]. Prophylactic antibiotics were administered prior to tourniquet inflation, with the tourniquet being released after deep closure. A medial Insall approach was utilized in all cases. The patella underwent removal of rim osteophytes, with a lateral patellar release only performed in cases were persistent patellar tilt or a mal-tracking was observed. In more severe cases (Sperner grade IV) a lateral facetectomy was performed [Fig. 1] [32]. No patellae underwent resurfacing. Thirty knees underwent lateral release and 1 required facetectomy.

All knees were closed in flexion and kept flexed on a pillow for 6 h to reduce blood loss [33]. Patients without a personal history of venous thromboembolism received oral aspirin 150 mg once daily for 6 weeks as thromboprophylaxis [34, 35]. Anesthesia consisted of a spinal anesthetic combined with regional femoral and sciatic nerve blocks. All patients were mobilized full weight-bearing on the first post-operative day.

Patients were reviewed by Arthroplasty Care Practitioners [36] with clinical and radiographic assessments at 3, 12, 60 and 120 months post-operatively.

Clinical outcome was assessed by comparison of pre and postoperative Oxford Knee Scores (OKS), American Knee Society Scores (AKSS) and Bartlett Patellar Scores (BPS). Quality of life was assessed using the 12 item Short Form Health Survey (SF-12).

Radiographic evaluation was performed by an independent external surgeon. Standardised erect anteroposterior (AP), lateral and skyline patellar views were obtained. Radiographs were assessed for the presence of radiolucent lines (RLLs) and osteolytic defects. A RLL was defined as a radiolucency of ≥1 mm in greater than 50% of a zone. The zones are illustrated in Fig. 2.

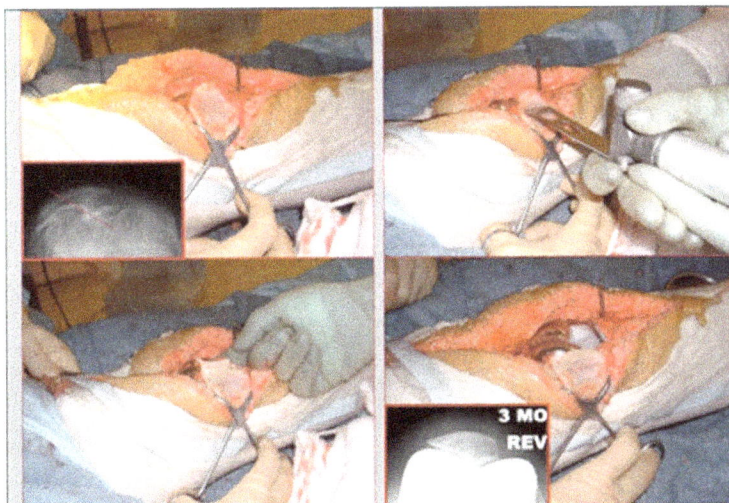

Fig. 1 Demonstrating the technique for patellar contouring with an inset showing preoperative and three-month skyline views

Revision for any reason was used as the end point for survivorship. Of the 237 patients enrolled in the study, 84 subjects were withdrawn at the end of 10 years: 70 Deceased, 2 Revisions, 12 lost to follow-up (7 due to ill-health, 3 moved away and 2 untraceable).

Statistical analysis
Survivorship was determined using the Kaplan-Meier method. Subjects who died or were lost to follow-up were included in the survivorship analysis and in the calculation of the 95% confidence intervals.

Results
The mean age of the patients at the time of surgery was 70.3 years (range 39–89). The series included 91 males and 146 females. One female and two males had bilateral staged knee replacements. Osteoarthritis was the indication for surgery in 94% of cases (226 knees). Other indications included inflammatory arthropathy 4.6% (11 knees) and post-traumatic arthritis 0.4% (1 knee). Four knees within this study underwent TKA for isolated patellofemoral disease [28]. Patient demographics are summarised in Table 1.

Pre-operative radiological alignment was predominantly varus with 165 (68.75%) knees being in varus alignment (Mean Hip Knee Ankle angle 10.2°) and 75 (31.25%) knees in valgus (Mean 7.9°). (Range 24° varus - 38° valgus).

Of the 240 knees in the study 186 (77.5%) were cementless, 53 (22.0%) were hybrid fixation with a cemented tibial component, and 1 (0.4%) was an all cemented knee. 81% of the patients were overweight or obese (Mean BMI 28.8 kg/m²). Of the 54 cemented tibias, 53 were female and of those 49 had either a neutral or valgus preoperative alignment. A cemented

component was used in the one male patient because a cementless component was unavailable.

Baseline & 10-year outcome measures
When comparing validated outcome scores from pre-operatively to those at 10-year review, a clinically and statistically significant improvement in all outcome measures was observed. Importantly this included patellar scores and pain scores (Table 2).

Radiographic analysis
Standardised post-operative AP and lateral radiographs were analysed using a modified Knee Society TKA Roentgenographic scoring system to determine the presence, width and location of any RLLs [37]. The AP radiograph was taken in approximately seven degrees of flexion to account for tibial resection slope and to ensure a proper view of the tibial-bone interface. The diagram in Fig. 2 shows the modified scoring system with femoral (1–4) and tibial (5–10) zones. Radiographic assessment showed no RLLs in femoral zones (1–4), suggesting excellent femoral component fixation.

Twenty-two tibial RLLs were observed in 12 subjects (12 knees) (see Table 3). Only one cemented tibial component had RLLs observed during the follow-up period (1/54(1.9%)). The total number of cementless tibial components with RLLs observed was 11/186 (5.9%), with RLLs being reported twice in one patient at two different time points and in different zones. The most common locations for RLLs were Zones 5 and 7 of the proximal tibia. No RLLs were progressive.

Two knees with documented RLLs at 3 months post-operatively showed full resolution at 1, 5 and 10-year review. Five knees had RLLs present for the first time at 1-year, and only 1 had RLLs visible at subsequent

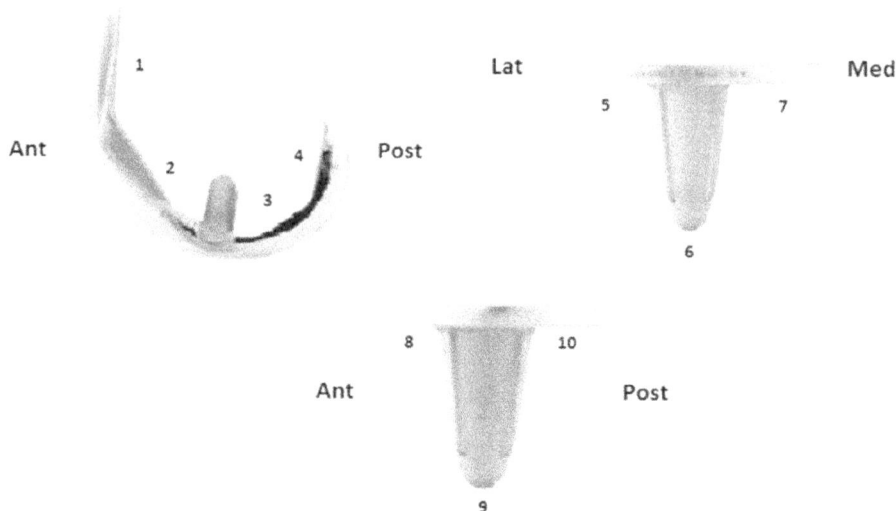

Fig. 2 Modified scoring system with femoral (1–4) and tibial (5–10) zones

Table 1 Demographics of Enrolled Patients

Patients/Knee (n)	237//240
Gender (Patients (%)	
Male	91 (38.4%)
Female	146 (61.6%)
Age at operations (years)	
Mean (years)	70.3
Minimum (years)	39
Maximum (years)	89
Age groups (knees) (%)	
< 50 years	7 (3%)
50–69 years	94 (39%)
70–79 years	110 (46%)
80–89 years	29 (12%)
Body Mass Index (kg/m^2)	
Mean	28.8
Minimum	18
Maximum	45
BMI groups (kg/m^2)	
Underweight (< 18.5)	1 (0.5%)
Normal (18.5–24.9)	45 (19%)
Overweight (25.0–29.9)	103 (43%)
Obese class 1(30.0–34.9)	71 (29.5%)
Obese class 2 (35–39.9)	17 (7%)
Morbidly obese ≥40	3 (1%)
Primary Diagnosis	
Osteoarthritis	226 (94.2%)
Post traumatic Arthritis	1 (0.4%)
Rheumatoid Arthritis	11 (4.6%)
Other	2 (0.8%)

5 or 10-year review and this occurred in a different location (Zone 10). Three knees had RLLs present for the first time at 5-year review, which were no longer apparent at 10-year review. Three knees had RLLs present for first time at 10-year review. There was no statistically significant difference in pain scores between cases with and without RLLs, (approximate t-test p-value of 0.77), suggesting neither pain nor revision was related to the presence of RLLs. Comparing RLL in cemented vs uncemented cases showed no statistical significance (Fisher's exact p-value = 0.308).

Patellofemoral alignment

Pre- and post-operative patellofemoral alignment was measured on Merchant skyline radiographs. Pre-operatively, the patella was centrally aligned in 61.9%, laterally aligned in 26.4%, and medially aligned in 11.7% of patients. At initial postoperative 3 month and final review (120 months) 99.5

and 98.9% of patellae respectively showed central patellar alignment. Patellar tilt was also evaluated on pre- and post-operative skyline radiographs. Preoperatively, 31.6% of patellae lay centrally (neutral tilt), 48.0% had lateral tilt and 20.4% had medial tilt. At the 3-month post-operative review 98.0% had neutral tilt. At 10-year follow-up, all reviewed knees exhibited neutral patellar tilt.

In this study, patients receiving cemented and uncemented tibial components were unmatched cohorts. There was no significant difference in Knee Society Pain Subscore or Knee Society Function Score between cemented and non-cemented knees at 10 years however there were fewer RLLs in the cemented tibial cohort.

Of the 240 knees in the study only 2 cementless implants underwent revision. The first case was a revision for late haematogenous infection at 9.2 years post primary surgery. The second case was for aseptic loosening at 8.3 years after primary surgery. X-rays showed anterior femoral cortical scalloping with osteolysis in femoral zones 1 and 4, and tibial zones 5 and 8. Intra-operatively, the femoral component was loose and only the tibial cone remained well fixed, both components were revised. Interestingly this patient had no RLLs at the time of 5-year review and was revised prior to 10-year review (Figs. 3 and 4). Ten additional patients had further surgery. Nine were early washouts without bearing exchange (6 for infection and 3 for non-infected haematoma) and the tenth was a late (109 months) periprosthetic fracture following a road traffic collision requiring internal fixation. There were no manipulations under anaesthetic, no cases of bearing spinout and no secondary patellar resurfacings [38].

Kaplan-Meier survivorship

The cumulative implant survivorship of the whole series using component revision for any reason as the endpoint was 98.9% (95% CI, 95.6 to 99.7%) at 10 years (Fig. 5). With revision due to infection excluded, cumulative implant survivorship increased to 99.4% (95% CI 96.1 to 99.9%) at 10 years.

Discussion

This paper encompasses three controversial issues within TKA. Firstly, the reported cohort is largely cementless; secondly all were non-posterior stabilized mobile-bearings and thirdly the patella was never resurfaced. The survivorship of this cohort is excellent.

Cementless fixation has the benefits of bone stock preservation, prevention of third body cement wear, and shorter surgical times. [11, 12] However the registry evidence in favour of cemented as opposed to cementless TKA is compelling, with the UK, Swedish, Australian and New Zealand registries all showing superior survivorship with cemented TKA [39–42]. In the 2014 UK

Table 2 Summary of baseline and last review outcome measures

Outcome Measure	Mean Score at Baseline	Mean Score at Final Review (10 years)	Change from Baseline	p-value
Total Knee Score	20.9	91.0	67.21	< 0.0001
Knee Function Scores	37.7	64.8	24.93	< 0.0001
Patella Score	9.6	25.3	15.16	< 0.0001
Oxford Knee Score	10.8	35.7	24.55	< 0.0001
SF-12 Physical Component	26.9	36.1	8.53	< 0.0001
SF-12 Mental Component	42.4	50.0	6.98	< 0.0001
Knee Pain Sub Score	2.8	46.1	43.20	< 0.0001
Range of Movement (Active)	101.4	105.9	3.67	0.0185

(Note- Mean baseline score subtracted from mean final review score does not equal change from baseline due to the reduction in numbers secondary to loss to follow-up at 10-years)

National Joint Registry (NJR) report [39] cementless use fell to 2.5% compared to 6.7% in 2003. Paradoxically in many areas of the world this minimal use of cementless TKA is in stark contrast to that of cementless total hip arthroplasty even though registry data also favours cement for that joint in terms of survivorship [39, 43] and the implants are more expensive.

Level I evidence in favour of cemented TKA is unconvincing. The prospective RCT by Park and Kim [44] has been used in support of cemented TKA [8]. Park and Kim's study [44] reported on 50 patients (100 knees) who had undergone bilateral, simultaneous cruciate retaining knee replacements with one cemented and the other cementless. At a minimum follow-up of 13 years, survival of the femoral components was 100% in both groups and there was one revision for aseptic loosening of a cementless tibial component that had occurred at 1 year. No osteolysis was identified in either group. Baker et al. [45] in their prospective RCT reported no difference in the survivorship of cemented versus uncemented

cruciate retaining knees at a mean follow-up of 9 years. However, cemented TKA demonstrated higher failure rates in younger, heavier men [45]. Our study population had an average BMI of 28.8, but a decade later the average BMI for patients presenting for TKA has risen to 31.8.

A meta-analysis by Gandhi et al. [10] suggested an improved survivorship of cemented as compared to uncemented implants when they looked at 15 studies selected from a total of 1292. Unfortunately, of the 15 studies only 5 were RCTs, with the other 10 being observational. Subgroup analysis of the 5 RCTs showed no survival difference. The authors noted that the patients in the cementless observational studies tended to be younger. In the absence of a clear advantage for either method of fixation the authors concluded that cement offered an economic advantage because of the reduced cost.

For both cemented and uncemented TKAs, aseptic loosening of the tibia is the most common reason for failure [14–16]. Although cement does have advantages

Table 3 Tibial RLL Zones identified during variable review periods

Subject #	Cemented/ Non-Cemented	Follow-up Interval	Tibial Radiolucencies (mm)					
			Zone 5	Zone 6	Zone 7	Zone 8	Zone 9	Zone 10
1–026	Non-cemented	5 years	4					
1–031	Non-cemented	3 months			1			
1–053	Non-cemented	5 years					1	
1–065	Non-cemented	12 months			1	1		
1–075	Non-cemented	5 years					1	
1–157	Non-cemented	12 months	1		1	1		
1–175	Non-cemented	10 years		1				
1–186	Cemented	10 years					1	
1–215*	Non-cemented	12 months	1		1			
1–215*	Non-cemented	10 years					1	
1–228	Non-cemented	3 months	1		1			1
1–232	Non-cemented	12 months	1			1		
1–241	Non-cemented	12 months	1		1	1		

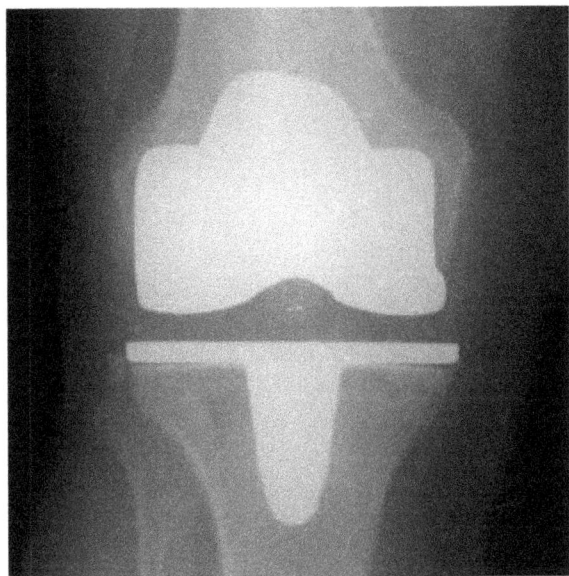

Fig. 3 Example of RLLs in Zones 5 & 7

such as augmenting bony defects or inaccurate bone cuts [46] its weakness and mode of failure is susceptibility to torsional and shear forces [47]. Posterior stabilized designs have higher stresses which hypothetically should impact on survivorship. This hypothesis is supported by results from the 2014 UK NJR [39] where cemented cruciate retaining TKAs have a better survivorship than posterior stabilized. Similarly for cementless fixed bearing (FB) TKAs these torsional and shear stresses could result in aseptic loosening if micromotion is present during early osteointegration [11]. Hypothetically if uncemented implants can survive these early threats to

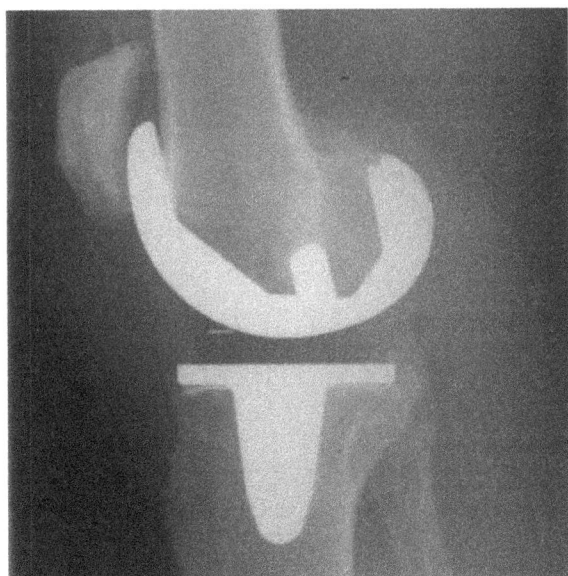

Fig. 4 Example of RLLs in Zone 8

osteointegration by forming a biological bond between bone and prosthesis this could improve long-term survivorship. This hypothesis is supported by a Cochrane review [17], however good results have been reported even with a posterior stabilized cementless TKA [47].

In contrast to the FB TKA the MB, as well as providing low contact stress and low wear [48], also reduces the stresses applied to the implant-bone interface. [3] This should reduce wear induced osteolysis and tibial loosening however these theoretical advantages over FB TKAs have not been confirmed in the literature [4–9] even though MB TKA has shown excellent medium to long-term results in function and survivorship [49, 50].

The reduced shear stress at the implant bone interface in cementless MB TKA should facilitate early osteointegration and may contribute to the survivorship in this study. One manifestation of failure of bony ingrowth is fibrous ingrowth presenting as a progressive RLL. A recognised concern with cementless porous coated tibial trays is the appearance and interpretation of RLLs. In a patient with unexplained pain this can lead to inappropriate revision. Two types of RLL have been described, physiological or pathological [51]. Physiological lines are usually < 2 mm with a sclerotic margin, and pathological lines are thicker, with a poorly defined border, and are usually progressive [52]. In this series only 1/54 cemented tibial components exhibited RLLs compared with 12/186 of the cementless tibias. Similar lines have undoubtedly resulted in unnecessary revision. We believe lines < 1 mm represent non-pathological fibro-osseous integration which is stable and non-progressive.

Paradoxically the cemented Oxford Uni-compartmental MB knee also suffers from inappropriate revisions due to the presence of lines below the tibial tray [53], but these are infrequent with the cementless HA coated version of the tibial tray [54].

The requirement for patellar resurfacing remains contentious and contradictory [19, 21, 23]. The geometry of the different femoral components observed between knee systems may play a role in this inconsistency [19–22]. In both resurfaced and non-resurfaced patellae, contact stresses within the trochlear sulcus are dictated by the component design [24]. With posterior stabilized designs traditionally having more patellofemoral problems [55]. The LCS system exhibits a common radius of curvature similar to that found in the native knee which allows it to accommodate the unresurfaced patella favorably [56]. However, the posterior stabilized LCS Complete was removed from the Australian market following higher than expected revision when the patella was not resurfaced [57]. With the benefits of patellar resurfacing unresolved within the literature, it is important to consider the associated risks of patellar fracture, avascular necrosis, implant loosening and instability

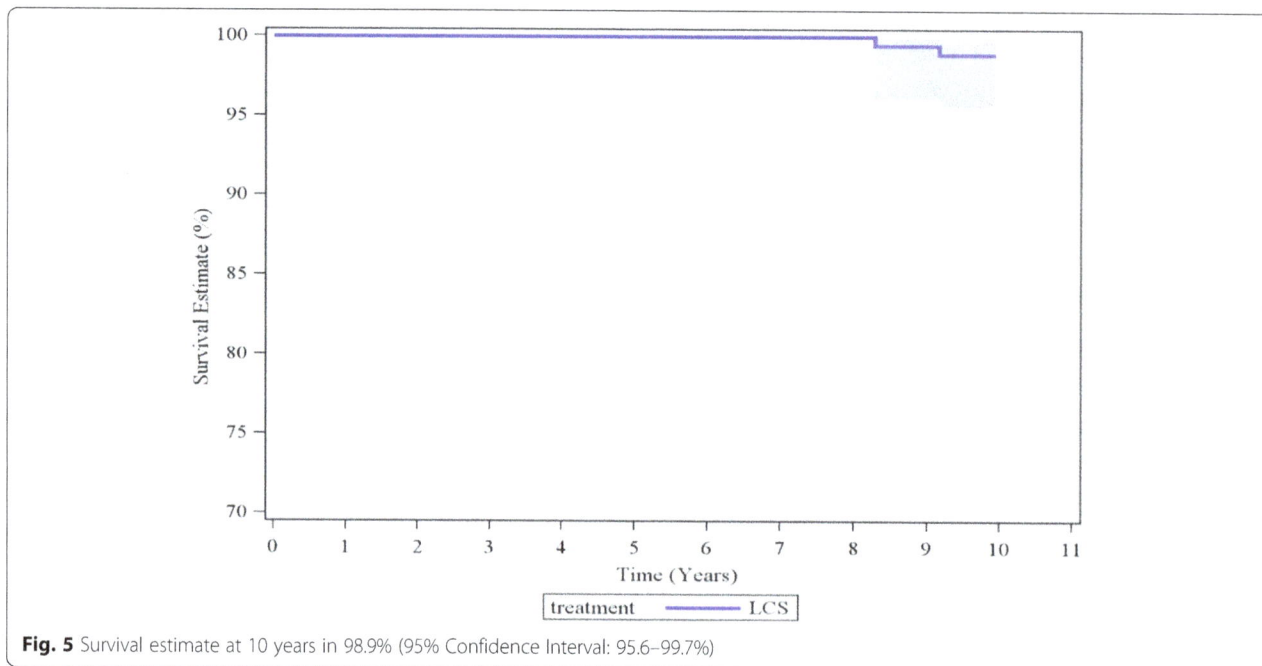

Fig. 5 Survival estimate at 10 years in 98.9% (95% Confidence Interval: 95.6–99.7%)

[27]. Intraoperatively, and irrespective of implant choice or decision to resurface, it is critical to achieve central patellofemoral tracking. Persistent anterior knee pain after TKA is common with and without patellar resurfacing [58, 59] and secondary resurfacing can be of questionable clinical value [18, 60].

Weaknesses of this study include the use of a number of cemented tibial components. Recruitment for this study had been on consecutive patients and the senior author's practice at the commencement of the study was to use hybrid fixation with a cemented tibia in females with valgus deformities due to perceived concerns about tibial insufficiency fractures [31]. Since the conclusion of this study, this practice has changed, with uncemented tibial components being implanted in all cases irrespective of age, gender, or deformity. We previously reported a series of 275 consecutive valgus knees with a pre-operative deformity of ≥10° which was completed after this study. Eighty three percent were female and of those 70% were cementless. At between 5.8 and 10.5 years follow-up, there has been only one revision, which was in a cemented tibia [31]. A further limitation was patients lost to follow-up being high. There were 84 subjects who had withdrawn from the study at the end of 10-years, 83% of these were deceased.

Conclusion

In terms of survivorship this study supports the use of non-cemented porous coated fixation without patellar resurfacing using a non-posterior stabilized mobile bearing TKA. It exhibits excellent survivorship at a minimum 10-year follow-up with the expectation that longer-term follow-up may be superior to cemented TKA. We believe lines < 1 mm represent non-pathological fibro-osseous integration which is stable and non-progressive. In the absence of definitive level-1 evidence the only clear advantage for cemented TKA is cost.

Abbreviations
AKSS: American Knee Society Scores; AP: Antero-posterior; BPS: Bartlett Patellar Scores; FB: Fixed Bearing; IRB : Institutional Review Board; MB: Mobile bearing; NJR: National Joint Registry; OKS: Oxford knee scores; RLLs: Radiolucent lines; SF-12 : 12 item Short Form Health Survey; TKA: Total Knee Arthroplasty

Authors' contributions
RJ Napier (Manuscript preparation/ Literature review/Radiographic Analysis). CO'N (Manuscript preparation/ Radiographic Analysis). SO'B (Data collection, patient assessment at follow-up). ED (Data collection, patient assessment at follow-up). BM (Data collection, patient assessment at follow-up). J B (Radiographic Analysis). DEB (Study design and implimentation, Manuscript preparation). All authors have read and approved this manuscript.

Consent for publication
Not applicable

Competing interests
The authors declare that they have no competing interests.

Author details
[1]Orthopaedic Outcomes Assessment Unit, Musgrave Park Hospital, Stockman's Lane, Belfast BT9 7JB, Northern Ireland. [2]Akutklinik Siloah, Worbstrasse 324, CH 3073 Guemligen, Switzerland.

References

1. Goodfellow JW, O'Connor J. The mechanics of the knee and prosthesis design. J Bone Joint Surg (Br). 1978;60B(3):358–68.

2. Buechel FF, Pappas MJ. The New Jersey low contact stress knee replacement system: biomechanical rationale and review of the first 123 cemented cases. Arch Orthop and Traumatic Surg. 1986;105:197–204.

3. Callaghan JJ, Insall JN, Greenwald AS, Dennis DA, Komistek RD, Murray DW, Bourne RB, Rorabeck CH, Dorr LD. Mobile-bearing knee replacement-concept and results. J Bone Joint Surg Am. 2000;82(7):1020.

4. Aglietti P, Baldini A, Buzzi R, Lup D, De Luca L. Comparison of mobile-bearing and fixed-bearing total knee arthroplasty: a prospective randomized study. J Arthroplasty. 2005;20(2):145–53.

5. Smith H, Jan M, Mahomed NN, Davey JR, Gandhi R. Meta-analysis and systematic review of clinical outcomes comparing mobile bearing and fixed bearing total knee arthroplasty. J Arthroplast. 2011;26(8):1205–13.

6. Kim YH, Kim JS, Choe JW, Kim HJ. Long-term comparison of fixed-bearing and mobile-bearing total knee replacements in patients younger than fifty-one years of age with osteoarthritis. J Bone Joint Surg Am. 2012;94(10):866–73.

7. Hofstede SN, Nouta KA, Jacobs W, van Hooff ML, Wymenga AB, Pijls BG, et al. Mobile bearing vs fixed bearing prostheses for posterior cruciate retaining total knee arthroplasty for postoperative functional status in patients with osteoarthritis and rheumatoid arthritis. Cochrane Database Syst Rev. 2015;2:CD003130.

8. Ranawat CS, Meftah M, Windsor EN, Ranawat AS. Cementless fixation in total knee arthroplasty: down the boulevard of broken dreams - affirms. J Bone Joint Surg Br. 2012;94(11 Suppl A):82–4.

9. Moskal JT, Capps SG. Rotating-platform TKA no different from fixed-bearing TKA regarding survivorship or performance: a meta-analysis. Clin Orthop Relat Res. 2014;472(7):2185–93.

10. Gandhi R, Tsvetkov D, Davey JR, Mahomed NN. Survival and clinical function of cemented and uncemented prostheses in total knee replacement: a meta-analysis. J Bone Joint Surg Br. 2009;91(7):889–95.

11. Drexler M, Dwyer T, Marmor M, Abolghasemian M, Sternheim A, Cameron HU. Cementless fixation in total knee arthroplasty: down the boulevard of broken dreams - opposes. J Bone Joint Surg Br. 2012; 94(11 Suppl A):85–9.

12. Yang JH, Yoon JR, Oh CH, Kim TS. Hybrid component fixation in total knee arthroplasty: minimum of 10-year follow-up study. J Arthroplast. 2012;27(6):1111–8.

13. Sharkey PF, Lichstein PM, Shen C, Tokarski AT, Parvizi J. Why are total knee arthroplasties failing today–has anything changed after 10 years? J Arthroplast. 2014;29(9):1774–8.

14. Sharkey PF, Hozack WJ, Rothman RH, Shastri S, Jacoby SM. Why are total knee arthroplasties failing today? Clin Orthop. 2002;404:7–13.

15. Gioe TJ, Killeen K, Grimm K, Mehle S, Scheltema K. Why are total knee replacements revised?: analysis of early revision in a community knee implant registry. Clin Orthop. 2004;428:100–6.

16. Fehring TK, Odum S, Griffin WL, Mason JB, Nadaud M. Early failures in total knee arthroplasty. Clin Orthop. 2001;392:315–8.

17. Nakama GY, Peccin MS, Almeida GJ, Lira Neto Ode A, Queiroz AA, Navarro RD. Cemented, cementless or hybrid fixation options in total knee arthroplasty for osteoarthritis and other non-traumatic diseases. Cochrane Database Syst Rev. 2012;10:CD006193.

18. O'Brien S, Spence DJ, Ogonda LO, Beverland DE. LCS mobile bearing total knee arthroplasty without patellar resurfacing. Does the unresurfaced patella affect outcome? Survivorship at a minimum 10-year follow-up. Knee. 2012; 19(4):335–8.

19. Waters TS, Bentley G. Patellar resurfacing in total knee arthroplasty: a prospective randomized study. J Bone Joint Surg Am. 2003;85(2):212–7.

20. Barrack RL, Wolfe MW, Waldman DA, Milicic M, Bertot AJ, Myers L. Resurfacing of the patella in total knee arthroplasty. A prospective randomized double-blind study. J Bone Joint Surg Am. 1997;79:1121–31.

21. Wood DJ, Smith AJ, Collopy D, White B, Brankov B, Bulsara MK. Patellar resurfacing in total knee arthroplasty: a prospective randomized study. J Bone Joint Surg Am. 2002;84(2):187 93.

22. Burnett RS, Haydon CM, Rorabeck CH, Bourne RB. Patella resurfacing versus non-resurfacing in total knee arthroplasty. Clin Orthop Relat Res. 2004;428:12–25.

23. Smith AJ, Wood DJ, Li MG. Total knee replacement with and without patellar resurfacing: a prospective randomised trial using the Profix total knee system. J Bone Joint Surg (Br). 2008;90(1):43–9.

24. Matsuda S, Ishinishi T, Whiteside LA. Contact stresses with an unresurfaced

patella in total knee arthroplasty. The effect of femoral component design. Orthopedics. 2000;23:213–8.

25. Chew JT, Stewart NJ, Hanssen AD, Luo ZP, Rand JA, An KN. Differences in patellar tracking and knee kinematics among three different total knee designs. Clin Orthop Relat Res. 1997;345:87–98.

26. Benjamin JB, Szivek JA, Hammond AS, Kubchandhani Z, Matthews Al Jr, Anderson P. Contact areas and pressures between native patellas and prosthetic femoral components. J Arthroplast. 1998;13:693–8.

27. He JY, Jiang LS, Dai LY. Is patellar resurfacing superior than nonresurfacing in total knee arthroplasty? A meta-analysis of randomized trials. Knee. 2011; 18(3):137–44.

28. Thompson NW, Ruiz AL, Breslin E, Beverland DE. Total knee arthroplasty without patellar resurfacing in isolated patellofemoral osteoarthritis. J Arthroplast. 2001;16(5):607–12.

29. Hamelynck KJ, Stiehl JB. Alternative technique of conservative distal femoral cut first. LCS mobile bearing knee arthroplasty 25 years of world wide experience. Revision total knee arthroplasty. New York: Springer; 2002. p. 183-94.

30. Thompson NW, McAlinden MG, Breslin E, Crone MD, Kernohan WG, Beverland DE. Periprosthetic tibial fractures after cementless low contact stress total knee arthroplasty. J Arthroplast. 2001;16(8):984–90.

31. Pagoti R, O'Brien S, Doran E, Beverland D. Unconstrained total knee arthroplasty in significant valgus deformity: a modified surgical technique to balance the knee and avoid instability. Knee Surg Sports Traumatol Arthrosc. 2017;25(9):2825-34.

32. Sperner G, Wantschek P, Benedetto KP, Glotzer W. Spatergebnisse bei Patellafrakturen. Akt Traumatol. 1990;20:24.

33. Napier RJ, Bennett D, McConway J, Wilson R, Sykes AM, Doran E, O'Brien S, Beverland DE. The influence of immediate knee flexion on blood loss and other parameters following total knee arthroplasty. BJJ. 2014;96-B(2):201–9.

34. Cusick LA, Beverland DE. The incidence of fatal pulmonary embolism after primary hip and knee replacement in a consecutive series of 4253 patients. J Bone Joint Surg Br. 2009;91(5):645–8.

35. Ogonda L, Hill J, Doran E, Dennison J, Stevenson M, Beverland D. Aspirin for thromboprophylaxis following primary lower limb arthroplasty: early thromboembolic events and 90-day mortality in 11 459 patients. Bone Joint J. 2016;98-B:341–8.

36. Arthroplasty Care Practitioners. Available at: http://www.acpa-uk.net. Accessed 27 Apr 2016.

37. Ewald FC. The knee society total knee arthroplasty roentgenographic evaluation and scoring system. Clin Orthop Relat Res. 1989;248:9–12.

38. Thompson NW, Wilson DS, Cran GW, Beverland DE, Stiehl JB. Dislocation of the rotating platform after low contact stress total knee arthroplasty. Clin Orthop Relat Res. 2004;425:207–11.

39. No authors listed. National Joint Registry for England and Wales: 12th Annual report, 2014. http://www.njrcentre.org.uk.

40. No authors listed. Australian Orthopaedic Association national joint replacement registry. Annual Report 2015. https://aoanjrr.sahmri.com.

41. No authors listed. The Swedish Knee Arthroplasty Register: annual report, 2014. http://myknee.se/pdf/SKAR2014_Eng_1.1.pdf.

42. Rothwell A, Hobbs T, Frampton C. New Zealand Orthopaedic association: New Zealand joint registry: 16th year report January 1999 to December 2014. 2015. http://www.nzoa.org.nz/system/files/Web_DH7657_NZJR2014Report_v4_12Nov15.pdf.

43. Hailer NP, Garellick G, Kärrholm J. Uncemented and cemented primary total hip arthroplasty in the Swedish hip arthroplasty register. Acta Orthop. 2010; 81(1):34–41.

44. Park JW, Kim YH. Simultaneous cemented and cementless total knee replacement in the same patients: a prospective comparison of long-term outcomes using an identical design of NexGen prosthesis. J Bone Joint Surg [Br]. 2011;93-B:1479–86.

45. Baker PN, Khaw FM, Kirk LM, Esler CN, Gregg PJ. A randomised controlled trial of cemented versus cementless press-fit condylar total knee replacement: 15-year survival analysis. J Bone Joint Surg [Br]. 2007;89-B:1608–14.

46. Lombardi AV Jr, Berasi CC, Berend KR. Evolution of tibial fixation in total knee arthroplasty. J Arthroplast. 2007;22(4 Suppl 1):25–9.

47. Harwin SF, Kester MA, Malkani AL, Manley MT. Excellent fixation achieved with cementless posteriorly stabilized total knee arthroplasty. J Arthroplast. 2013;28(1):7–13.

48. McEwen HM, Fisher J, Goldsmith AA, Auger DD, Hardaker C, Stone MH. Wear of fixed bearing and rotating platform mobile bearing knees

subjected to high levels of internal and external tibial rotation. J Mater Sci Mater Med. 2001;12(10–12):1049–52.

49. Hopley CD, Crossett LS, Chen AF. Long-term clinical outcomes and survivorship after total knee arthroplasty using a rotating platform knee prosthesis: a meta-analysis. J Arthroplasty. 2013;28(1):68–77. e1–3

50. Carothers JT, Kim RH, Dennis DA, Southworth C. Mobile-bearing total knee arthroplasty: a meta-analysis. J Arthroplasty. 2011;26(4):537–42.

51. Tibrewal SB, Grant KA, Goodfellow JW. The radiolucent line beneath the tibial components of the Oxford meniscal knee. J Bone Joint Surg Br. 1984; 66(4):523e8.

52. Mukherjee K, Pandit H, Dodd CA, Ostlere S, Murray DW. The Oxford unicompartmental knee arthroplasty: a radiological perspective. Clin Radiol. 2008;63(10):1169–76.

53. Gulati A, Chau R, Pandit HG, et al. The incidence of physiological radiolucency following Oxford unicompartmental knee replacement and its relationship to outcome. J Bone Joint Surg (Br). 2009;91-B:896–902.

54. Liddle AD, et al. Cementless fixation in Oxford unicompartmental knee replacement - a multicentre study of 1000 knees. BJJ. 2013;95-B(2):181–7.

55. Hozack WJ, Rothman RH, Booth RE Jr, Balderston RA. The patellar clunk syndrome. A complication of posterior stabilized total knee arthroplasty. Clin Orthop Relat Res. 1989;241:203–8.

56. Ma HM, Lu YC, Kwok TG, Ho FY, Huang CY, Huang CH. The effect of the design of the femoral component on the conformity of the patellofemoral joint in total knee replacement. J Bone Joint Surg (Br). 2007;89(3):408–12.

57. Medical Devices safety update. DEVICE CORRECTION NOTICE for the LCS COMPLETE™ RPS Knee System. Australian Orthopaedic Association national joint replacement registry. Annual Report 2015. https://www.tga.gov.au/alert/lcs-complete-rps-knee-system-used-knee-replacements.

58. Pilling RW, Moulder E, Allgar V, Messner J, Sun Z, Mohsen A. Patellar resurfacing in primary total knee replacement: a meta-analysis. J Bone Joint Surg Am. 2012;94(24):2270–8.

59. Feng B, Weng X, Lin J, Jin J, Qian W, Wang W, Qiu G. Long term follow up of clinical outcome between patellar resurfacing and nonresurfacing in total knee arthroplasty: Chinese experience. Chin Med J. 2014;127(22):3845–51.

60. Mockford BJ, Beverland DE. Secondary resurfacing of the patella in mobile-bearing total knee arthroplasty. J Arthroplast. 2005;20(7):898–902.

11

Revisiting patient satisfaction following total knee arthroplasty

Stirling Bryan[1,2]* ⓘ, Laurie J. Goldsmith[1,3], Jennifer C. Davis[1,4], Samar Hejazi[5], Valerie MacDonald[6], Patrick McAllister[7], Ellen Randall[1,2], Nitya Suryaprakash[1], Amery D. Wu[8] and Richard Sawatzky[9,10]

Abstract

Background: Total knee arthroplasty (TKA) is the most common joint replacement surgery in Canada. Earlier Canadian work reported 1 in 5 TKA patients expressing dissatisfaction following surgery. A better understanding of satisfaction could guide program improvement. We investigated patient satisfaction post-TKA in British Columbia (BC).

Methods: A cohort of 515 adult TKA patients was recruited from across BC. Survey data were collected preoperatively and at 6 and 12 months, supplemented by administrative health data. The primary outcome measure was patient satisfaction with outcomes. Potential satisfaction drivers included demographics, patient-reported health, quality of life, social support, comorbidities, and insurance status. Multivariable growth modeling was used to predict satisfaction at 6 months and change in satisfaction (6 to 12 months).

Results: We found dissatisfaction rates ("very dissatisfied", "dissatisfied" or "neutral") of 15% (6 months) and 16% (12 months). Across all health measures, improvements were seen post-surgery. The multivariable model suggests satisfaction at 6 months is predicted by: pre-operative pain, mental health and physical health (odds ratios (ORs) 2.65, 3.25 and 3.16), and change in pain level, baseline to 6 months (OR 2.31). Also, improvements in pain, mental health and physical health from 6 to 12 months predicted improvements in satisfaction (ORs 1.24, 1.30 and 1.55).

Conclusions: TKA is an effective intervention for many patients and most report high levels of satisfaction. However, if the TKA does not deliver improvements in pain and physical health, we see a less satisfied patient. In addition, dissatisfied TKA patients typically see limited improvements in mental health.

Keywords: Total knee arthroplasty, Patient satisfaction, Longitudinal observational study, Survey research

Background

Total knee arthroplasty (TKA) is the most commonly performed joint replacement surgery in Canada where there were over 67,000 TKAs in 2016/17 [1]. TKA is typically performed on people with osteoarthritis, the prevalence of which increases with age, and so demand for TKA can be expected to continue to rise given population demographic trends [2–4]. Through 2015/16, Canada saw a 5-year increase in TKA procedures of 16%

[1]. A commonly cited and troubling statistic is that approximately 1 in 5 TKA patients express some dissatisfaction with their outcomes following surgery [5, 6]. The concern is magnified when placed in the contemporary context of health system commitments to patient-centred care, with consideration of traditionally ignored outcomes such as patient satisfaction and quality of life [7, 8]. Using a patient-centred lens, a dissatisfied TKA patient has not had a successful surgery, and a rate of 20% dissatisfied patients points to a need for improvement. A better understanding of patient satisfaction drivers could guide program improvement initiatives.

Previous studies have explored the relationship between post-TKA patient satisfaction and various combinations of

* Correspondence: stirling.bryan@ubc.ca
[1]Centre for Clinical Epidemiology & Evaluation, Vancouver Coastal Health Research Institute, West 10th Avenue, Vancouver, BC V5Z 1M9, Canada
[2]School of Population & Public Health, University of British Columbia, 2206 E Mall, Vancouver, BC V6T 1Z3, Canada
Full list of author information is available at the end of the article

pre- and post-surgery clinical and patient-reported mea-sures. Factors found to be related to patient dissatisfaction across multiple studies include: knee-related factors (e.g., pain, functioning, stiffness and inflammation), self-rated factors (e.g., physical and mental health status, and quality of life), pre-surgery expectations not met, complications, pain catastrophizing, and patient demographics (e.g., age, gender and employment status) [5, 9–19]. The existing lit-erature typically reports analyses of post-TKA patient sat-isfaction at a single time, even if repeated measurements (most commonly at 6- and 12-months) were made, and so contributes very little to understanding changes in satis-faction over time [20–23]. For example, are the concerns of patients in the early post-operative period different from those dealing with longer-term dissatisfaction? That requires a longitudinal analysis which simultaneously ad-justs for correlations between repeated measures [24].

The longitudinal observational study reported in this paper was designed to understand patient satisfaction with TKA at 6 and 12-months post-surgery, as well as changes in satisfaction over time. The paper reports the quantitative work from a multiphase, longitudinal, mixed methods study investigating patient satisfaction follow-ing TKA surgery [25]. Using a patient-centred perspec-tive, we investigated patient satisfaction rates post-TKA in British Columbia (BC), with exploration of the pri-mary drivers of variation in the level of, and change in, patient satisfaction following TKA.

Methods
Setting, sample and data collection
A cohort of 515 patients was recruited from six hospital sites spanning all regional health authorities in BC. Con-secutive patients (aged 19 years or older) with a primary or secondary diagnosis of osteoarthritis, and scheduled to undergo primary TKA at one of the six sites, were in-vited to participate during mandatory pre-surgical total joint replacement education sessions. Patients scheduled to undergo revision surgery, bilateral knee replacement, unicompartmental knee replacement, or TKA due to an accident were excluded. The participation rate was 57% (515/808) out of all invited patients. Approval was ob-tained from research ethics boards of all health author-ities and universities in the study.

Much of the study data were collected using a pre-operative survey questionnaire (administered up to 3 months before surgery) and two post-operative survey questionnaires (at 6 and 12 months post-surgery). The questionnaires were self-administered in English, with family members or caregivers serving as translators for non-English speaking patients. All non-respondents re-ceived reminders. Retention rates were 91% (466/515) and 88% (455/515) at 6 and 12 months, respectively. In

addition, health administrative data were obtained from medical records of consenting patients (93%, 479/515).

Measurements and outcomes
The primary outcome measure was patient satisfaction with the results of their knee surgery, collected at 6 and 12 months. These intervals were chosen to mirror previous work in TKA [5], and endorsed by clinical experts on our team. Participants were asked to re-spond to a single-item measuring satisfaction with the outcomes of knee surgery based on a 5-point Likert rating (varying from "very satisfied" through "very dis-satisfied"), which was previously used in a large Can-adian cohort study of knee arthroplasty outcomes [4]. For analysis purposes, the primary satisfaction out-come variable was collapsed into a binary variable with values 0 ("very satisfied" or "satisfied") and 1 ("very dissatisfied", "dissatisfied" or "neutral").

Potential patient-centred drivers of satisfaction ex-plored in our analyses, based on the literature review, in-cluded demographic variables, patient-reported health status (SF-12 [26], EQ-5D-5 L [27], WOMAC [28], SLANSS [29]), depression and anxiety (HADS [30]), so-cial support (MOS-SSS [31]), patient expectations, co-morbidities (Charlson [32]), health insurance, and global quality of life (Cantril [33]). All selected instruments have been used previously in TKA patients, with strong evidence for their validity [26–33].

In addition to patient-reported measures, administra-tive data were extracted from in-patient medical records to measure hospital length of stay during the surgical period, complications following surgery, re-admissions and presence of co-morbidity during the inpatient stay. The patient's postal code information was used to classify rural/urban residence and to measure distances from the patient's home to the hospital where they had their TKA surgery, and the nearest hospital where TKA is offered.

Analyses
Multivariable growth modeling was conducted using the M*Plus* software (version 7.4) [34] to predict individual differences in satisfaction at 6 months (intercepts) and change (slopes) in satisfaction from 6 to 12 months [35, 36]. The model was specified as a logistic regression, with satisfaction as a binary variable and random effects for the intercepts and slopes. Accordingly, the results are presented as odds ratios (ORs) pertaining to the in-tercepts and slopes associated with the independent vari-ables. To minimize collinearity issues resulting from high correlations over time, the time-varying predictor variables were represented as pre-surgery scores, the change from pre-surgery to 6 months post-surgery, and the change from 6 to 12 months post-surgery. All continuous

predictor variables were rescaled to vary from 0 to 10 to enhance interpretability and comparisons for the odds ratios. Full information maximum likelihood estimation was applied to accommodate for missing data.

The model was built sequentially where the selection of variables was informed by prior studies, findings from our qualitative analysis [37], and emerging statistical results, including changes in overall model fit and parameter estimates [38, 39]. First, the patient-reported outcome variables (WOMAC subscales, SF-12 mental and physical health component scores, the EQ-5D valuation score) were examined. To avoid multicollinearity, variable selection at this step was guided by identifying a set of variables that were correlated with satisfaction and least correlated with one another. Second, demographic variables (age, sex, health region, marital status, education, ethnicity, and urban versus rural) were entered into the model. The third and final step involved examining other health-related predictors, including neuropathic pain (SLANSS), depression and anxiety (HADS), social support (MOS SSS), comorbidities (Charlson), health insurance, and global quality of life (Cantril). At each of steps 2 and 3, all variables were first entered simultaneously and the models were subsequently trimmed by sequentially removing variables that were not statistically significant predictors ($p < .05$) while monitoring the impact on overall model fit, based on the Bayesian Information Criterion (BIC), and changes in parameter estimates.

Results

The characteristics of the patient cohort at the time of recruitment into the study are reported in Table 1. The cohort had a mean age of 66 years, was predominantly female (61%), over one-quarter was still working and over half waited longer than 12 months for surgery. Almost one-third of patients had no supplementary health insurance to cover the costs of additional health care services such as privately-financed physiotherapy over and above the standard series of publicly provided physiotherapy.

Table 2 reports the results of the primary outcome variable, satisfaction with outcomes (at both 6 and 12 months post-surgery). Our data indicate an overall dissatisfaction rate ("very dissatisfied", "dissatisfied" or "neutral") of 15% at 6 months and 16% at 12 months post-surgery. The vast majority of participants (78%) were satisfied or very satisfied with their outcomes at both time points, and 8% indicating some level of dissatisfaction (or neutrality) at both time points.

Self-reported patient health outcomes over time are reported in Table 3. Our data point to major improvements in patient health post-surgery; a finding seen across all outcome instruments. The improvement is most clearly seen from baseline to 6 months, with very

Table 1 Time Invariant Variables at Baseline

Variable	Mean (SD) / Frequency (%)
Age in years ($n = 515$)	66.5 (9.0)
Sex ($n = 511$)	
Male	200 (39)
Female	311 (61)
Marital Status ($n = 509$)	
Married or Common law	353 (69)
Widowed	54 (11)
Separated or Divorced or Single	102 (20)
Working Status ($n = 510$)	
No	375 (74)
Yes	135 (26)
Annual Household Income ($n = 471$)	
< $40 k	168 (36)
$40 k - $60 k	122 (26)
$60 k - $80 k	60 (13)
> $80 k	121 (26)
Education ($n = 464$)	
< High school	72 (16)
High school	144 (31)
College/Technical	136 (29)
University degree undergraduate	112 (24)
Other	37 (8)
Ethnicity ($n = 505$)	
North American	309 (61)
European	134 (27)
South Asian Indian Pakistani Bangladesh	29 (6)
Pacific Asian Chinese Japanese Korean	17 (3)
Other	16 (3)
Supplementary insurance ($n = 459$)	
No	148 (32)
Yes	311 (68)
Expected pain 3 months after surgery ($n = 502$)	
Not at all painful	150 (30)
Slightly painful	238 (47)
Moderately painful	101 (20)
Very painful	13 (3)
Expected limitation in usual activity 3 months after surgery ($n = 501$)	
Not at all limited	124 (25)
Slightly limited	246 (49)
Moderately limited	117 (23)
Very limited	14 (3)
Urban or rural ($n = 497$)	
Urban	445 (86)
Rural	52 (10)

Table 2 Distribution of satisfaction with outcomes at 6 and 12 months

Satisfaction at 6 months	Satisfaction at 12 months					Missing	Total
	Very dissatisfied	Dissatisfied	Neutral	Satisfied	Very satisfied		
Very dissatisfied	2	0	0	1	4	3	10
Dissatisfied	4	3	4	5	1	0	17
Neutral	1	9	11	13	2	7	43
Satisfied	0	8	16	85	37	9	155
Very satisfied	7	0	2	39	176	14	238
Missing	1	0	4	5	11	31	52
Total	15	20	37	148	231	64	515

little further improvement beyond 6 months. Improvements were seen in quality of life, pain, physical function and mental health.

The final multivariable model predictors of satisfaction are shown in Table 4. This represents the best fitting and most parsimonious model predicting satisfaction and change in satisfaction scores. The multilevel multivariable regression results suggest that self-reported pre-operative pain, based on the WOMAC, as well as the difference in pain at 6 months were predictive of satisfaction at 6 months. In addition, pre-operative mental and physical health are both predictive of satisfaction at 6 months (ORs 3.25 and 3.16, respectively). Change in pain from 0 to 6 months was also predictive of satisfaction at 6 months (OR = 2.31). However, changes in mental and physical health from 0 to 6 months were not. Further, a change in any of the three variables (pain, mental health and physical health) from 6 to 12 months was predictive of a change in satisfaction; people experiencing improved pain, mental health or physical health were more likely also to experience

improved satisfaction from 6 to 12 months (ORs 1.30, 1.55 and 1.24, respectively).

Different combinations of the core patient-reported outcome variables (including the SF-36 component scores, the WOMAC subscales, and EQ-5D) were explored, but none resulted in additional statistically significant parameter estimates and improved model fit (based on the BIC). The addition of individual time-invariant variables (marital status, age, gender, comorbidity, and having additional health insurance) also did not result in any improvement in model fit, regardless of whether the variables were entered individually or in combination with one or more other time-invariant variables. Model fit was also not improved by any of the other patient-reported outcome variables (global quality of life, neuropathic pain, anxiety, depression and social support) when entered into the model as pre-operative scores and their difference scores at 6 and 12 months.

In summary, a key driver of patient satisfaction post-surgery is pain (both pre-surgery and the change in pain levels over time). The other factors associated with patient satisfaction post-surgery are both physical health

Table 3 Time varying variables

Instrument	Component	Mean (SD)		
		Baseline (n = 515)	6 months (n = 463)	12 months (n = 451)
EQ-5D	Visual Analogue Scale (0–100; higher score is better)	69.2 (17.7)	78.3 (15)	78.2 (14.5)
EQ-5D utility	Utility score (−0.148 to 1; higher positive score is better)	0.59 (0.21)	0.82 (0.14)	0.82 (0.14)
SF-12	Physical Composite Scale (PCS) Score (0–100; higher score is better)	34.3 (7.5)	43.2 (12.6)	44.9 (9.2)
	Mental Health Composite Scale (MCS) Score (0–100; higher score is better)	51.6 (10.7)	54.0 (8.8)	54.0 (8.7)
WOMAC	Pain (0–20; higher score, more pain)	10.1 (3.6)	3.4 (3.0)	2.9 (3.2)
	Stiffness (0–8; higher score, more stiffness)	4.2 (1.7)	2.1 (1.6)	1.7 (1.5)
	Physical Function (0–68; higher score, more limitations)	33.8 (11.9)	13.2 (11.2)	12.4 (11.5)
HADS	Anxiety (0–21; higher score, more anxiety)	5.6 (3.9)	4.0 (3.4)	4.1 (3.6)
	Depression (0–21; higher score, more depression)	4.8 (3.3)	3.1 (3.2)	3.3 (3.1)
SLANSS	Neuropathic pain (0–24; score > =12, pain of neuropathic origin)	7.0 (6.6)	6.4 (6.9)	5.7 (6.4)

Table 4 Final multivariable model results

Variable	Time	Estimate	SE	p	OR[1] (95%CI)
Predictors of the intercept					
SF-MCS	1	0.118	0.034	0.001	3.25 (1.67–6.34)*
	2–1	0.01	0.026	0.686	1.11 (0.66–1.84)
SF-PCS	1	0.115	0.038	0.002	3.16 (1.50–6.65)*
	2–1	0.026	0.036	0.473	1.30 (0.64–2.63)
WOMAC PAIN[2]	1	0.418	0.111	< 0.001	2.65 (1.76–4.01)*
	2–1	0.488	0.105	< 0.001	2.31 (1.49–3.56)*
Predictors of the slope					
SF-MCS	3–2	0.026	0.011	0.014	1.30 (1.05–1.61)*
SF-PCS	3–2	0.044	0.016	0.005	1.55 (1.13–2.12)*
WOMAC PAIN[2]	3–2	0.109	0.034	0.001	1.24 (1.09–1.42)*
Correlation intercept and slope		−1.161	2.184	0.595	
slope (mean)		−0.334	0.433	0.441	
intercept (threshold)		2.244	2.384	0.346	
Residual variance: intercept		8.851	9.003	0.326	
Residual variance: slope		0.159	0.417	0.703	

Notes Time 1 is baseline, Time 2 is 6 months, and Time 3 is 12 months. *Log likelihood* – 227.67, *BIC* 548.03, [1]*OR* odds ratio pertaining to a 10% difference in scores of the continuous independent variables comparing the odds of being in a higher satisfaction category relative to a lower satisfaction category. [2]Reverse-scored, such that higher score indicates less pain

(over and above pain) and mental health. Many other factors were found not to have an association with patient satisfaction, notably socio-demographic characteristics of patients, patient expectations and level of support.

Discussion

Summary of main findings
Our data indicate that TKA is an effective intervention for many recipients, with major gains in health-related quality of life reported by those who receive the procedure. Further, most patients report high levels of satisfaction post-surgery: we found an overall dissatisfaction rate among Canadian TKA patients of approximately 16% at 12 months post-surgery. Although this dissatisfaction rate, in aggregate, remains stable from 6 to 12 months post-surgery, we do see movement over time; some patients indicating increasing dissatisfaction and others moving in the opposite direction. When looking to understand factors associated with patient satisfaction, the longitudinal nature of our data and analyses allow us to tease out the impact of pre-surgery measurements and changes over time. Our results indicate three key satisfaction drivers: pain, physical health and mental health. Pre-surgery levels of all three variables were found to be important predictors of satisfaction at 6 months; and changes in the levels of all three (from 6 to 12 months post-surgery) were strongly associated with changes in satisfaction. In summary, if the TKA procedure has positive impacts on a patient's pain levels and

overall physical health, we are likely to see a satisfied patient. However, and more surprisingly, we also see that satisfied TKA patients are also likely to have seen some improvements in relation to mental health too.

Comparison with previous work
Our study resembles others in finding knee pain to be a key predictor of post-TKA satisfaction [13, 16, 40, 41]. This common finding holds for both pre-surgical pain and post-surgery pain improvement. Our study also reinforces findings by others that pre-surgical physical and mental health are positively related to post-TKA patient satisfaction [13, 16, 19, 41, 42]. However, given our longitudinal analysis, our study departs from the existing literature in being able to comment on contributors to change in satisfaction rates over time. As far as we know, our principal findings of a relationship between changes in pain, physical health status and mental health status and changes in patient satisfaction have not been shown previously.

Strengths and weaknesses of our study
One of the main strengths of our research is the longitudinal design and analysis of the research. Ours is not the first study of knee replacement experience to measure satisfaction longitudinally, but it is the first to employ methods that directly incorporate the longitudinal data into the analysis. Another major strength is the retention rates achieved; approximately 90% of the cohort returned surveys at both 6 and 12 months, with very

little loss over time. However, we also recognize that many patients invited to participate in this research chose not to do so, the consequence being a challenge to the representativeness of the sample.

The limited ethnic diversity in our sample is a weakness, resulting in part from the fact that we were able only to use English language surveys and study materials. Further work is required to establish the generalizability of our findings to other major ethnic groups in British Columbia and Canada more generally. We selected a measure of patient satisfaction used previously in a Canadian TKA context, in part to facilitate direct comparison with earlier Canadian work [5]. We do, however, acknowledge weaknesses with the satisfaction measure, notably its focus on satisfaction with results only, as opposed to a broader measure of patient experience. Our sample of patients all received care in BC, with recruitment from all regions of the province, reflecting both urban and more rural settings. To facilitate the recruitment process, we targeted pre-surgery education sessions and so we were only able to recruit from hospital sites that offered such education. Finally, other variables not measured in this study may explain some variation in satisfaction. For example, we had data on supplementary health insurance status but not on which patients might have augmented the standard series of publicly-provided physiotherapy with additional privately-financed physiotherapy or on the total number of private physiotherapy sessions received. We would encourage future research on this topic to consider gathering additional clinical data (e.g., clinical indication for surgery such as pain or joint surface destruction; clinical outcomes such as knee alignment; services provided such as number of physiotherapy sessions, and patient out of pocket costs) that might point directly to actions for improvement.

Conclusions

Our research confirms the importance of pain and functioning post-surgery as key drivers of patient satisfaction. Ongoing monitoring of such patient-reported factors, and intervention in cases where such symptoms persist, is central to patient satisfaction. Another key finding of our work is that a patient's mental health also heavily influences satisfaction post-TKA. Both the level of self-reported mental health and changes in that level over time predict satisfaction rates. This important finding points to the need for broad clinical review of patients, before and after surgery that encompasses both physical and mental health aspects. Screening for and addressing mental health concerns will likely be a new domain for many surgical orthopedic programs. The priority research implications of this work are two-fold. First, we need to explore the robustness of our results across more ethnically diverse British Columbian and Canadian patient populations. Second, the effectiveness and cost-effectiveness of any new interventions targeting the drivers of dissatisfaction uncovered in our work will need to be tested empirically. For example, a response to our findings might be to consider new interventions to promote mental health and wellness amongst patients receiving TKA but this should, of course, be subjected to evaluation of its costs and benefits before implementation.

Abbreviations

BC: British Columbia; BIC: Bayesian Information Criterion; CIHI: Canadian Institutes for Health Information; EQ-5D-5 L: Euroqol 5 dimension, 5 level instrument; HADS: Hospital Anxiety and Depression Scale; MOS-SSS: Medical Outcomes Study Social Support Survey; OR: Odds ratio; SF-12: Short-form 12 instrument; SLANSS: Self-completed Leeds Assessment of Neuropathic Symptoms and Signs pain scale; TKA: Total knee arthroplasty; WOMAC: Western Ontario and McMaster Universities Osteoarthritis Index

Acknowledgements

We thank the TKA patients who participated in this research study, and acknowledge the data collection contributions from Jessica Shum, Faith Furlong, Heidi Howay, Christine Morrison, Valerie Oglov and Christina Parkin. Study guidance was provided by our collaborators and advisory team members, including Ramin Mehin, Susann Camus, Susan Chunick, Alison Dormuth, Denise Dunton, Vivian Giglio, Charlie Goldsmith, David Nelson, Cindy Roberts, Magdelena Newman, Joan Vyner, Mike Wasdell, Robert Bourne, and many others.

Funding

The study "Why are so many patients dissatisfied with knee replacement surgery? Exploring variations of the patient experience" was funded through support from the Canadian Institutes of Health Research Partnerships for Health System Improvement (CIHR PHSI) operating grant (number 114106), the Michael Smith Foundation for Health Research (MSFHR; number PJ HSP 00004 [10–1]), and the BC Rural & Remote Health Research Network. Funding and in-kind support were received from Vancouver Coastal Health Authority and Fraser Health Authority. Dr. Sawatzky holds a Canada Research Chair (CRC) in Patient-Reported Outcomes from the Government of Canada CRC program. Dr. Davis held postdoctoral funding from CIHR and MSFHR during this study. Assistance with the pre-funding study design was provided through in-kind support from the Fraser Health Authority. Otherwise, no funder of this study was involved in the design of the study and collection, analysis and interpretation of data and in writing the manuscript.

Authors' contributions

SB led and participated in the design, conduct and analysis of this study and the drafting of this manuscript. RS and LJG participated in the design, conduct and analysis of the study and helped draft the manuscript. JD, SH, VM, PM, ER, NS, and AW participated in the design, conduct and analysis of the study and revised the manuscript critically for important intellectual content. SB also led the overall mixed methods study within which this quantitative study was embedded. All authors read and approved the final manuscript.

Consent for publication

All study participants provided written informed consent for the information collected to be used for publication where no information that disclosed their identity was released or published.

Competing interests

The authors declare that they have no competing interests.

Author details

[1]Centre for Clinical Epidemiology & Evaluation, Vancouver Coastal Health Research Institute, West 10th Avenue, Vancouver, BC V5Z 1M9, Canada. [2]School of Population & Public Health, University of British Columbia, 2206 E Mall, Vancouver, BC V6T 1Z3, Canada. [3]Faculty of Health Sciences, Simon Fraser University, 8888 University Drive, Burnaby, BC V5A 1S6, Canada. [4]Faculty of Management, University of British Columbia – Okanagan Campus, EME 4145 3333 University Way, Kelowna, BC V1V 1V7, Canada. [5]Department of Evaluation & Research Services, Fraser Health Authority, Suite 400, Central City Tower, 13450 102 Avenue, Surrey, BC V3T 0H1, Canada. [6]Burnaby Hospital & Surgical Network, Fraser Health Authority, 3935 Kincaid St, Burnaby, BC V5G 2X6, Canada. [7]Rebalance MD, 3551 Blanshard St, Victoria, BC V8Z 0B9, Canada. [8]Educational and Counselling Psychology, and Special Education, University of British Columbia, 2125 Main Mall, Vancouver, BC V6T 1Z4, Canada. [9]School of Nursing, Trinity Western University, 7600 Glover Rd, Langley, BC V2Y 1Y1, Canada. [10]Centre for Health Evaluation & Outcomes Sciences, Providence Health Care Research Institute, 588 – 1081 Burrard Street, St. Paul's Hospital, Vancouver, BC V6Z 1Y6, Canada.

References

1. Canadian Institute for Health Information (CIHI). Hip and Knee Replacements in Canada, 2016-2017: Canadian joint replacement registry annual report. Ottawa: CIHI; 2018 [Available from: https://www.cihi.ca/en/canadian-joint-replacement-registry-cjrr].

2. Mahomed NN, Barrett J, Katz JN, Baron JA, Wright J, Losina E. Epidemiology of total knee replacement in the United States Medicare population. J Bone Joint Surg Am. 2005;87(6):1222–8.

3. Kopec JA, Rahman MM, Sayre EC, Cibere J, Flanagan WM, Aghajanian J, et al. Trends in physician-diagnosed osteoarthritis incidence an an administrative database in British Columbia, Canada, 1996-1997 through 2003-2004. Arthrit Rheum-Arthr. 2008;59(7):929–34.

4. Kopec JA, Rahman MM, Berthelot JM, Le Petit C, Aghajanian J, Sayre EC, et al. Descriptive epidemiology of osteoarthritis in British Columbia. Canada J Rheumatol. 2007;34(2):386–93.

5. Bourne RB, Chesworth BM, Davis AM, Mahomed NN, Charron KD. Patient satisfaction after total knee arthroplasty: who is satisfied and who is not? Clin Orthop Relat Res. 2010;468(1):57–63.

6. Gandhi R, Davey JR, Mahomed NN. Predicting patient dissatisfaction following joint replacement surgery. J Rheumatol. 2008;35(12):2415–8.

7. Saha S, Beach MC, Cooper LA. Patient centeredness, cultural competence and healthcare quality. J Natl Med Assoc. 2008;100(11):1275–85.

8. Association OM. Patient-Centred care. Ontario; 2010.

9. Barlow T, Clark T, Dunbar M, Metcalfe A, Griffin D. The effect of expectation on satisfaction in total knee replacements: a systematic review. Springerplus. 2016;5:167.

10. Choi Y-J, Ra HJ. Patient satisfaction after Total knee arthroplasty. Knee Surgery & Related Research. 2016;28(1):15.

11. Culliton SE, Bryant DM, Overend TJ, MacDonald SJ, Chesworth BM. The relationship between expectations and satisfaction in patients undergoing primary total knee arthroplasty. J Arthroplast. 2012;27(3):490–2.

12. Dunbar MJ, Haddad FS. Patient satisfaction after total knee replacement: new inroads. Bone Joint J. 2014;96 - B(10):1285–6.

13. Gibon E, Goodman MJ, Goodman SB. Patient satisfaction after Total knee arthroplasty: a realistic or imaginary goal? Orthop Clin North Am. 2017;48(4):421–31.

14. Hamilton DF, Lane JV, Gaston P, Patton JT, Macdonald D, Simpson AH, et al. What determines patient satisfaction with surgery? A prospective cohort study of 4709 patients following total joint replacement. BMJ Open. 2013;3(4):e002525.

15. Jones CA, Beaupre LA, Johnston DW, Suarez-Almazor ME. Total joint arthroplasties: current concepts of patient outcomes after surgery. Rheum Dis Clin N Am. 2007;33(1):71–86.

16. Lau RL, Gandhi R, Mahomed S, Mahomed N. Patient satisfaction after total knee and hip arthroplasty. Clin Geriatr Med. 2012;28(3):349 65.

17. Nam D, Nunley RM, Barrack RL. Patient dissatisfaction following total knee replacement: a growing concern? Bone Joint J. 2014;96 - B(11 Supple A):96–100.

18. Schulze A, Scharf HP. Satisfaction after total knee arthroplasty. Comparison of 1990-1999 with 2000-2012. Orthopade. 2013;42(10): 858–65.

19. Vissers MM, Bussmann JB, Verhaar JA, Busschbach JJ, Bierma-Zeinstra SM, Reijman M. Psychological factors affecting the outcome of total hip and knee arthroplasty: a systematic review. Semin Arthritis Rheum. 2012;41(4):576–88.

20. Adie S, Dao A, Harris IA, Naylor JM, Mittal R. Satisfaction with joint replacement in public versus private hospitals: a cohort study. ANZ J Surg. 2012;82(9):616–24.

21. Dickstein R, Heffes Y, Shabtai EI, Markowitz E. Total knee arthroplasty in the elderly: patients' self-appraisal 6 and 12 months postoperatively. Gerontology. 1998;44(4):204–10.

22. Harris IA, Harris AM, Naylor JM, Adie S, Mittal R, Dao AT. Discordance between patient and surgeon satisfaction after total joint arthroplasty. J Arthroplast. 2013;28(5):722–7.

23. Nilsdotter AK, Toksvig-Larsen S, Roos EM. Knee arthroplasty: are patients' expectations fulfilled? A prospective study of pain and function in 102 patients with 5-year follow-up. Acta Orthop. 2009;80(1):55–61.

24. Verbeke G, Fieuws S, Molenberghs G, Davidian M. The analysis of multivariate longitudinal data: a review. Stat Methods Med Res. 2014;23(1):17.

25. Leech N, Onwuegbuzie A. A typology of mixed methods research designs. Qual Quant. 2007;43(2):10.

26. Ware J Jr, Kosinski M, Keller SD. A 12-item short-form health survey: construction of scales and preliminary tests of reliability and validity. Med Care. 1996;34(3):220–33.

27. Brooks R. EuroQol: the current state of play. Health Policy. 1996;37(1):53–72.

28. McConnell S, Kolopack P, Davis AM. The Western Ontario and McMaster universities osteoarthritis index (WOMAC): a review of its utility and measurement properties. Arthritis Rheum. 2001;45(5):453–61.

29. Bennett MI, Smith BH, Torrance N, Potter J. The S-LANSS score for identifying pain of predominantly neuropathic origin: validation for use in clinical and postal research. J Pain. 2005;6(3):149–58.

30. Zigmond AS, Snaith RP. The hospital anxiety and depression scale. Acta Psychiatr Scand. 1983;67(6):361–70.

31. Sherbourne CD, Stewart AL. The MOS social support survey. Soc Sci Med. 1991;32(6):705–14.

32. Charlson ME, Pompei P, Ales KL, MacKenzie CR. A new method of classifying prognostic comorbidity in longitudinal studies: development and validation. J Chronic Dis. 1987;40(5):373–83.

33. Cantril H. The Pattern of Human Concerns. New Brunswick: Rutgers University Press; 1965.

34. Muthén B, Muthén L. MPlus (version 7.4). Statmodel: Los Angeles; 2015.

35. Heck RH, Thomas SL. An introduction to multilevel modeling techniques : MLM and SEM approaches using Mplus. 3rd ed. Routledge, Taylor & Francis Group: New York; 2015.

36. Bolger N, Laurenceau J-P. Intensive longitudinal methods : an introduction to diary and experience sampling research. New York: Guilford Press; 2013. p. 256.

37. Goldsmith LJ, Suryaprakash N, Randall E, Shum J, MacDonald V, Sawatzky R, et al. The importance of informational, clinical and personal support in patient experience with total knee replacement: a qualitative investigation. BMC Musculoskelet Disord. 2017;18(1):127.

38. Hosmer DW, Lemeshow S, Sturdivant RX. Applied logistic regression. Hoboken: Wiley; 2013.

39. Wu W, West SG, Taylor AB. Evaluating model fit for growth curve models: integration of fit indices from SEM and MLM frameworks. Psychol Methods. 2009;14(3):183–201.

40. Dunbar MJ, Richardson G, Robertsson O. I can't get no satisfaction after my total knee replacement: rhymes and reasons. Bone Joint J. 2013;95 - B(11 Suppl A):148–52.

41. Husain A, Lee GC. Establishing realistic patient expectations following Total knee arthroplasty. J Am Acad Orthop Surg. 2015;23(12):707–13.

42. Khatib Y, Madan A, Naylor JM, Harris IA. Do psychological factors predict poor outcome in patients undergoing TKA? A systematic review. Clin Orthop Relat Res. 2015;473(8):2630–8.

12

Analysis of total knee arthroplasty revision causes

Anne Postler*, Cornelia Lützner, Franziska Beyer, Eric Tille and Jörg Lützner

Abstract

Background: The number of revision Total Knee Arthroplasty (TKA) is rising in many countries. The aim of this study was the prospective assessment of the underlying causes leading to revision TKA in a tertiary care hospital and the comparison of those reasons with previously published data.

Methods: In this study patients who had revision TKA between 2010 and 2015 were prospectively included. Revision causes were categorized using all available information from patients' records including preoperative diagnostics, intraoperative findings as well as the results of the periprosthetic tissue analysis. According to previous studies patients were divided into early (up to 2 years) and late revision (more than 2 years). Additional also re-revisions after already performed revision TKA were included.

Results: We assessed 312 patients who underwent 402 revision TKA, 89.6% of them were referred to our center for revision surgery. In 289 patients (71.9%) this was the first revision surgery after primary TKA. Among the first revisions the majority was late revisions (73.7%). One hundred thirteen patients (28.1%) had already had one or more revision surgeries before. Overall, the most frequent reason for revision was infection (36.1%) followed by aseptic loosening (21.9%) and periprosthetic fracture (13.7%).

Conclusions: In a specialized arthroplasty center periprosthetic joint infection (PJI) was the most common reason for revision and re-revision TKA. This is in contrast to population-based registry data and has consequences on costs as well as on success rates in such centers.

Keywords: Total knee arthroplasty, Failure, Revision, Complication, Re-revision

Background

Total knee arthroplasty (TKA) is one of the most frequent surgical procedures and a very effective treatment option for advanced osteoarthritis of the knee, which decreases pain and improves function [1]. Nevertheless, some patients achieve poor results after surgery or the implant fails and a revision surgery is required. The number of revision TKA is rising in many countries, with 22,403 procedures in the United States [2], 15,232 in Australia [3], 5873 in the UK [4] and 17,677 in Germany in 2015 [5].

Previous studies investigated the failure causes after total knee arthroplasties and differed between early (within the first 2 years after primary TKA) and late revision (thereafter). They found polyethylene wear and accordingly aseptic loosening as most common causes

for late revisions [6, 7]. Infection and instability were the most common revision causes in the early failure groups [8]. Over the last decade failure mechanisms have changed and polyethylene wear as revision cause decreased. Infection on the contrary was increasing [9, 10]. General information on TKA survival and revision causes in large populations can be obtained from Arthroplasty registries or health care provider data. However, these data are not very specific and provided from many different persons who might have different judgements for categorizing the revision causes [2–4, 11]. Therefore single- or multi-center studies with the possibility to review the patients' records give a more detailed picture of the revision causes.

The aim of this study was therefore the prospective assessment of causes for revision TKA, and comparison of those reasons with previously published data.

* Correspondence: Anne.Postler@uniklinikum-dresden.de
University Center of Orthopaedics and Traumatology, University Medicine Carl Gustav Carus Dresden, TU Dresden, Fetscherst. 74, 01307 Dresden, Germany

Methods

After receiving institutional review board approval, all revision surgeries of TKA from January 2010 to December 2015 in our department were prospectively included. According to previous studies we defined revision TKA as replacement of at least one component (femur, tibia or patella), patients with isolated exchange of the polyethylene insert were excluded. Additional and in contrast to other studies we did not only include first revisions, as we intended to present the complete perspective of a tertiary care hospital. The cause of revision was based on analysis of x-rays, Computed tomography (CT) scans, blood tests, joint aspiration, intraoperative findings, culture and histology results. The revision cause was determined by the surgeon in the OR report but was reviewed by the authors using all available data and the below described definitions. Causes were assessed in detail and categorized into infection, aseptic loosening, polyethylene wear, instability, periprosthetic fracture, pain, restricted range of motion/fibrosis, extensor mechanism insufficiency, implant failure and allergy against implant materials. In case of more than one causes for revision the leading cause was reported. The following hierarchy was used: infection, fracture, implant failure, loosening, osteolysis, wear, instability, restricted range of motion, extensor mechanism insufficiency, allergy and pain.

The diagnosis of PJI was based on the Musculoskeletal Infection Society criteria [12]: as two positive periprosthetic cultures with phenotypically identical organisms, or a sinus tract communicating with the joint or having three of the following minor criteria: elevated serum c-reactive protein (CRP), elevated synovial fluid white blood cell count, elevated synovial fluid polymorphonuclear neutrophil percentage, positive histological analysis of periprosthetic tissue or a single positive culture. A two- or multiple-stage revision with temporary placement of an antibiotic-loaded bonecement spacer was always performed and considered as one surgery. Periprosthetic fractures, mechanical implant failure and aseptic loosening were assessed radiographically and if necessary with computed tomography. Polyethylene wear was assessed by macroscopic findings on the insert and microscopic report according to criteria described by Krenn et al. [13]. Instability, pain and extensor mechanism insufficiency were clinical diagnoses by positive history and suitable physical examination. Pain was used as a revision cause only if no other reason could be determined. Fibrosis was defined as a limited range of motion (ROM) in flexion and/or extension, that is not attributable to an osseous or prosthetic block to movement from malaligned, malpositioned or incorrectly sized components, metal hardware, ligament reconstruction, infection, pain, chronic regional pain syndrome (CRPS) or other specific causes, but due to soft-tissue fibrosis that was not present pre-operatively [14].

Allergy against implant materials was considered as revision cause if other reasons could be ruled out (especially PJI), the patients had a positive patch test and the microscopic report described it as likely [13].

Revisions were categorized into two groups: first revision after primary TKA and re-revision after already performed revision surgery. The interval from primary TKA to the first revision surgery was recorded and the patients were categorized into early and late failure groups. An interval between primary TKA and revision procedure of 2 years was considered as the cut-off between early and late failures [7]. In case of more than one revision surgeries (re-revisions) the total number of previous revisions and the time from the last revision was recorded.

Patients demographics, age and gender were documented, as well as Body Mass Index (BMI) and comorbidities (ASA score). Previous surgeries and additional reoperations between implant removal and re-implantation PJI were recorded, too.

Data description is based on means, standard deviations (SD) and ranges for continuous values and absolute and relative frequencies for categorical values. Differences between groups were analyzed using t-test for continuous values and chi-square test for categorical values. A p-value of 0.05 results was considered statistically significant. All data analyses were carried out using SPSS (release 22.0 for Windows).

An ethics approval for this study was obtained from the Ethics Committee of the University Medicine Carl Gustav Carus, TU Dresden in 2011 (EK 288082011).

Results

The study group consisted of 402 cases in 312 patients who had revision TKA between January 2010 and December 2015.The primary TKA was performed in only 42 patients (10.4%) at our department, 360 patients (89.6%) were referred to our center for revision.

There were 402 TKA revisions in 312 patients. Thirty-two patients have been revised bilaterally (64 surgeries) and 25 knees have been revised more than one time during the investigation period. Three hundred thirteen patients had just one surgery. However, we analyzed TKA.

In 289 surgeries (71.9%) this was the first revision surgery in mean 6.2 years (range 0.1 – 24.2 years) after primary TKA. Among the first revisions the majority were late revisions after 2 years (n = 207; 73.7%). Three hundred thirteen patients (28.1%) had already had one to 18 (median 1) revision surgeries before. In these patients the time between primary implantation and current re-revision was 3.9 years (range 0.1 – 17.6 years). The overall time to revision 5.5 years (range 0.03 – 24.2 years).

Our patients were in mean 72.3 years old (SD 9.7, range 48.2 – 95.4 years), the majority (64.4%) had severe systemic diseases (ASA grade III and IV) and a mean

BMI of 30.6, see Table 1. The 146 patients (36.3%) suffering from infection (72.8 ± 8.8 years; range 48.2 – 92.4 years) were in mean 3 years older than those with aseptic reasons (72.8 vs 69.9 years, $p = 0.06$).

The most frequent reason for revision was infection (overall 36.1%, first early revisions 51.3%, first late revisions 26.8%, re-revisions 44.2%) followed by aseptic loosening (overall 21.9%, first early revisions 9.2%, first late revisions 23.0%, re-revisions 27.4%) and periprosthetic fracture (overall 13.7%, first early revisions 5.3%, first late revisions 21.1%, re-revisions 5.3%), see Fig. 1 and Table 2 for details. Forty-five patients (11.2%) had just one cause of failure, 356 patients (88.6%) more than one.

If the cause for re-revision was PJI (49 patients) the majority (40 patients, 81.6%) had already had one or more revision surgeries due to previous infection.

Discussion

Total Knee Arthroplasty is a very effective and safe treatment option for advanced osteoarthritis of the knee [15]. Revision rates are generally low, the revision risk at 10 years as reported in the major Arthroplasty registries is about 5%: the Australian Joint Replacement Report stated 5.5% revision rate after 10 years [3], for the UK reported rates are below 5% [4] and slightly more than 5.5% for Sweden [11]. Caused by a growing number of TKA overall, a shift towards younger patients and technical developments of revision implants the number of revisions is growing. While primary TKA is a standard procedure revision TKA is a complex surgery which is often performed in specialized centers. The majority of all revisions in this study (90%) were referred to our center after primary TKA performed elsewhere. Through the concentration of difficult surgeries the causes for revision in specialized centers are likely to be different from population based registries.

In this study the mean time between index surgery and revision TKA of the late revision group was 8.1 years. This is consistent with previous studies, Sharkey et al. reported in 212 with late revisions (more than 2 years) an average time to failure of 7 years (range, 2.2

– 28 years) [7]. Thiele et al. reported a mean time to failure of 7.9 years in patients with a revision of at least 3 years after primary surgery in overall 358 patients [10].

The revision causes however, are different to published data, see Fig. 2. In 2002 Sharkey et al. found polyethylene wear (25%) as the most prevalent mechanism for TKA revision [7] and in 2014 aseptic loosening (39.9%) was the most common failure mechanism [9]. Thiele et al. identified aseptic loosening (21.8%), instability (21.8%) and malalignement (20.7%) as the most common indications for revision [10]. In the registries of the US (18.6%), Sweden (about 26%) and Australia (38.3%) aseptic loosening is the most frequent reason for revision, followed by infection (9.1%, about 26%, 25.6%). In our center PJI was the most common reason for revision TKA. The reason for the high frequency of PJI in our patients (146, 36.3%) might be that this is the most difficult to treat and most expensive complication after TKA. Aseptic loosening and other mechanical revision causes might have been considered as "simple" revisions and performed in smaller hospitals whereas PJI were more frequently referred to our department. This has implications on success rates as well as on costs. Success rates for revision TKA for PJI are generally lower than for aseptic revisions [16, 17]. Additionally these revisions have a higher risk of complications with significantly higher length of hospitalization, higher number of readmission and higher rates of mortality [16, 18, 19]. This could be a problem for such centers in pay-for-performance programs which are already in place or intended from different health care providers. Furthermore, revisions for PJI need much more resources and, depending on the health care system, costs are not always completely compensated. Therefore centers performing many revisions for PJI might have disadvantages in public reports on success rates and complications as well as financially. However, PJI are the most challenging complications after TKA and should be treated in specialized centers with experience and sufficient resources [12, 18, 20].

With regard to early surgeries (within 2 years) in the first revisions, the main reason for revision was again infection followed by aseptic loosening, restriction of ROM/arthrofibrosis and extensor mechanism insufficiency just as reported

Table 1 Comparison of patients characteristics between first and re-revisions

Patients		All revision surgeries (n = 402)	First revision surgeries (n = 289)	Re-revision surgeries (n = 113)	p
Gender	Male	157 (39.1%)	109 (37.7%)	48 (42.5%)	n.s.
	Female	245 (60.9%)	180 (62.3%)	65 (57.5%)	n.s.
Age [years]		72.3 (48.2 – 95.4)	72.2 (48.2 - 95.4)	72.6 (54.4 - 92.5)	n.s.
ASA classification	1	3 (0.7%)	3 (1.0%)	0 (0%)	n.s.
	2	140 (34.8%)	107 (37.0%)	33 (29.2%)	
	3	249 (61.9%)	170 (58.8%)	79 (69,9%)	
	4	10 (2.5%)	9 (3.1%)	1 (0.9%)	
BMI [kg/m^2]		30.6 (SD 5.7)	30.5 (SD 5.8)	30.9 (5.4)	n.s.

ASA classification of the American Society of Anesthesiologists, *BMI* body mass index

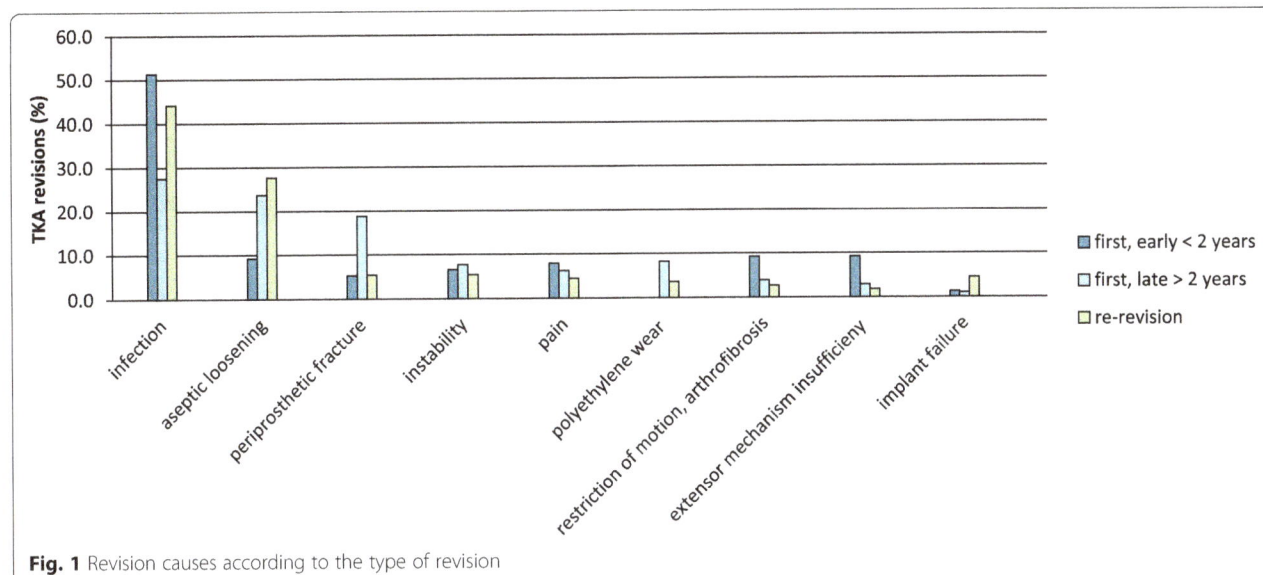

Fig. 1 Revision causes according to the type of revision

by Sharkey [9] and Thiele [10] for the early revisions. Early loosening of the prosthesis could be related to TKA component fixation methods including cementing technique [9]. Reasons for loosening change with time, which means loosening in the first few years most likely reflects failure to gain fixation. Loosening reported in later years is often due to loss of fixation by secondary bone resorption [3].

For the re-revisions infection (44.2%) and aseptic loosening (27.4%) were the major causes of failure, too. Leta reported about 145 re-revisions after 1016 aseptic revisions in the Norwegian Arthroplasty Register and found deep infection the most frequent cause (28%) because of increased risk after multiple operations, longer operative time, previous scars, larger implants, comorbidities and poorly vascularized tissue [21]. Mortazavi [13] included 499 patients with TKA revisions with a 20.4% re-revision rate and found infection to be the major reason for re-operation or re-revision of the failed TKA (44.1%). Of

Table 2 causes and time to revision

Failure mechanism	Total [n (%)] n = 402	Time to revision[a] (yr)	Primary revision [n (%)]				Re-revision	
			Early n = 76	Time to revision[a] (yr)	Late n = 207	Time to revision[a] (yr)	[n (%)]	Time to revision[a] (yr)
Infection	146 (36.3)	4.2 ± 4.4 (0.06 - 20.1)	39 (51.3)	1.0 ± 0.6 (0.06 - 2.0)	57 (27.5)	7.3 ± 4.8 (2.1 - 20.1)	50 (44.2)	3.3 ± 3.3 (0.1 - 13.0)
Aseptic loosening	87 (21.6)	6.5 ± 5.4 (0.4 - 21.6)	7 (9.2)	1.6 ± 0.2 (1.4 - 2.0)	49 (23.7)	8.6 ± 5.6 (2.1 - 21.6)	31 (27.7)	4.3 ± 3.8 (0.4 - 17.1)
Periprosthetic fracture	55 (13.7)	8.5 ± 5.4 (0.04 - 24.2)	4 (5.3)	0.5 ± 0.6 (0.04 - 1.4)	39 (18.8)	9.5 ± 5.1 (2.6 - 24.2)	6 (5.4)	7.9 ± 4.9 (3.9 - 17.6)
Instability	27 (6.7)	5.4 ± 4.1 (0.08 - 15.2)	5 (6.6)	1.3 ± 0.2 (1.1 - 1.6)	16 (7.7)	6.9 ± 4.1 (2.2 - 15.2)	6 (5.4)	4.9 ± 3.3 (0.1 - 9.2)
Pain	24 (6.0)	3.6 ± 3.0 (1.1 - 11.1)	6 (7.9)	1.4 ± 0.2 (1.1 - 1.6)	13 (6.3)	5.6 ± 3.1 (2.0 - 11.1)	5 (4.5)	1.9 ± 0.4 (1.4 - 2.2)
Polyethylene wear	21 (5.2)	10.5 ± 5.8 (1.6 - 19.5)	0 (0)		17 (8.2)	11.9 ± 5.3 (3.7 - 19.5)	4 (3.6)	4.8 ± 4.2 (1.6 - 10.8)
Restriction of motion, arthrofibrosis	18 (4.5)	2.6 ± 2.3 (0.04 - 9.6)	7 (9.2)	0.9 ± 0.6 (0.04 - 0.9)	8 (3.9)	4.1 ± 2.6 (2.1 - 9.6)	3 (2.7)	2.6 ± 1.9 (0.6 - 4.3)
Extensor mechanism insufficiency	15 (3.7)	2.9 ± 3.6 (0.03 - 11.8)	7 (9.2)	0.7 ± 0.8 (0.03 - 1.8)	6 (2.9)	5.6 ± 4.4 (2.0 - 11.8)	2 (1.8)	2.9 ± 1.9 (1.6 - 4.2)
Mechanically defect	8 (2.0)	5.5 ± 2.8 (1.4 - 9.8)	1 (1.3)	1.4	2 (1.0)	8.5 ± 1.8 (7.2 - 9.8)	5 (4.5)	5.1 ± 2.1 (2.6 - 7.9)
Allergy	1 (0.2)	1.2	0 (0)		0 (0)		1 (0.9)	1.2
Total		5.5 ± 5.0 (0.03 - 24.2)		1.0 ± 0.6 (0.03 - 2.0)		8.1 ± 5.1 (2.0 - 24.2)		3.9 ± 3.5 (0.08 - 17.6)

[a] values are given as mean ± SD (range)

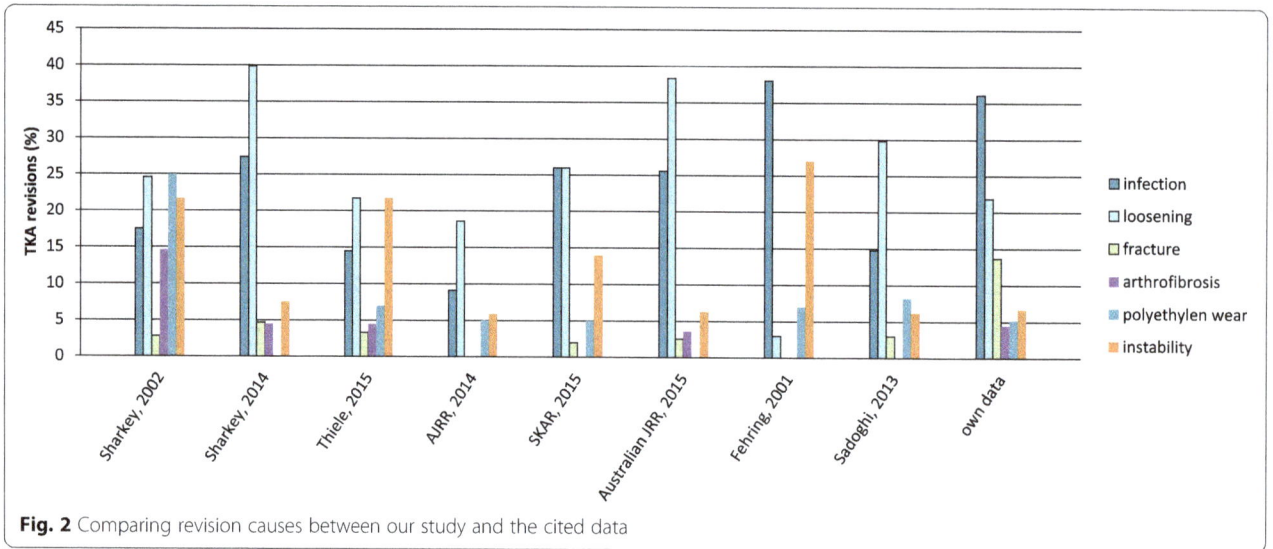

Fig. 2 Comparing revision causes between our study and the cited data

these periprosthetic joint infections only 32% had no history of infection before, 58% had already had revision due to infection. In our patients 81.6% of patients with re-revision due to PJI had already had revision due to PJI before. These numbers emphasize the difficulties in the treatment of PJI. These patients with re-revisions are more difficult to treat for several reasons. There are often compromised soft-tissues which increases the risk of wound healing problems, because of the restricted circulation. Even adequate exposure might be a problem due to contracture, patella baja and intraarticular scarring. In many of these patients there are already relevant bone defects and consecutively large revision implants sometimes even mega-prostheses are needed. Again, this needs to be taken into consideration when success rates between centers are compared and pay-for-performance programs are being implemented.

We acknowledge some limitations of this study. Most patients were referred to our department and we had therefore not always complete baseline information on the primary TKA. Furthermore we did not always know the precise time to failure. Time to failure is usually less. However, patients with an indication for revision are usually efficiently referred to our center and time between recognized failure and revision is usually less than 3 month. We were not in all cases able to get detailed information about all previous revisions. In some cases, more than one reason lead to revision and we categorized the patients into the leading revision cause. Finally, this is a selection of probably more complicated revision TKA and therefore the frequencies differ from other studies and joint replacement registries. However, this is a more detailed description because we had not only limited information like in registries or from health care provider data. We believe that our data are representative for tertiary care centers.

Conclusions

Most patients which are revised in a specialized arthroplasty center were referred from other hospitals. PJI was the most common reason for revision and re-revision TKA. This is in contrast to population-based registry data and has consequences on costs as well as on success rates in such centers.

Abbreviations
ASA score: Physical classification system of the American society of anesthesiologists; BMI: Body mass index; CRP: C-reactive protein; CRPS: Chronic regional pain syndrome; CT: Computed tomography; PJI: Periprosthetic joint infection; ROM: Range of motion; SD: Standard deviations; TKA: Total Knee Replacement

Acknowledgments
We thank Brit Brethfeld and Anne Schützer for her valuable assistance during patient recruitment.

Funding
There was no funding of this study.

Authors' contributions
CL and JL made substantial contributions to conception and design of the study. AP, CL, FB, ET and JL made substantial contributions in acquisition of data. AP, CL, FB, ET and JL in the analysis and interpretation of data. AP and JL have been involved in drafting the manuscript and all authors revised it critically for important intellectual content. All authors gave final approval of the version to be published. Each author have participated sufficiently in the work to take public responsibility for appropriate portions of the content and agreed to be accountable for all aspects of the work in ensuring that questions related to the accuracy or integrity of any part of the work are appropriately investigated and resolved.

Consent for publication
Not applicable.

Competing interests

Research support and other financial or material support have been received from the following companies: Arthrosehilfe, Aesculap, Mathys, Smith&Nephew, Stryker and Zimmer.

ReferenceS

1. Carr AJ, Robertsson O, Graves S, Price AJ, Arden NK, Judge A, et al. Knee replacement. Lancet. 2012;379(9823):1331–40.

2. Registry AJR. American Joint Replacement Registry. ISSN 2375-9119 (online). Annual Report 2014. 2014. www.ajrr.net.

3. Australian Orthopaedic Association National Joint Replacement Registry. Annual Report. Adelaide: AOA; 2015.

4. Registry NJ. National Joint Registry. ISSN 2054-183X (Online). 12th Annual Report 2015 - National Joint Registry for England, Wales, Northern Ireland and the Isle of Man. 2015. www.njrreports.org.uk.

5. IQTIG. Institut für Qualitätssicherung und Transparenz im Gesundheitswesen, Berlin. ISBN 978-3-9818131-0-4. Qualitätsreport 2015. 2015. www.iqtig.org.

6. Khan M, Osman K, Green G, Haddad FS. The epidemiology of failure in total knee arthroplasty: avoiding your next revision. Bone Joint J. 2016;98-B(1 Suppl A):105–12.

7. Sharkey PF, Hozack WJ, Rothman RH, Shastri S, Jacoby SM. Insall Award paper. Why are total knee arthroplasties failing today? Clinical orthopaedics and related research. 2002;404:7-13.

8. Fehring TK, Odum S, Griffin WL, Mason JB, Nadaud M. Early failures in total knee arthroplasty. Clin Orthop Relat Res. 2001;392:315–8.

9. Sharkey PF, Lichstein PM, Shen C, Tokarski AT, Parvizi J. Why are total knee arthroplasties failing today–has anything changed after 10 years? J Arthroplast. 2014;29(9):1774–8.

10. Thiele K, Perka C, Matziolis G, Mayr HO, Sostheim M, Hube R. Current failure mechanisms after knee arthroplasty have changed: polyethylene wear is less common in revision surgery. J Bone Joint Surg Am. 2015;97(9):715–20.

11. Registry SKA. The Swedish Knee Arthroplasty Register. ISBN 978-91-88017-04-8. Annual Report 2015. 2015. www.knee.se.

12. Parvizi J, Gehrke T. International consensus on periprosthetic joint infection: let cumulative wisdom be a guide. J Bone Joint Surg Am. 2014;96(6):441.

13. Morawietz L, Krenn V. The spectrum of histomorphological findings related to joint endoprosthetics. Pathologe. 2014;35(Suppl 2):218–24.

14. Kalson NS, Borthwick LA, Mann DA, Deehan DJ, Lewis P, Mann C, et al. International consensus on the definition and classification of fibrosis of the knee joint. Bone Joint J. 2016;98-B(11):1479–88.

15. Lohmander LS, Roos EM. Clinical update: treating osteoarthritis. Lancet. 2007;370(9605):2082–4.

16. Choi HR, Bedair H. Mortality following revision total knee arthroplasty: a matched cohort study of septic versus aseptic revisions. J Arthroplast. 2014; 29(6):1216–8.

17. van Kempen RW, Schimmel JJ, van Hellemondt GG, Vandenneucker H, Wymenga AB. Reason for revision TKA predicts clinical outcome: prospective evaluation of 150 consecutive patients with 2-years followup. Clin Orthop Relat Res. 2013;471(7):2296–302.

18. Kapadia BH, McElroy MJ, Issa K, Johnson AJ, Bozic KJ, Mont MA. The economic impact of periprosthetic infections following total knee arthroplasty at a specialized tertiary-care center. J Arthroplast. 2014;29(5): 929–32.

19. Saleh KJ, Dykes DC, Tweedie RL, Mohamed K, Ravichandran A, Saleh RM, et al. Functional outcome after total knee arthroplasty revision: a meta-analysis. J Arthroplast. 2002;17(8):967–77.

20. Sadoghi P, Liebensteiner M, Agreiter M, Leithner A, Bohler N, Labek G. Revision surgery after total joint arthroplasty: a complication-based analysis using worldwide arthroplasty registers. J Arthroplast. 2013;28(8):1329–32.

21. Leta TH, Lygre SH, Skredderstuen A, Hallan G, Furnes O. Failure of aseptic revision total knee arthroplasties. Acta Orthop. 2015;86(1):48–57.

13

Cementless unicompartmental knee replacement allows early return to normal activity

Benjamin Panzram, Ines Bertlich, Tobias Reiner, Tilman Walker, Sébastien Hagmann and Tobias Gotterbarm[*] (iD)

Abstract

Background: Physical activity and regular participation in recreational sports gain importance in patients' lifestyle after knee arthroplasty. Cementless unicompartimental Knee replacement with the Oxford System has been introduced into clinical routine. Currently there is no data reporting on the physical activity, return to sports rate and quality of live after medial cementless Oxford Unicompartimental Knee Replacement (OUKR).

Methods: This retrospective cohort study reports on the functional outcome of the first 27 consecutive patients (30 knees) that were consecutively treated with a cementless medial OUKR between 2007 and 2009 in our hospital. Physical activity and quality of life were measured using the Tegner-Score, the UCLA-Activity Score, the Schulthess Clinical Activity Questionnaire and the SF-36 Score. The patients' satisfaction with the outcome was measured using a visual analogue scale.

Results: Mean age at surgery was 62.5 years. Patients showed a rapid recovery with 17 out of 27 patients returning to sports within 3 months, 24 within 6 months after surgery. The Return-to-activity-rate was 100%. 10 out of 27 patients showed a high activity level (UCLA ≥7 points) with a mean postoperative UCLA-Score of 6.1 points.

Conclusions: Patients recover rapidly after cementless OUKR with a return to sports rate of 100% and patients are able to participate in high impact sports disciplines.

Keywords: Cementless UKR, OUKR, Oxford medial, Physical activity, Sports, Return-to-activity, Knee arthroplasty

Background

As life expectancy is increasing and the incidence of osteoarthritis (OA) rises with age, there is a high demand of joint replacement for people of middle and advanced age. While the mean age of patients receiving UKR is 63.6 years, several studies show that patients perform high levels of activities up until after 70 years of age [1–3].

Therefore, physical functioning and participation in sports after surgery are important outcome measures of a successful joint replacement. To allow high levels of activity, UKR provides more physiological knee kinematics, a higher range of motion, a more natural perception of the knee, shorter hospital stay, faster recovery with a lower rate of complication when compared to Total Knee Replacement [4–6]. UKR has shown to have excellent long-term survival rates compared to TKR [7–9]. As the cemented UKR is a reliable treatment option for antero medial OA, its' widespread use has been recommended for the elderly as well as for younger OA patients (e.g. patients <60 years) [4, 10–13].

For further improvement of the clinical outcome, implant survival and to eliminate complications associated with cementation, a cementless medial OUKR has been developed. Cementless fixation may offer several advantages compared to cemented OUKR. Reduced operation time, the absence of possible cement related tissue reactions, inefficient cementation which might influence the fixation or lead to early wear, clinical symptoms or even revision due to foreign bodies. Furthermore, radiographic radiolucent lines are less common suggesting a superior biological fixation [14]. Especially for patients at younger age with higher demands of sports activity

* Correspondence: Tobias.Gotterbarm@med.uni-heidelberg.de
Clinic of Orthopaedic and Trauma Surgery, University of Heidelberg, Schlierbacher Landstr. 200a, 69118 Heidelberg, Germany

these benefits seem to be desirable. However, cementless fixation is associated with a higher risk of intra and postoperative tibial plateau fractures and tibial valgus subsidence. Particularly an extended sagittal saw cut, a low bone density might lower the fracture load which may lead to tibial plateau fractures in combination with the firm impaction to achieve the desired press fit [15]. Valgus subsidence in cementless OUKR may be caused by extensive vertical saw cuts and or laterally implanted femoral components, causing impingement of the inlay against the medial tibial wall during flexion [16].

So far, there are promising short- to medium-term results published by the developing centres as well as registry data, indicating good clinical outcome and survival rates with a lower revision rate compared to the cemented version [17–20]. So far there are no published data reporting on the physical activity level after cementless OUKR. We therefore report in this study on the physical activity, return to sports rate and quality of life of our first consecutive 30 cementless medial OUKR.

Methods

In this retrospective study we evaluated the first 27 patients (30 knees) who were treated consecutively with a cementless medial OUKR in our hospital. The study was assessed and approved by the ethics committee of the University of Heidelberg (S-546/2013). Surgery was performed by three experienced surgeons between 2007 and 2009 using the Oxford III System. The patient cohort was described in our previous work analysing the incidence of radiolucent lines in cementless fixation [21].

Patients were examined before surgery and at final follow-up. The level of physical activity before and after surgery was measured using Tegner and UCLA Activity Score. Detailed information about physical activity was obtained using the Schulthess Clinical Activity Questionnaire, which compares the state at follow-up with the last time point before the onset of OA symptoms. The SF-36 Score determines the self-perception of the patients' quality of life, compared to a healthy cohort and a standard group suffering from osteoarthritis/ rheumatoid arthritis. The patient's satisfaction with the operated knee was measured using a visual analogue scale (0–10).

The indication for operation in all cases was anteromedial osteoarthritis (OA) with intact lateral knee compartment. The anterior cruciate ligament (ACL) and the collateral ligaments were intact and the varus deformity was fully correctable manually. A flexion deformity >15° or previous osteotomy were contraindications for the procedure, while cartilage loss in the femoro-patellar joint, age and obesity were not considered as contraindications [22]. Indications were concordant with the recommendations by Goodfellow et al. [23]. After surgery, the patients followed a three-week rehabilitation scheme with full weight-bearing.

Data analysis
SPSS Version 21 was applied to analyse the data. We used the Pearson's Chi Square Test for categorial and ordinal variables. Comparison of Pre-and post-operative scores were performed utilising the Wilcoxon signed-rank test. To compare differences between two independent groups with ordinal or continuous variables we used the Mann-Whitney U test. P-values of 0.05 or smaller were considered as significant.

Results
Demographics and study group
The study group consisted of the first 27 consecutive patients (15 male, 12 female, 30 knees) that were consecutively treated with cementless OUKR in our institution. Patient age at surgery ranged from 49 to 76 years with a mean of 62.5 years. Mean follow-time after surgery was 60 months, raging from 47 to 69 months (SD 8.3).

No patient died during follow up. Overall 3 knees were excluded from the study. In one case the reason was a major deviation from the recommended surgical technique. One patient suffered a periprosthetic tibial fracture within the first month after initial operation with consecutive revision of the tibial component to a cemented version and ORIF. The third patient was excluded after total knee replacement following progressive OA of the lateral and the patellofemoral joint (PFJ). The remaining 27 knees (24 patients) were included in the clinical and functional assessment. We observed one reoperation due to dislocation of the mobile-bearing 21 months postoperative and consecutive exchange of the inlay to a thicker one. In one case OA of the PFJ resulted in additional patello femoral arthroplasty (PFA).

Return to activity
Twenty-four out of 27 patients were physically active before surgery and all have returned to sports at final-follow up (see Table 1).

Seventeen patients (18 knees) returned to sports within 3 months after surgery (see Fig. 1). There were no age- and gender-related differences.

Most popular activities before and after surgery were cycling, hiking and long walks (see Fig. 2). Altogether, 18 types of sport were performed pre- or postoperatively. There were 5 types of high-impact sports practised before the onset of OA symptoms as well as after surgery. There was a notable shift from giving up sports such as soccer or jogging and starting volleyball and mountaineering. The main cause for the change was "pain" (3 patients, 4 knees). The Change did not reach statistical significance. ($p = 0.202$).

Table 1 Return to activity

| | | After surgery | | Total |
		Active (patients/ knees)	Inactive (patients/ knees)	(patients/ knees)
Before surgery	Active	24/27	0/0	24/27
	Inactive	2/2	1/1	3/3
Total		26/29	1/1	27/30

Amount of activities

There was no significant difference ($p = 0.132$) regarding the number of sports disciplines before the onset of OA symptoms and after surgery. During sports, 20 patients (22 knees) did not experience pain and 4 patients (4 knees) practised although feeling pain. One patient (one knee) did not participate in sports after surgery.

The quantitative assessment of sports participation was done using either the total number of patients that practised sports at least three times per week or the number of patients that practised at least 1 h per training session. There was no statistically significant difference comparing the state before OA onset and at follow-up in both parameters ($p = 0.146$).

While practicing sports, 19 patients (19 knees) felt excellent and did not report on any limitation or discomfort. Three patients (four knees) described a feeling of insecurity or fear of damaging the knee implant, three patients (three knees) felt they had a limit in the range of motion, and two patients each (two knees each) reported that they were not in a good physical condition or had a limited general flexibility.

Scores and satisfaction

All 24 patients (27 knees) showed a significant improvement in both Tegner and UCLA-Scores after surgery ($p = 0.042$ each, see Fig. 3). UCLA–Score was 4.9 (SD 2.3) preoperatively and increased significantly to 6.1 after surgery (SD 1.8), with a mean change of 1.2 points (SD 1.8). Tegner Score improved by 0.5 points (SD 0.2) from 2.9 points before surgery (SD

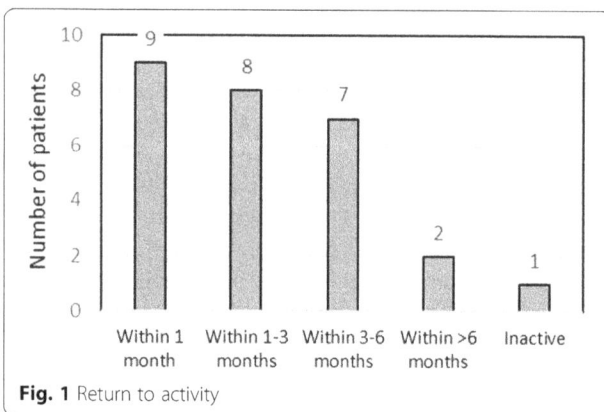

Fig. 1 Return to activity

1.4) to 3.4 points postoperatively (SD1.0). We classified the pre- and postoperative UCLA-Scores into three categories: ≥7 points: high activity levels, 4–6 points: moderate activity and ≤3 points: low activity [24]. At follow-up, 10 patients (11 knees) were highly active and 14 patients (12 knees) showed moderate activity. Three patients (4 knees) showed low activity levels.

The SF-36 Score showed high score values in all patients with cementless OUKR at final follow-up (see Fig. 4). The Results compared to the two reference groups are shown in Fig. 4. Overall 23 patients were extremely and very satisfied with the outcome, 4 patients were satisfied.

Discussion

This retrospective study assessed the physical activity and satisfaction in the first 27 consecutive patients (15 male, 12 female, 30 knees) that were treated with cementless OUKR in our institution between 2007 and 2009. Mean follow-up time was 60.0 months (47–69; SD 8.3) and mean age at surgery was 62.5 years (range 49–76).

Our main finding was that patients showed a high level of activity after cementless OUKR. Return-to-activity rate was 100% and the extent of activity did not differ from the time point before the onset of OA symptoms. The postoperative mean UCLA of 6.1 points and the predominant number of patients achieving 7 points or more in the UCLA-Score (10/26 patients) displayed that patients after cementless medial OUKR were able to reach a high level of impact sports.

In a meta-analysis by Witjes et al., the postoperative activity in 8 studies of patients receiving cemented UKR and 13 studies of patients receiving TKR was analysed. They found that the postoperative return-to-activity-rate as well as the level of activity were higher after cemented UKR than after TKR. They reported return-to-activity-rates between 75 - >100% in the UKR group and 36–89% in the TKR group. Our results indicate that cementless OUKR also allows patients high return- to-activity-rates compared to cemented UKR [25]. Although other authors presume that the effects of the learning curve, regarding the implantation of Oxford UKR, might affect the postoperative outcome and therefore the physical activity, our results show similar physical activity compared to cemented implantation [26, 27].

Our return-to-activity-rate showed higher values compared to studies about Oxford medial UKR, which range between 80.1% and 97% [3, 11, 28, 29]. In a retrospective study on the activity after cemented OUKR with a follow-up of 4.2 years, Pietschmann et al. reported a return-to-activity rate of 80.1% [3]. Possible reasons include the larger patient cohort and the high age of

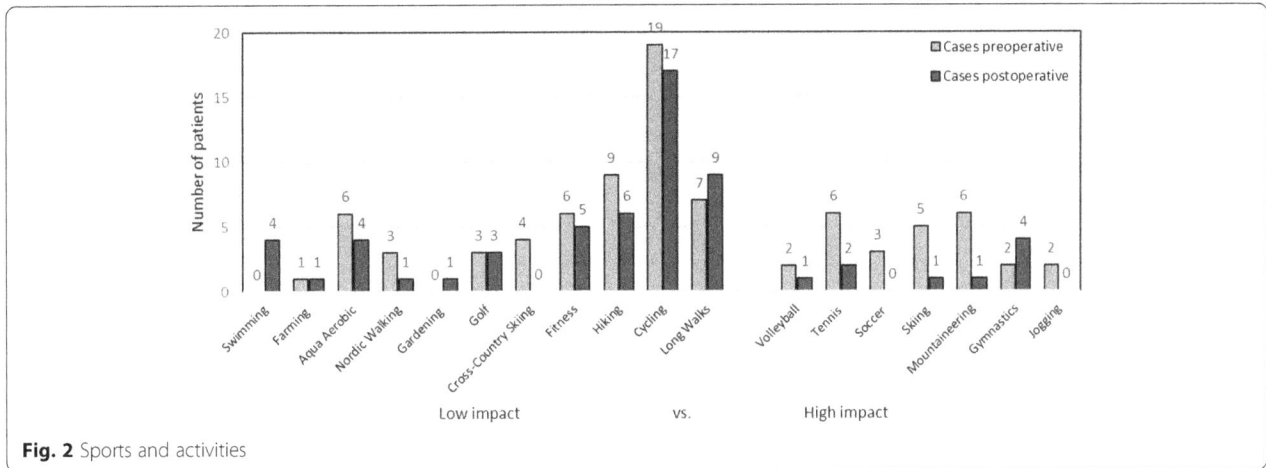

Fig. 2 Sports and activities

treated patients (131 patients with a mean age of 65.3 years compared to 27 patients with a mean age of 62.5 years). They split the patient collective into an active and an inactive group and found the active group to be significantly younger than the inactive group. They referred to the results of the "German Health Survey" 2006, which showed that activity decreased significantly in patients over 70 years of age. At five-year follow-up, the average patient in our study was 67.5 years old, compared to 69.5 years in Pietschmann's study. Walker et al. reported a return-to-activity rate of 93% in patients of sixty years or younger after medial UKR. Almost two thirds reached postoperative UCLA-Scores >7 [11]. This matches the excellent outcome of our study with almost half of the collective being younger than sixty years. However, we did not detect a significant difference in the activity levels of patients older and younger than median age (data not shown).

In our study, patients did recover quickly after cementless OUKR, which supports literature findings [25, 30]. Price et al. showed minimal-invasive OUKR patients to recover twice as fast as standard incision UKR patients and three times as fast as TKR patients [31]. More than 60% of the patients in our study had picked up sports already during 3 months after surgery and 90% within the first 6 months.

Another finding of the present study is the high rate of patients without pain during sports (22 out of 26, 85%). Others have reported on the amount of patients being pain-free during activity ranging between 57% and 76% after cemented OUKR [11, 29]. A possible explanation for these different findings might be a shorter follow-up time of approximately 2 years compared to the five-year follow-up in our study.

In our study, UCLA-Score improved significantly from 4.9 points preoperatively to 6.1 points postoperatively ($p = 0.042$). This matches the findings of other studies: Fisher et al. reported an improvement from 4.2 to 6.5 points [28]. Generally, postoperative UCLA-Scores range from 6.1 to 6.8 points [11, 25, 32, 33]. Tegner-Score values are the only activity-related item that was published so far on cementless medial OUKR. In the randomized controlled trial, Pandit et al. compared cementless- with cemented OUKR. They reported an improvement from 1.9 points preoperatively to 3.1 points 2 years after implantation and 2.9 points at five-year follow-up in the cementless group. At 2 years follow-up, the Tegner-Score was significantly higher in the cementless group compared to the cemented group, but the difference did not persist until 5 years after surgery [19]. Tegner Score in our study was 2.9 points preoperatively and 3.4 points postoperatively at a mean follow up of 5 years, with a significant improvement ($p = 0.042$).

Concerning the extent, frequency and length of activities in our study, we found that there was no significant decrease after surgery compared to the time before the onset of OA symptoms. Our findings match the results

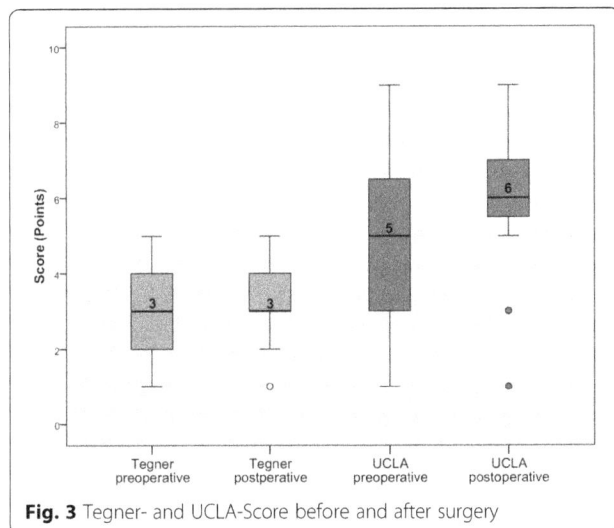

Fig. 3 Tegner- and UCLA-Score before and after surgery

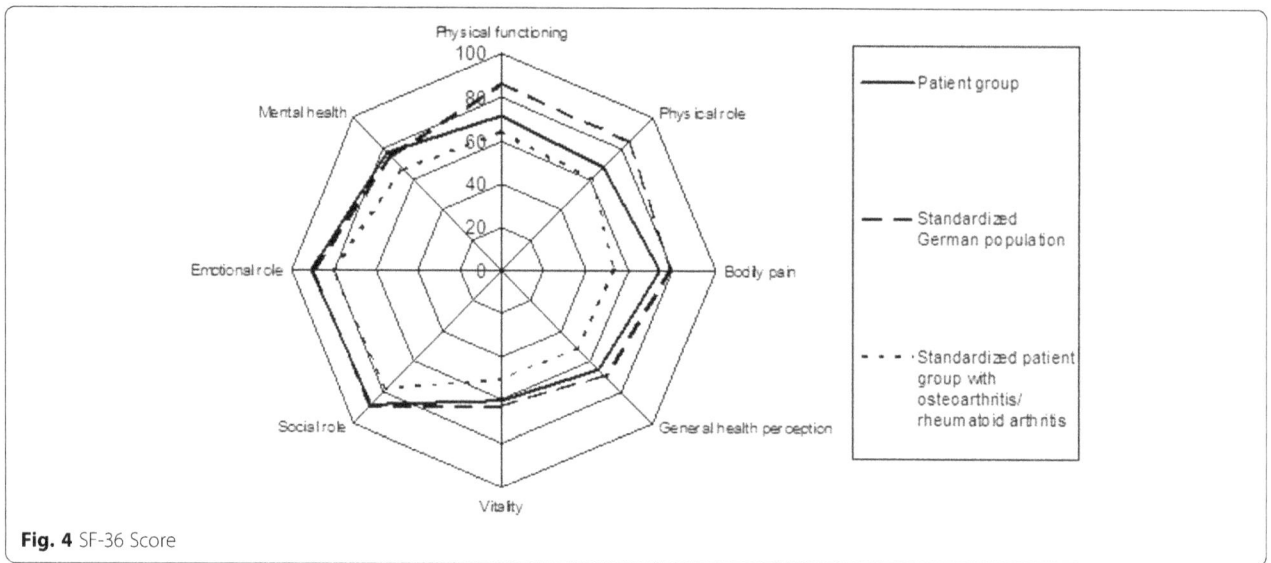

Fig. 4 SF-36 Score

of other authors assessing activity after cemented OUKR as well as activity after cementless Total Hip Arthroplasty [11, 34].

Sports were divided into high-impact (with high peak loads in the joints) and low-impact forms (with constant low joint loads). In contrast to other authors assessing postoperative activity after UKR, we did not find a significant increase or decrease in any type of sports after surgery. There are several authors reporting a significant decrease of high-impact sports after surgery, while low-impact sports tend to increase [2, 3, 11, 35]. The reason for this is might be attributed to multiple causes such as the surgeon's recommendations, lack of function, feeling of insecurity, pain, comorbidities etc. Asked for their reasons to abandon high-impact sports, the majority of patients in a study by Walker et al. named "precaution" (59%) and "less motivation" (20%), while pain only followed fourth with 9% [30]. Although there is no final conclusion on the best type of sports for patients after joint replacement, there seems to be a general consensus from surgeons to discourage patients from high-impact sports such as soccer and tennis [36]. Supporting this position, there is indication that high-impact sports lead to high joint loads and can thereby increase implant wear followed by a higher rate of complications and revisions [36, 37]. Mobile-bearing devices such as the cementless OUKR are known to minimize wear due to the fully congruent mobile bearing [38, 39]. In accordance with these findings, although the postoperative level of activity was high, there were no revisions due to implant wear in this five-year follow-up study. Pietschmann et al. report that although they noticed a significant decrease in high-impact sports, they did not detect a correlation between high impact sports and complication. General activity is necessary to maintain

cardiovascular fitness and bone density. There are several studies indicating that bone density depends on frequency of activity as well as on the imposed skeletal forces, indicating that impact up to a certain level has positive effects on bone density and should not generally be discouraged [40–42].

Assessing the quality of life, our patients reported excellent results. Regarding the physical dimensions, they accomplished higher values than the reference group suffering from OA/ rheumatoid arthritis. In the emotional-social domains of SF-36, they reached the same or better scores than the healthy reference population. Naal et al. compared the findings of their population to a matched reference group and they achieved significantly higher scores in every domain [2]. A possible explanation for the higher scores could be higher preoperative scores of their collective or the short time between surgery and questioning (18 months). Recently operated patients tend to remember their state before surgery more easily. Both studies showed high SF-36 Scores and were comparable with the findings of Walker et al., who investigated activity after cemented OUKR in patients ≤60 years of age [11].

In the present study, in accordance with literature, patients reported a high satisfaction rate with the outcome of the joint replacement [3, 11].

Superior radiological osseointegration and no cement associated complications seem to be a clear advantage of cementless fixation, especially desirable for young and active patients. However, possible early intra and postoperative complications associated with cementless OUKR like periprosthetic fractures and valgus subsidence might impair early return to sports and activity. Overall these complications are rare and appear to be rather influenced by mistakes in the surgical technique [15, 16].

Main limitation of this study is the small number of patients. We did not collect preoperative SF-36 data which makes the efficacy of cementless OUKR hard to compare to other author's findings, but as we aimed to compare the postoperative quality of life with a healthy reference group, we think that the conclusions are not impaired.

Furthermore, although the scores and questionnaires used in our study (Tegner, UCLA, Schulthess Clinical Activity Questionnaire) are validated for the evaluation of physical activity, it is a difficult to quantify and compare the results as many parameters can only be answered using a free text, which makes subcategorization difficult. Activity cannot be reduced to one parameter only, thus comparison of many aspects of activity is necessary. However, patients' subjective perceptions of sports capability may be an outcome measure that outweighs the supposed objective parameters of physical activity.

Another major weakness of this study besides the retrospective design might be selection bias since the patients were recruited within a 3-year time period (2007–2009) between the first and last inclusion.

The strength of this study is its detailed information at a mean follow-up of 5 years. Not only UCLA- and Tegner Score were measured, but also individual information about sports disciplines, frequency and length of activity. This is the first study to give detailed information about sports and activity after cementless medial OUKR. No patient died or was lost to follow-up.

Conclusions

This study demonstrates that patients treated with cementless OUKR achieve high activity levels after surgery. Furthermore, patients seem to participate in the same sports activities than before onset of OA. Cementless OUKR allows fast recovery and a high return-to-activity rate. Quality of life was excellent compared to the healthy reference group.

Abbreviations
ACL: Anterior Cruciate Ligament; OA: Osteoarthritis; OUKR: Oxford Unicompartimental Knee Replacement; PFA: Patello Femoral Arthroplasty; PFJ: Patello Femoral Joint; UKR: Unicompartimental Knee Replacement

Acknowledgements
Not applicable

Funding
This research did not receive any specific grant from funding agencies in the public, commercial, or not-for-profit sectors.

Authors' contributions
BP, IB, TG and SH contributed to study conception and design. BP, IB, TR and TW contributed to the acquisition of data. BP, IB, TG, TW and SH contributed to analysis and interpretation of data. BP, IB, TG drafted the manuscript. All authors critically revised the manuscript. All authors read and approved the final manuscript.

Consent for publication
Not applicable

Competing interests
TG and TW received payment from Zimmer Biomet as a Principal Investigator outside of this submitted work.

References
1. No authors listed (c) (2013) National Joint Registry for England, Wales and Northern Ireland: 10th Annual Report 2013.. http://www.njrcentre.org.uk/njrcentre/Portals/0/Documents/England/Reports/10th_annual_report/NJR%2010th%20Annual%20Report%202013%20B.pdf.
2. Naal FD, Fischer M, Preuss A, et al. Return to sports and recreational activity after unicompartmental knee arthroplasty. Am J Sports Med. 2007;35(10):1688–95.
3. Pietschmann MF, Wohlleb L, Weber P et al. (2013) Sports activities after medial unicompartmental knee arthroplasty Oxford III-what can we expect? Int Orthop 37 (1):31-37.
4. Amin AK, Patton JT, Cook RE, et al. Unicompartmental or total knee arthroplasty?: results from a matched study. Clin Orthop Relat Res. 2006;451:101–6.
5. Brown NM, Sheth NP, Davis K, et al. Total knee arthroplasty has higher postoperative morbidity than unicompartmental knee arthroplasty: a multicenter analysis. J Arthroplast. 2012;27(8 Suppl):86–90.
6. Laurencin CT, Zelicof SB, Scott RD, et al. Unicompartmental versus total knee arthroplasty in the same patient. A comparative study. Clin Orthop Relat Res. 1991;273:151–6.
7. Price AJ, Waite JC, Svard U. Long-term clinical results of the medial Oxford unicompartmental knee arthroplasty. Clin Orthop Relat Res. 2005;435:171–80.
8. Pandit H, Jenkins C, Barker K, et al. The Oxford medial unicompartmental knee replacement using a minimally-invasive approach. J Bone Joint Surg Br. 2006;88(1):54–60.
9. Lisowski LA, van den Bekerom MP, Pilot P, et al. Oxford phase 3 unicompartmental knee arthroplasty: medium-term results of a minimally invasive surgical procedure. Knee Surg Sports Traumatol Arthrosc. 2011;19(2):277–84.
10. Price AJ, Dodd CA, Svard UG, et al. Oxford medial unicompartmental knee arthroplasty in patients younger and older than 60 years of age. J Bone Joint Surg Br. 2005;87(11):1488–92.
11. Walker T, Streit J, Gotterbarm T, et al. Sports, physical activity and patient-reported outcomes after medial Unicompartmental knee Arthroplasty in young patients. J Arthroplasty. 2015;30(11):1911–6. https://doi.org/10.1016/j.arth.2015.05.031.
12. Kort NP, van Raay JJ, van Horn JJ. The Oxford phase III unicompartmental knee replacement in patients less than 60 years of age. Knee Surg Sports Traumatol Arthrosc. 2007;15(4):356–60.
13. Price AJ, Svard U. A second decade lifetable survival analysis of the Oxford unicompartmental knee arthroplasty. Clin Orthop Relat Res. 2011;469(1):174–9.
14. Pandit H, Jenkins C, Beard DJ, et al. Cementless Oxford unicompartmental knee replacement shows reduced radiolucency at one year. J Bone Joint Surg Br. 2009;91(2):185–9.
15. Seeger JB, Haas D, Jager S, et al. Extended sagittal saw cut significantly reduces fracture load in cementless unicompartmental knee arthroplasty compared to cemented tibia plateaus: an experimental cadaver study. Knee Surg Sports Traumatol Arthrosc. 2012;20(6):1087–91.
16. Liddle AD, Pandit HG, Jenkins C, et al. Valgus subsidence of the tibial component in cementless Oxford unicompartmental knee replacement. Bone Joint J. 2014;96-B(3):345–9.
17. Akan B, Karaguven D, Guclu B, et al. Cemented versus Uncemented Oxford Unicompartimental knee Arthroplasty: is there a difference? Adv Orthop. 2013;2013:245915.

18. Liddle AD, Pandit H, O'Brien S, et al. Cementless fixation in Oxford unicompartmental knee replacement: a multicentre study of 1000 knees. Bone Joint J. 2013;95-B(2):181–7.

19. Pandit H, Liddle AD, Kendrick BJ, et al. Improved fixation in cementless unicompartmental knee replacement: five-year results of a randomized controlled trial. J Bone Joint Surg Am. 2013;95(15):1365–72.

20. Rothwell A, Hobbs, T., Frampton, C. (2012) The New Zealand joint registry. Thirteen year report: New Zeeland Orthopaedic Association. January 1999 to December 2011http://nzoa.org.nz/system/files/ NJR%2013%20Year%20Report.pdf.

21. Panzram B, Bertlich I, Reiner T, et al. Results after Cementless medial Oxford Unicompartmental knee replacement - incidence of radiolucent lines. PLoS One. 2017;12(1):e0170324.

22. Pandit H, Jenkins C, Gill HS, et al. Unnecessary contraindications for mobile-bearing unicompartmental knee replacement. J Bone Joint Surg Br. 2011; 93(5):622–8.

23. Goodfellow JW, Kershaw CJ, Benson MK, et al. The Oxford knee for unicompartmental osteoarthritis. The first 103 cases. J Bone Joint Surg Br. 1988;70(5):692–701.

24. Chang MJ, Kim SH, Kang YG, et al. Activity levels and participation in physical activities by Korean patients following total knee arthroplasty. BMC Musculoskelet Disord. 2014;15:240.

25. Witjes S, Gouttebarge V, Kuijer PP, et al. Return to sports and physical activity after Total and Unicondylar knee Arthroplasty: a systematic review and meta-analysis. Sports Med. 2016;46(2):269–92.

26. Robertsson O, Knutson K, Lewold S, et al. The routine of surgical management reduces failure after unicompartmental knee arthroplasty. J Bone Joint Surg Br. 2001;83(1):45–9.

27. Rees JL, Price AJ, Beard DJ, et al. Minimally invasive Oxford unicompartmental knee arthroplasty: functional results at 1 year and the effect of surgical inexperience. Knee. 2004;11(5):363–7.

28. Fisher N, Agarwal M, Reuben SF, et al. Sporting and physical activity following Oxford medial unicompartmental knee arthroplasty. Knee. 2006;13(4):296–300.

29. Hopper GP, Leach WJ. Participation in sporting activities following knee replacement: total versus unicompartmental. Knee Surg Sports Traumatol Arthrosc. 2008;16(10):973–9.

30. Walker T, Gotterbarm T, Bruckner T, et al. Return to sports, recreational activity and patient-reported outcomes after lateral unicompartmental knee arthroplasty. Knee Surg Sports Traumatol Arthrosc. 2015;23(11):3281–7.

31. Price AJ, Webb J, Topf H, et al. Rapid recovery after oxford unicompartmental arthroplasty through a short incision. J Arthroplast. 2001;16(8):970–6.

32. Jahnke A, Mende JK, Maier GS, et al. Sports activities before and after medial unicompartmental knee arthroplasty using the new Heidelberg sports activity score. Int Orthop. 2015;39(3):449–54.

33. Felts E, Parratte S, Pauly V, et al. Function and quality of life following medial unicompartmental knee arthroplasty in patients 60 years of age or younger. Orthop Traumatol Surg Res. 2010;96(8):861–7.

34. Innmann MM, Weiss S, Andreas F, et al. Sports and physical activity after cementless total hip arthroplasty with a minimum follow-up of 10 years. Scand J Med Sci Sports. 2016;26(5):550–6. https://doi.org/10.1111/sms.12482.

35. Wylde V, Blom A, Dieppe P, et al. Return to sport after joint replacement. J Bone Joint Surg Br. 2008;90(7):920–3.

36. Swanson EA, Schmalzried TP, Dorey FJ. Activity recommendations after total hip and knee arthroplasty: a survey of the American Association for hip and Knee Surgeons. J Arthroplast. 2009;24(6 Suppl):120–6.

37. Ollivier M, Frey S, Parratte S, et al. Does impact sport activity influence total hip arthroplasty durability? Clin Orthop Relat Res. 2012;470(11):3060–6.

38. Price AJ, Short A, Kellett C, et al. Ten-year in vivo wear measurement of a fully congruent mobile bearing unicompartmental knee arthroplasty. J Bone Joint Surg Br. 2005;87(11):1493–7.

39. Kendrick BJ, Longino D, Pandit H, et al. Polyethylene wear in Oxford unicompartmental knee replacement: a retrieval study of 47 bearings. J Bone Joint Surg Br. 2010;92(3):367–73.

40. Bassey EJ, Ramsdale SJ. Increase in femoral bone density in young women following high-impact exercise. Osteoporos Int. 1994;4(2):72–5.

41. Whalen RT, Carter DR, Steele CR. Influence of physical activity on the regulation of bone density. J Biomech. 1988;21(10):825–37.

42. Scerpella TA, Davenport M, Morganti CM, et al. Dose related association of impact activity and bone mineral density in pre-pubertal girls. Calcif Tissue Int. 2003;72(1):24–31.

14

Comparison between autologous blood transfusion drainage and closed-suction drainage/ no drainage in total knee arthroplasty

Kun-hao Hong[1†], Jian-ke Pan[2†], Wei-yi Yang[2†], Ming-hui Luo[2], Shu-chai Xu[2] and Jun Liu[2*]

Abstract

Background: Autologous blood transfusion (ABT) drainage system is a new unwashed salvaged blood retransfusion system for total knee replacement (TKA). However, whether to use ABT drainage, closed-suction (CS) drainage or no drainage in TKA surgery remains controversial. This is the first meta-analysis to assess the clinical efficiency, safety and potential advantages regarding the use of ABT drains compared with closed-suction/no drainage.

Methods: PubMed, Embase, and the Cochrane Library were comprehensively searched in March 2015. Fifteen randomized controlled trials (RCTs) were identified and pooled for statistical analysis. The primary outcome evaluated was homologous blood transfusion rate. The secondary outcomes were post-operative haemoglobin on days 3–5, length of hospital stay and wound infections after TKA surgery.

Results: The pooled data included 1,721 patients and showed that patients in the ABT drainage group might benefit from lower blood transfusion rates (16.59 % and 37.47 %, OR: 0.28 [0.14, 0.55]; 13.05 % and 16.91 %, OR: 0.73 [0.47,1.13], respectively). Autologous blood transfusion drainage and closed-suction drainage/no drainage have similar clinical efficacy and safety with regard to post-operative haemoglobin on days 3–5, length of hospital stay and wound infections.

Conclusions: Autologous blood transfusion drainage offers a safe and efficient alternative to CS/no drainage with a lower blood transfusion rate. Future large-volume high-quality RCTs with extensive follow-up will affirm and update this system review.

Keywords: Knee arthroplasty, Knee replacement, Autologous blood transfusion, Closed-suction, Drainage, Drains

Background

Total knee arthroplasty (TKA) is a highly successful standard procedure for patients who suffer serious knee arthralgia, instability and deformity. It is used after non-surgical treatments are exhausted, especially in advanced knee osteoarthritis [1, 2]. However, TKA can result in significant blood loss, reduction in haemoglobin (Hb) and other clinical risks [3, 4]. Reports of blood transfusion rates of 39 %–50 % have been published [5–7].

Autologous blood transfusion (ABT) drainage system is a new unwashed salvaged blood retransfusion system for primary TKA. However, whether to use ABT drainage, closed-suction (CS) drainage or no drainage in TKA surgery is still controversial. Some studies have found that ABT significantly reduced the need for homologous blood [8, 9], but other research has questioned the benefits of this method [10, 11] or demonstrated that post-TKA ABT had a limited effect on blood conservation [12, 13]. While gaining worldwide acceptance [14] for effectively decreasing hematoma formation [15, 16], conventional suction drains have been theoretically thought to decrease postoperative pain, swelling and incidence of infection [17]. However, a closed suction drainage system

* Correspondence: liujun.gdtcm@hotmail.com
Kun-hao Hong, Jian-ke Pan and Wei-yi Yang are co-first author
†Equal contributors
[2]Department of Orthopedic Surgery, Second School of Clinical Medicine, Guangzhou University of Chinese Medicine, No. 111 Dade Road,, Guangzhou, Guangdong 510120, China
Full list of author information is available at the end of the article

inevitably increases bleeding because the tamponade effect of a closed undrained wound is eliminated [14].

Until now, no systematic reviews incorporating meta-analyses (SRMA) have found sufficient evidence to recommend ABT drainage or no drainage in primary TKA. This is the first SRMA to systematically compare the clinical results of ABT drainage with closed-suction (CS)/no drainage in patients undergoing TKA. Previous SRMAs comparing ABT drainage versus CS drainage and CS drainage versus no drainage were published as the standard in evidence-based medicine with conflicting results [6, 18, 19]. Quinn et al. [19] showed that ABT drainage was superior to CS drainage for reducing blood transfusion rate (OR: 0.25 [0.13, 0.47]; $P < 0.0001$), and length of hospital stay (WMD: -0.25 [-0.48, -0.01]; $P = 0.04$). However, data extraction errors occurred in two included studies [20, 21] when extracting the number of patients requiring homologous blood transfusion for the meta-analysis. Another flaw is that in meta-analysis extracted data without intention-to-treat (ITT) analysis, treatment effectiveness may be exaggerated. The previous meta-analysis also did not evaluate other outcome measures like wound complication and post-operative haemoglobin on days 3–5. The aim of this SRMA was to pool extracted data from available published RCTs to provide a directly substantiated judgment regarding the use of ABT drainage following TKA surgery.

Methods

In accordance with Preferred Reporting Items for Systematic Reviews and Meta-analysis (Additional file 1) [22], we made a prospective protocol of objectives, literature-search strategies, inclusion and exclusion criteria, outcome measurements and methods of statistical analysis before the research began.

Data sources and search strategies

The following databases were searched in March 2015 without restriction to regions and publication types: Pubmed (1950–March 2015), Embase (1974–March 2015) and Cochrane Library (March 2015 Issue 3) (Additional file 2). The MeSH terms and their combinations searched in [Title/Abstract] was as follows: "total knee replacement" OR "total knee arthroplasty" OR "total knee prosthesis" OR "unicompartmental" OR "unicondylar" OR "arthroplasty, replacement, knee" [MeSH term] AND ("autologous blood transfusion" OR "autotransfusion" OR "blood transfusion, autologous" [MeSH Terms] OR "intra-operative blood salvage" OR "intraoperative blood" OR "postoperative blood salvage" OR "intraoperative blood cell salvage" OR "operative blood salvage" [MeSH Terms]). The reference lists of related reviews and original articles identified for any relevant studies, including randomized controlled trials (RCTs) involving adult humans

were reviewed. The search also included the Controlled Trials Register (http://www.controlled-trials.com). Only articles originally written in English or translated into English were considered. When multiple reports describing the same situation were published, the most recent or complete report was used.

Inclusion and exclusion criteria

Two independent researchers (Pan and Yang) identified studies that met the defined inclusion criteria, with disagreements resolved by consensus (Hong and Liu). Inclusion criteria were: (1) the comparison was between ABT drainage and CS/no drainage post TKA; (2) at least one of the quantitative outcomes we determined to evaluate was reported; (3) study design was a RCT; and (4) full text was published in English. Non-original research (e.g. review article, editorials, letter to the editor), case reports, animal experimental studies and duplicated publications were excluded.

Data extraction and analysis

The data from eligible studies were extracted by two researchers (Hong and Pan) independently to minimize errors and reduce potential biases. In cases of disagreement, a consensus was reached by the adjudicating senior authors (Yang and Liu). The extracted data was input into a computerized spreadsheet, including sample size, study design, patient age, gender, preoperative/postoperative Hb levels, number of patients transfused with homologous blood, length of hospital stay and wound infection. The primary outcome was homologous blood transfusion rate. The secondary outcomes were postoperative haemoglobin on days 3–5, length of hospital stay and wound infection.

Quality assessment and data synthesis

The RCTs were graded according to criteria of the Centre for Evidence-Based Medicine in Oxford, UK [23]. The quality of the RCTs; methodology was evaluated by the Cochrane risk of bias tool [24].

The statistical analysis was conducted with Cochrane Collaboration Review Manager 5.3.5 (Cochrane Collaboration, Oxford, UK). Our analyses were based on ITT or modified ITT data. Odds risk (OR) with 95 % confidence intervals (CIs) was calculated for dichotomous data and weighted mean differences (WMD) with 95 % CIs for continuous data. Statistical heterogeneity was assessed by using the chi-square test and I2 statistic. A random-effects model was used when significant heterogeneity was detected between studies without clinical diversity ($P < 0.10$; I2 > 50 %). Otherwise, a fixed-effect model was performed [24]. In cases with I^2 values greater than 50 % for outcome measures, sensitivity analyses were conducted for

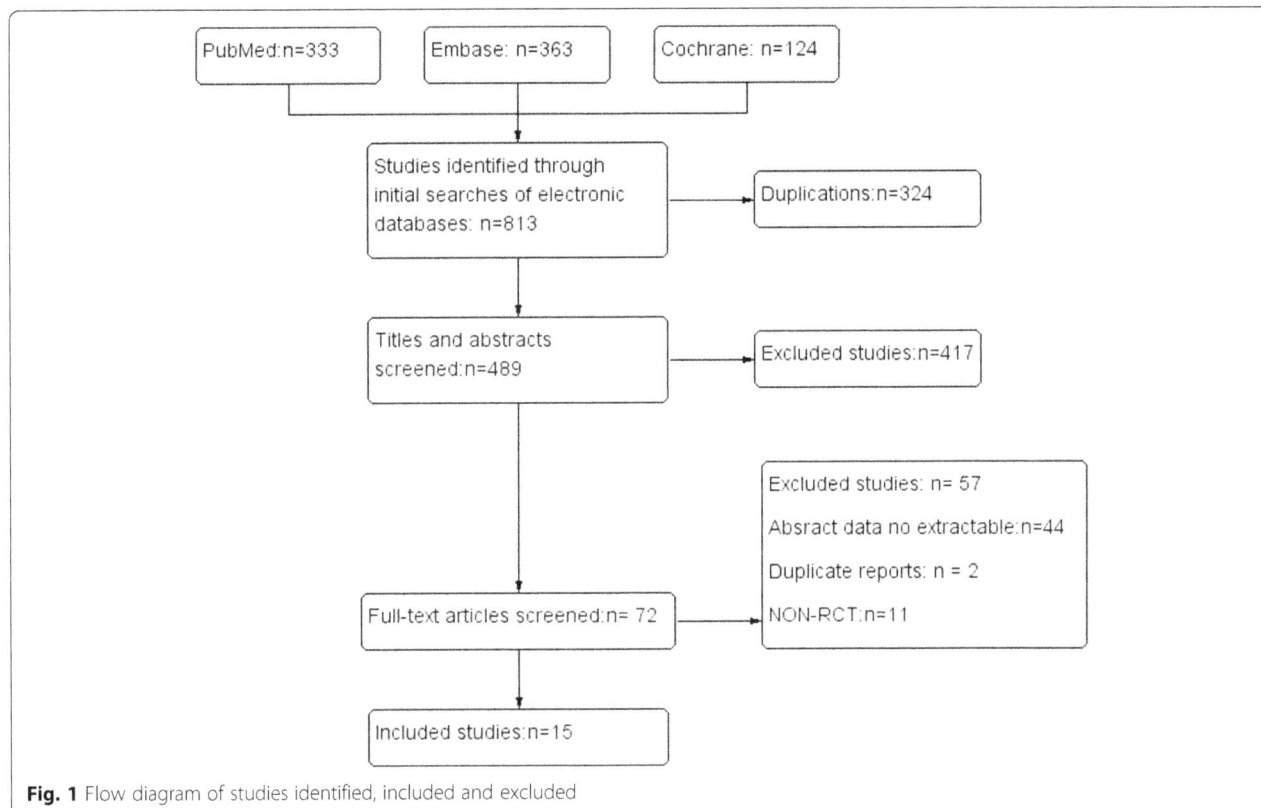

Fig. 1 Flow diagram of studies identified, included and excluded

Table 1 Characteristics of included studies

Study	LOE[a]	Patients, no.			Surgical method	Age[a]			M:F ratio			Pre-op Hb[a]		
		A	B	C		A	B	C	A	B	C	A	B	C
Amin A 2008 [11]	1b	92	86	—	SU-TKA	70.3	70.4	—	43:49	39:47	—	13.2 (1.2)	13.4(1.3)	—
Zacharopoulos A 2007 [25]	2b	30	30	—	SU-TKA	69.2	70.2	—	6:24	7:23	—	NA	NA	—
Abuzakuk T 2007 [10]	1b	52	52	—	SU-TKA	NA	NA	—	21:31	22:30	—	13.6(1.5)	13.5(1.2)	—
Kirkos JM 2006 [27]	2b	78	77	—	SU-TKA	69.1(5.5)	68.9(5.1)	—	18:60	10:67	—	13.0(1.4)	13.1(1.4)	—
Dramis A 2006 [26]	2b	25	24	—	SU-TKA	NA	NA	—	NA	NA	—	NA	NA	—
Cheng SC 2005 [28]	1b	26	34	—	SU-TKA	72	69.6	—	6:20	12:22	—	12.4	12.8	—
Thomas D 2001 [29]	1b	115	116	—	SU-TKA	NA	NA	—	44:71	55:61	—	NA	NA	—
Adalberth G 1998 [20]	1b	30	30	30	SU-TKA	71(5.4)	72(8)	71(1.3)	NA	NA	NA	13.8(1.1)	14.3(1.3)	14.2(2.6)
Newman J 1997 [30]	2b	35	35	—	SU-TKA	NA	NA	—	NA	NA	—	13.4 ± 1.2	13.2 ± 1.4	—
Heddle NM 1992 [21]	1b	39	40	—	SU-TKA	69.3(6.9)	71(9)	—	25:14	26:14	—	NA	NA	—
Majkowski RS 1991 [31]	1b	20	20	—	SU-TKA	71.3	70.3	—	6:14	6:14	—	13.2	12.7	—
Horstmann W 2014 [33]	1b	59	—	56	SU-TKA	68(9)	—	69(8)	17:24		39:17	14(1.4)	—	14(1.4)
Dutton T 2012 [34]	2b	23	—	25	SU-TKA	68.7	—	70.5	10:13		10:15	NA	—	NA
Thomassen BJ 2014 [32]	1b	88	—	87	SU-TKA	68.9	—	69.5	NA	NA	NA	14.2	—	14.2
Ritter MA 1994 [35]	2b	128	—	123	SU-TKA	NA	—	NA	NA	NA	NA	13.0	—	13.1

LOE Level of evidence, *SU-TKA* selective unilateral total knee replacement, *B-TKA* bilateral total knee replacement
A autologous blood transfusion drainage, *B* conventional suction drain, *C* No drainage, *NA* data not available;. — = without this group ; [a]Mean or Mean(SD)

heterogeneity. When overall results and conclusions are not affected by the different decisions that could be made during the review process, the results of the review can be regarded with a higher degree of certainty [24]. Funnel plots were used to identify potential publication bias.

Results

Fifteen studies [10, 11, 20, 21, 25–35], all full-text articles in English including 1,721 cases (840 ABT drainage, 544 closed-suction drainage and 337 no drainage), were selected for synthesis analysis (Fig. 1, Table 1).

Characteristics of included studies

The demographic characteristics of the 15 studies are presented in Table 1.

The majority of the RCTs reviewed were moderate-quality studies. Among the included studies, there were nine RCTs [10, 11, 20, 21, 28, 29, 31–33] with a 1b level of evidence and six RCTs [25–27, 30, 34, 35] with a 2b level of evidence. Figures 2 and 3 showed the methodological quality of RCTs assessed by the Cochrane risk of bias tool. True randomization was used in only nine RCTs [10, 11, 20, 21, 28, 30, 32, 34, 35], while five RCTs [25, 26, 29, 31, 32] did not mention the method of randomization and one RCT [27] used quasi-randomization. Five studies [20, 28, 32–34] mentioned the method of allocation concealment. One study [28] provided information about blinding for participants. One study [33] mentioned the blinding of outcome assessments. Fourteen studies [10, 11, 20, 21, 25–29, 31–35] reported the complete analysis. One study [30] was at high risk on selective reporting.

Primary outcomes

Homologous blood transfusion rate

Fourteen studies [10, 11, 20, 21, 25, 26, 28–35] compared the effect of ABT drainage versus closed-suction drainage/no drainage according to changes in the number of patients requiring homologous blood transfusion. The meta–analysis of ABT versus CS drainage groups [10, 11, 20, 21, 25, 26, 28–31] showed substantial heterogeneity in the consistency of results (Chi^2 = 34.04, $P < 0.0001$; I^2 = 74 %). Sensitivity analyses were conducted with different decisions of excluding a study. When excluding the study [30] without clinical diversity detected, the heterogeneity was reduced (I^2 = 59 %, $P = 0.01$). The result of sensitivity analysis was similar to the total analysis. Therefore, the random effects model showed a significant beneficial effect of ABT compared to CS drainage in reducing the blood transfusion rate (16.59 % and 37.47 %, OR: 0.28 [0.14, 0.55]; Z = 3.67, $P < 0.0001$) (Fig. 4). The meta-analysis of ABT versus no drainage groups [20, 32–35] showed no heterogeneity in the consistency of results (Chi^2 = 1.22, $P = 0.87$; I^2 = 0 %) and no significant difference in reducing the

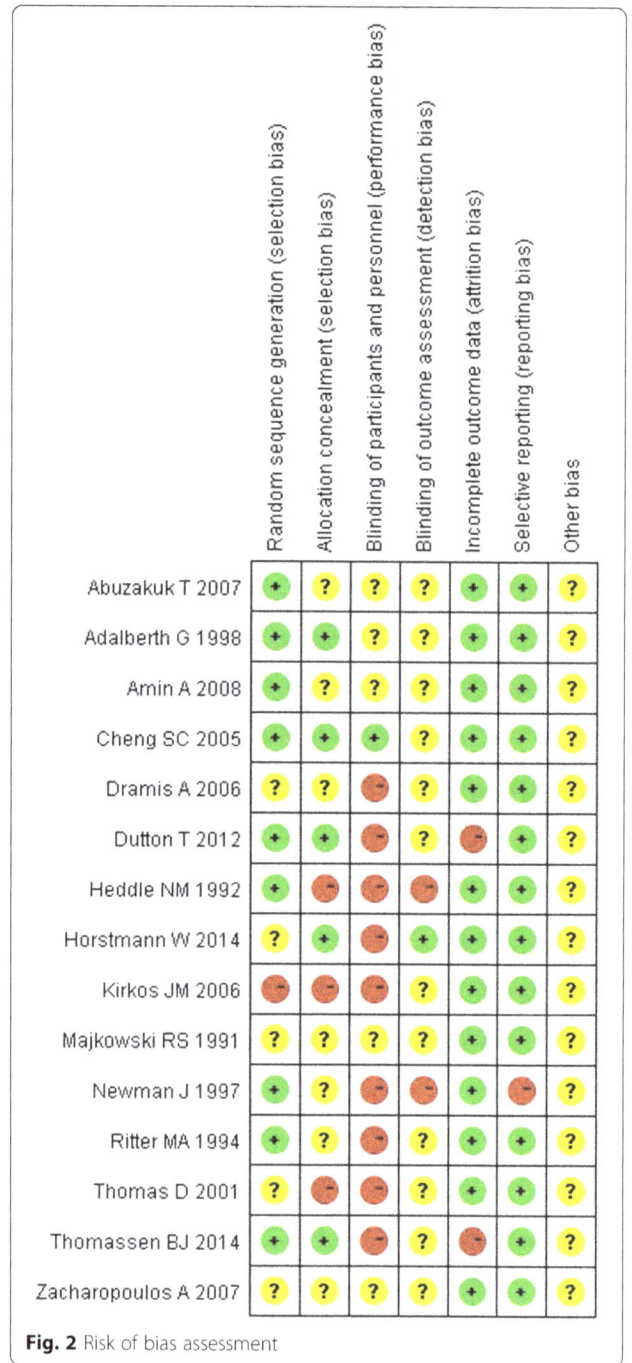

Fig. 2 Risk of bias assessment

blood transfusion rate (13.05 % and 16.91 %, OR: 0.73 [0.47, 1.13], Z = 1.41, $P = 0.16$) (Fig. 4). However, a 3.86 % reduction in blood transfusion rate when comparing ABT drainage directly to no drainage should be given attention.

Secondary outcomes

Post-operative haemoglobin on days 3–5

Four studies [10, 11, 20, 33] reported post-operative haemoglobin on days 3–5. Among them, one study [10]

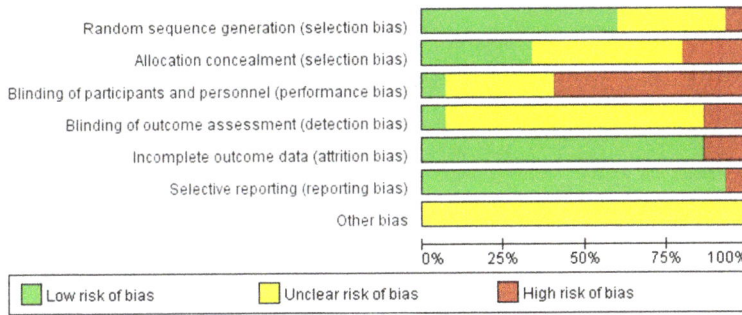

Fig. 3 Risk of bias summary

only reported haemoglobin on the fifth day post-operation, while the other study reported haemoglobin only on the third day post-operation. Pooling the data of the 342 patients in the ABT versus CS drainage groups showed no significant difference (WMD: 0.25 [−0.06, 0.56] ; Z = 1.56, P = 1.2) (Fig. 5). No significant heterogeneity in this group was detected (P = 0.42, I^2 = 0 %). The meta-analysis of ABT versus no drainage group showed substantial heterogeneity in the consistency of results (Chi^2 = 2.50, P = 0.11; I^2 = 60 %). For two studies, sensitivity analyses were not necessary with no clinical diversity identified. The random effects model of meta-analysis in the group showed no significant beneficial effect of ABT drainage compared with

no drainage in post-operative haemoglobin on days 3–5 (WMD: 0.41 [−0.26, 1.09] ; Z = 1.20, P = 0.23).

Length of hospital stay

Pooling the data from four studies [10, 20, 30, 33] that assessed length of hospital stay in 339 patients showed no significant difference in the ABT versus CS drainage and ABT versus no drainage groups (WMD: −0.962 [−2.09, 0.17]; Z = 1.67, P = 0.01; WMD: 0.07 [−0.67, 0.81], Z = 0.19, P = 0.85, respectively). The comparison of ABT versus CS drainage group showed substantial heterogeneity in the consistency of trial results (Chi^2 = 4.14, P = 0.13; I^2 = 52 %). Owing to marked heterogeneity within the evaluated length of hospital stay, sensitivity analyses were conducted by

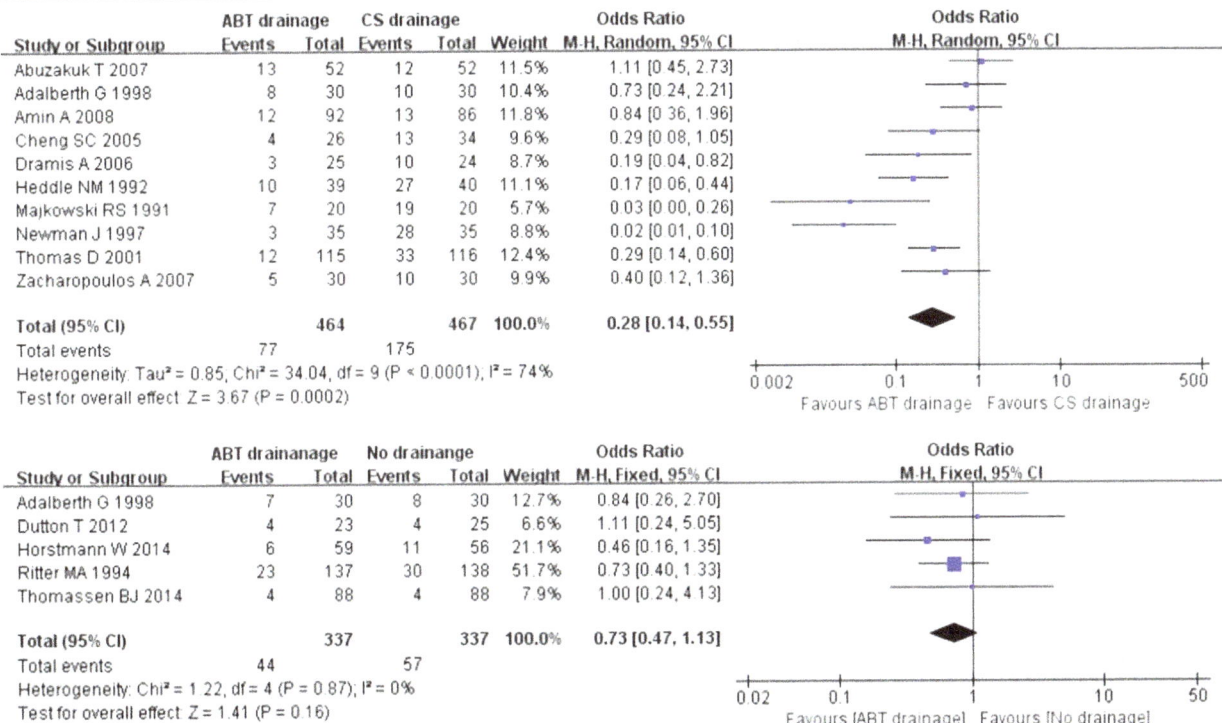

Fig. 4 Forest plot and meta-analysis of homologous blood transfusion rate

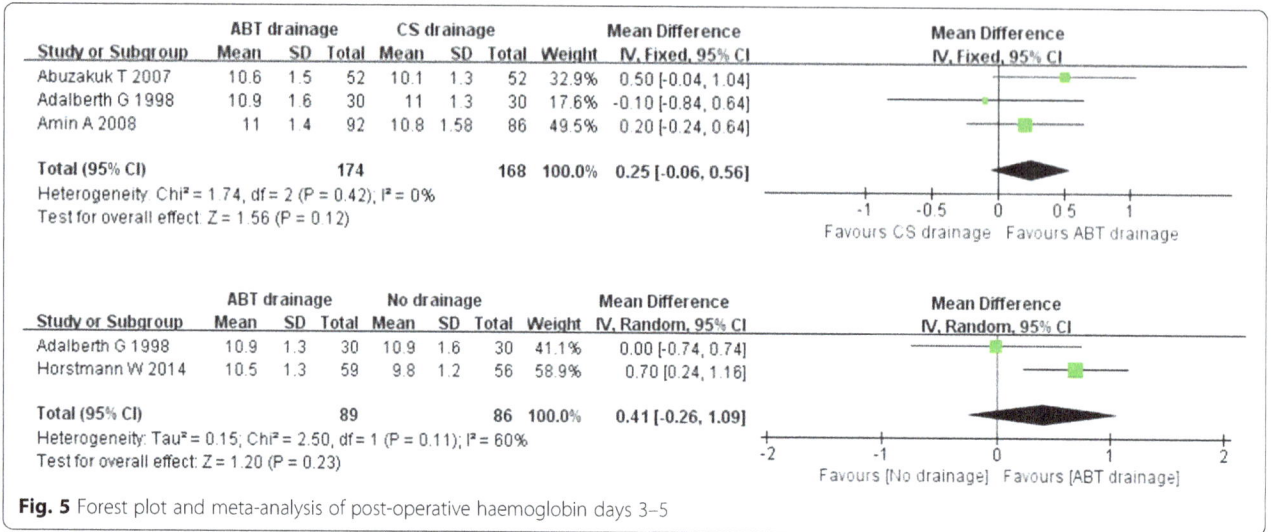

Fig. 5 Forest plot and meta-analysis of post-operative haemoglobin days 3–5

excluding one study [10] with lower quality. Then, no significant heterogeneity was detected ($P = 0.32$, $I^2 = 0$ %) and there was also no significant difference between the ABT and CS drainage groups in length of hospital stay (WMD: -0.52 [-1.30, 0.25]; $Z = 1.33$, $P = 0.18$). However, no significant heterogeneity was detected in the ABT drainage versus no drainage groups ($Chi^2 = 0.01$, $P = 0.90$, $I^2 = 0$ %). (Fig. 6).

Wound infection

Four studies [11, 29, 31, 35] reported the complication of wound infection. The result showed no heterogeneity in the consistency of results in ABT versus CS drainage groups ($Chi^2 = 0.80$, $P = 0.66$; $I^2 = 0$ %). Pooling the data of the 444 patients in the ABT versus CS drainage group and the 275 patients in the ABT versus no drainage group showed no significant difference

between ABT drainage and closed-suction/no drainage (OR: -0.98 [0.40, 2.38] ; $Z = 0.04$, $P = 0.97$; OR: 1.01 [0.06, 16.27] , $Z = 0.01$, $P = 1.00$, respectively) (Fig. 7).

Publication bias

Figure 8 shows a funnel plot of the included studies that reported homologous blood transfusion rates. All studies lie inside the 95 % CIs except two studies, with an asymmetric distribution around the vertical indicating presence of obvious publication bias. This obvious publication bias is for the beneficial effect of lowering blood transfusion rate.

Discussion

This SRMA of 15 studies including 1,721 patients comparing the clinical efficacy and safety of ABT drainage and closed-suction/no drainage showed significant statistical

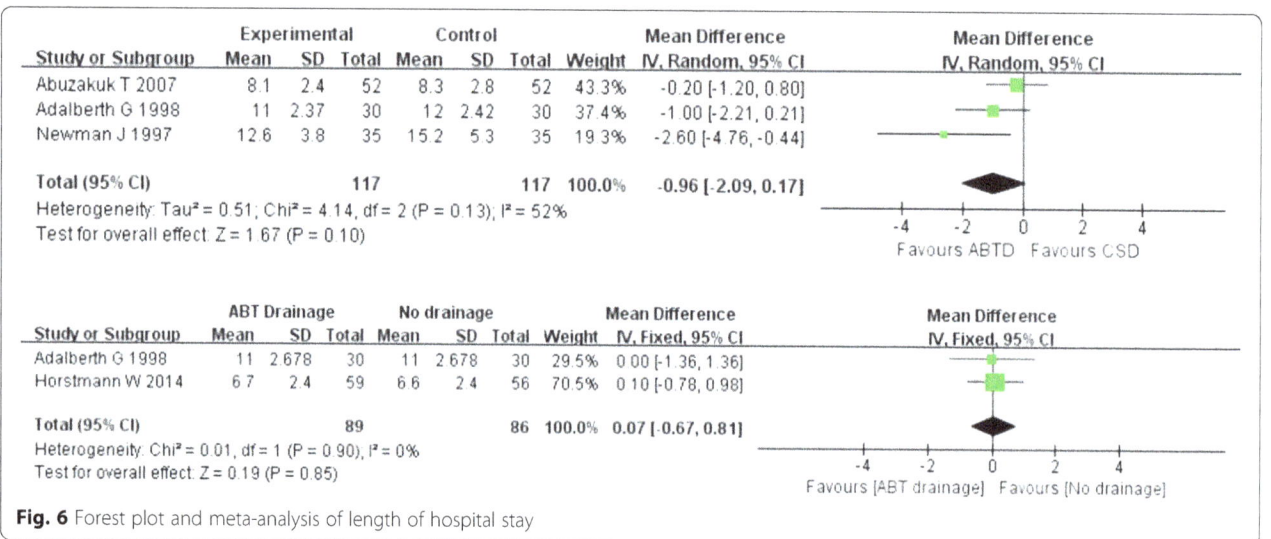

Fig. 6 Forest plot and meta-analysis of length of hospital stay

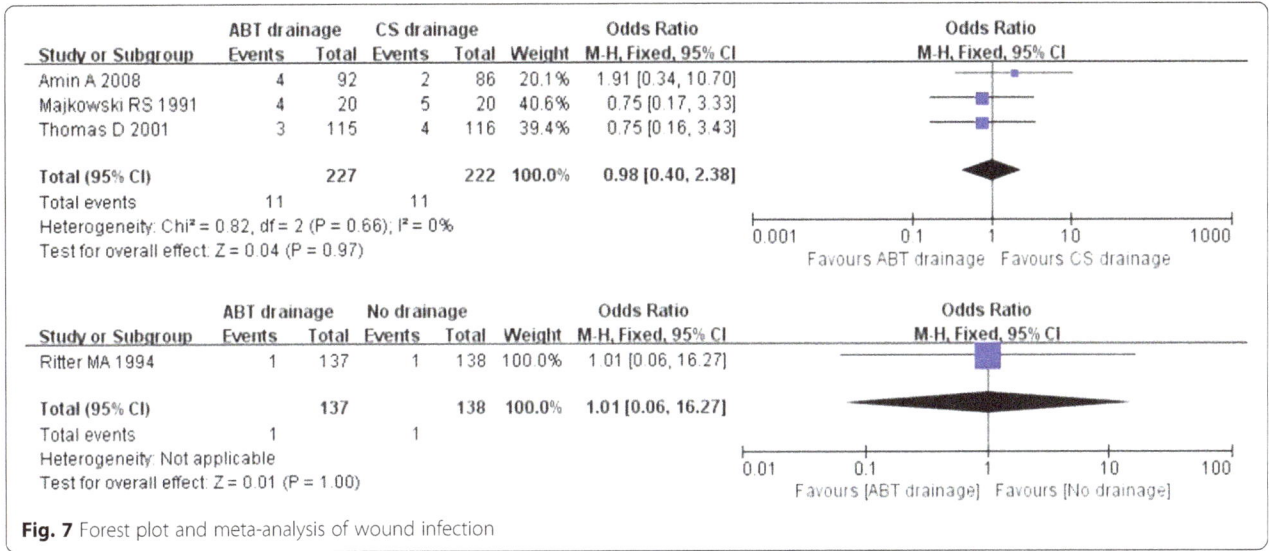

Fig. 7 Forest plot and meta-analysis of wound infection

differences in homologous blood transfusion rates and similar clinical efficacy and safety in post-operative haemoglobin on days 3–5, length of hospital stay and wound infection in post-TKA patients.

With recent techniques, ABT drainage post TKA manifests the attractive concept of retransfusing collected drainage blood and continues to be a controversial issue in TKA surgery. Some studies have published considerable doubt with respect to its advantages [16, 36]. Despite the advantageous results, including reduced homologous blood transfusion rates shown in some studies [29, 37, 38], some authors have suggested insufficient efficiency for ABT

[10, 39]. In spite of the paucity of consistent evidence, for many years the majority of orthopaedic procedures were followed by the use of ABT drainage post TKA to reduce the blood transfusion rate. However, the present systematic review and meta-analysis demonstrate a significant beneficial effect of ABT drainage in reducing the blood transfusion rate. The result of this meta-analysis showed no significant difference in post-operative haemoglobin on days 3–5. As those patients who received allogenic blood were not excluded from this analysis and there was a higher rate of allogenic blood transfusion in the closed suction drainage group compared with the

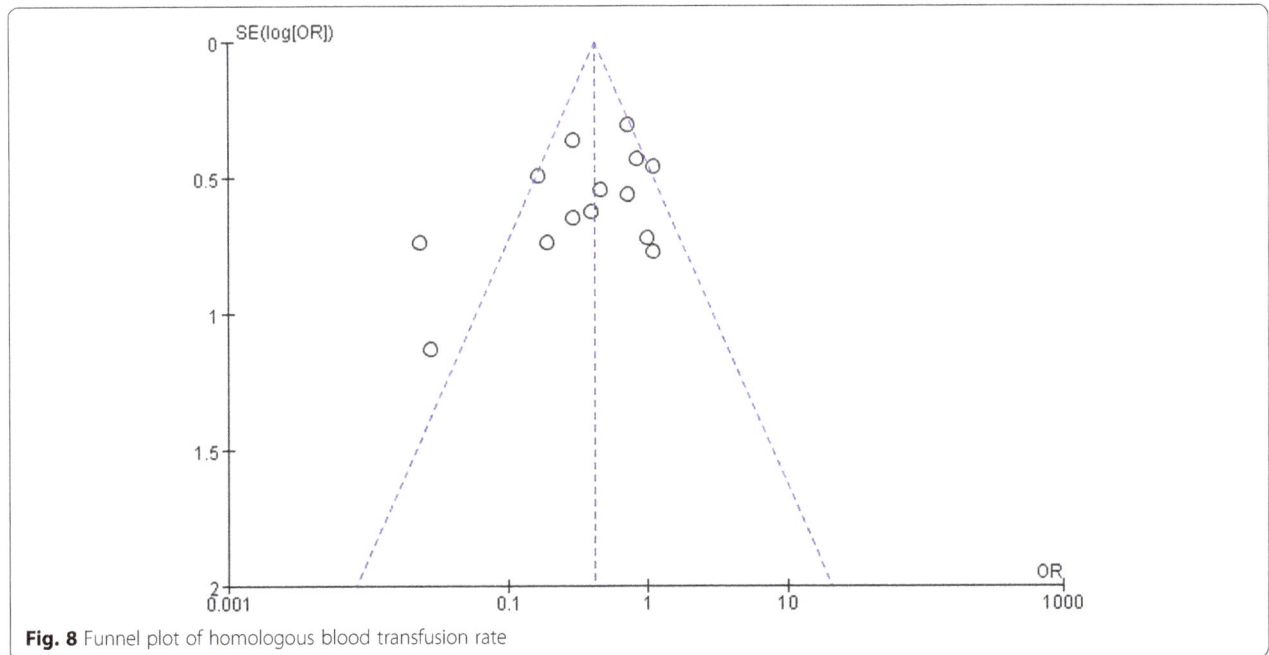

Fig. 8 Funnel plot of homologous blood transfusion rate

ABT drainage group, it cannot be ascertained whether this is owing to a failure in ABT drainage to produce a beneficial effect on post-operative haemoglobin or to the positive nature of allogenic blood on haemoglobin levels. With the application of any new medical device, the safety of the patients is always of paramount importance. Acting as a channel for the introduction of infection, drainage may increase infection risk by impairing host resistance and allowing pathogens access to a sterile field [16, 17, 40]. The demands on nursing care and physiotherapy are increased to accommodate the presence of drainage. In orthopaedic surgery, wound infection is a devastating complication. However, the pooled data of postoperative outcomes indicated that the ABT drainage equipment was safe and effective for TKA. There was no significant difference in wound complication and length of hospital stay. This finding indicates that ABTD is as safe and efficient as CS/no drainage.

Some possible limitations of this meta-analysis and future research directions should be noted. The primary limitation is that the selected RCTs in this meta-analysis were moderate-quality studies with small sample sizes. With fewer included studies in the outcome analysis, the statistical heterogeneity assessments, including I^2 text, were able to make false negative errors. Future systematic reviews should evaluate the indications from literature from sufficient, larger multi-centre clinical studies. In addition, this meta-analysis limited the included articles to those published in English. There might be selection bias in language. Finally, no long-term outcome measures were assessed, which is most pertinent to patients [41]. Therefore, other outcomes like range of movement, deep joint infection and component loosening, which are manifested after many years, should be considered.

Conclusions

To our knowledge, this is the first SRMA to systematically compare the results of ABT drainage with closed-suction drainage/no drainage in patients undergoing TKA. The pooled results demonstrated that ABT drainage was more efficacious than CS drainage in clinically reducing blood transfusion rate. This meta-analysis also indicated that ABT drainage and closed-suction drainage/no drainage had similar clinical efficacy and safety with regard to post-operative haemoglobin on days 3–5, length of hospital stay and wound infection. Nevertheless, in spite of our rigorous methodology, the inherent limitations of eligible studies prevented us from reaching definitive conclusions. Based on the above clinical equipoise and potential benefit, future large-volume high-quality RCTs with long-term measures are awaited to affirm and update this system review.

Abbreviations

TKA: total knee arthroplasty; ABT: autologous blood transfusion; CS: closed-suction; SRMA: systematic reviews incorporating meta-analyses; RCT: randomized controlled trial; ITT: intent-to-treat; OR: odds risk; WMD: weighted mean differences; CI: confidence interval.

Competing interests

The authors declare that they have no competing interests.

Authors' contributions

Conceived and designed the SRMA: JL. Performed the SRMA: KHH, JKP, WYY. Analyzed the data: KHH, JKP, WYY, MHL, SCX, JL. Contributed reagents/materials/analysis tools: KHH, JKP, WYY, JL. Drafting the manuscript: KHH. All authors read and approved the final manuscript.

Acknowledgements

This study was funded by National Natural Science Foundation of China (No. 81473698, No. 81273781), TCM Standardization Projects of State Administration of Traditional Chinese Medicine of China (No. SATCM-2015-BZ115, SATCM-2015-BZ173), Project of Guangdong Provincial Department of Finance (No. [2014] 157), Science and Technology Research Project of Guangdong Provincial Hospital of Chinese Medicine (No. YK2013B2N19).

Author details

Department of Orthopedic Surgery, Guangdong Second Traditional Chinese Medicine Hospital, No. 60 Hengfu Road, Guangzhou, Guangdong 510095, China. ²Department of Orthopedic Surgery, Second School of Clinical Medicine, Guangzhou University of Chinese Medicine, No. 111 Dade Road,, Guangzhou, Guangdong 510120, China.

References

1. Visser AW, de Mutsert R, Bloem JL, Reijnierse M, Kazato H, le Cessie S, den Heijer M, Rosendaal FR, Kloppenburg M. Knee osteoarthritis and fat free mass interact in their impact on health-related quality of life in men: The Netherlands Epidemiology of Obesity study. Arthrit Care Res. 2015;67(7): 981–8.
2. Alkan BM, Fidan F, Tosun A, Ardicoglu O. Quality of life and self-reported disability in patients with knee osteoarthritis. Mod Rheumatol. 2014;24(1):166–71.
3. Keating EM, Meding JB, Faris PM, Ritter MA. Predictors of transfusion risk in elective knee surgery. Clin Orthop Relat Res. 1998;357:50–9.
4. Torres-Claramunt R, Hinarejos P, Pérez-Prieto D, Gil-González S, Pelfort X, Leal J, Puig L. Sealing of the intramedullary femoral canal in a TKA does not reduce postoperative blood loss: A randomized prospective study. Knee. 2014;21(4):853–7.
5. Bidolegui F, Arce G, Lugones A, Pereira S, Vindver G. Tranexamic acid reduces blood loss and transfusion in patients undergoing total knee arthroplasty without tourniquet: a prospective randomized controlled trial. Open Orthop J. 2014;8:250–4.
6. Markar SR, Jones GG, Karthikesalingam A, Segaren N, Patel RV. Transfusion drains versus suction drains in total knee replacement: meta-analysis. Knee Surgery Sports Traumatol Arthrosc. 2012;20(9):1766–72.
7. Bierbaum BE, Callaghan JJ, Galante JO, Rubash HE, Tooms RE, Welch RB. An analysis of blood management in patients having a total hip or knee arthroplasty. J Bone Joint Surg Am. 1999;81(1):2–10.
8. Tsumara N, Yoshiya S, Chin T, Shiba R, Kohso K, Doita M. A prospective comparison of clamping the drain or post-operative salvage of blood in reducing blood loss after total knee arthroplasty. J Bone Joint Surg Br. 2006;88(1):49–53.
9. Steinberg EL, Ben-Galim P, Yaniv Y, Dekel S, Menahem A. Comparative analysis of the benefits of autotransfusion of blood by a shed blood collector after total knee replacement. Arch Orthop Traum Su. 2004;124(2):114–8.

10. Abuzakuk T, Senthil Kumar V, Shenava Y, Bulstrode C, Skinner JA, Cannon SR, Briggs TW. Autotransfusion drains in total knee replacement. Are they alternatives to homologous transfusion? Int Orthop. 2007;31(2):235–9.

11. Amin A, Watson A, Mangwani J, Nawabi DH, Ahluwalia R, Loeffler M. A prospective randomised controlled trial of autologous retransfusion in total knee replacement. J Bone Joint Surg Br. 2008;90(4):451–4.

12. Strümper D, Weber E, Gielen Wijffels S, Van Drumpt R, Bulstra S, Slappendel R, Durieux M, Marcus M. Clinical efficacy of postoperative autologous transfusion of filtered shed blood in hip and knee arthroplasty. Transfusion. 2004;44(11):1567–71.

13. So-Osman C, Nelissen RGHH, Eikenboom HCJ, Brand A. Efficacy, safety and user-friendliness of two devices for postoperative autologous shed red blood cell re-infusion in elective orthopaedic surgery patients: a randomized pilot study. Transfusion Med. 2006;16(5):321–8.

14. Tai T, Chang C, Yang C. The role of drainage after total knee arthroplasty. INTECH Open Access Publisher; 2012

15. Drinkwater CJ, Neil MJ. Optimal timing of wound drain removal following total joint arthroplasty. J Arthroplasty. 1995;10(2):185–9.

16. Holt BT, Parks NL, Engh GA, Lawrence JM. Comparison of closed-suction drainage and no drainage after primary total knee arthroplasty. Orthopedics. 1997;20(12):1121–4. 1124-1125.

17. Kim YH, Cho SH, Kim RS. Drainage versus nondrainage in simultaneous bilateral total knee arthroplasties. Clin Orthop Relat Res. 1998;347:188–93.

18. Haien Z, Yong J, Baoan M, Mingjun G, Qingyu F. Post-operative auto-transfusion in total hip or knee arthroplasty: a meta-analysis of randomized controlled trials. Plos One. 2013;8(1):e55073.

19. Quinn M, Bowe A, Galvin R, Dawson P, O'Byrne J. The use of postoperative suction drainage in total knee arthroplasty: a systematic review. Int Orthop. 2015;39(4):653–8.

20. Adalberth G, Bystrom S, Kolstad K, Mallmin H, Milbrink J. Postoperative drainage of knee arthroplasty is not necessary: a randomized study of 90 patients. Acta Orthop Scand. 1998;69(5):475–8.

21. Heddle NM, Brox WT, Klama LN, Dickson LL, Levine MN. A randomized trial on the efficacy of an autologous blood drainage and transfusion device in patients undergoing elective knee arthroplasty. Transfusion. 1992;32(8):742–6.

22. Liberati A, Altman DG, Tetzlaff J, Mulrow C, Gotzsche PC, Ioannidis JP, Clarke M, Devereaux PJ, Kleijnen J, Moher D. The PRISMA statement for reporting systematic reviews and meta-analyses of studies that evaluate healthcare interventions: explanation and elaboration. BMJ. 2009;339:b2700.

23. Phillips B, Ball C, Sackett D, Badenoch D, Straus S, et al. Levels of evidence and grades of recommendation. Oxford Centre for Evidence-based Medicine Web site http://www.cebm.net/index.aspx?o=1025. Accessed April 22,2015.

24. Higgins JPT, Green S. Cochrane Handbook for Systematic Reviews of Interventions Version 5.1.0 [updated March 2011]. The Cochrane Collaboration, 2011. Available from. http://handbook.cochrane.org/.

25. Zacharopoulos A, Apostolopoulos A, Kyriakidis A. The effectiveness of reinfusion after total knee replacement. A prospective randomised controlled study. Int Orthop. 2007;31(3):303–8.

26. Dramis A, Plewes J. Autologous blood transfusion after primary unilateral total knee replacement surgery. Acta Orthop Belg. 2006;72(1):15.

27. Kirkos JM, Krystallis CT, Konstantinidis PA, Papavasiliou KA, Kyrkos MJ, Ikonomidis LG. Postoperative re-perfusion of drained blood in patients undergoing total knee arthroplasty: is it effective and cost-efficient? Acta Orthop Belg. 2006;72(1):18–23.

28. Cheng SC, Hung TS, Tse PY. Investigation of the use of drained blood reinfusion after total knee arthroplasty: a prospective randomised controlled study. J Orthop Surg (Hong Kong). 2005;13(2):120–4.

29. Thomas D, Wareham K, Cohen D, Hutchings H. Autologous blood transfusion in total knee replacement surgery. Br J Anaesth. 2001;86(5):669–73.

30. Newman JH, Bowers M, Murphy J. The clinical advantages of autologous transfusion. A randomized, controlled study after knee replacement. J Bone Joint Surg Br. 1997;79(4):630–2.

31. Majkowski RS, Currie IC, Newman JH. Postoperative collection and reinfusion of autologous blood in total knee arthroplasty. Ann Roy Coll Surg. 1991;73(6):381–4.

32. Thomassen BJ, den Hollander PH, Kaptijn HH, Nelissen RG, Pilot P. Autologous wound drains have no effect on allogeneic blood transfusions in primary total hip and knee replacement: a three-arm randomised trial. Bone Joint J. 2014;96-B(6):765–71.

33. Horstmann W, Kuipers B, Ohanis D, Slappendel R, Kollen B, Verheyen C. Autologous re-transfusion drain compared with no drain in total knee arthroplasty: a randomised controlled trial. Blood Transfus. 2014;12 Suppl 1:s176–81.

34. Dutton T, De-Souza R, Parsons N, Costa ML. The timing of tourniquet release and 'retransfusion' drains in total knee arthroplasty: A stratified randomised pilot investigation. Knee. 2012;19(3):190–2.

35. Ritter MA, Keating EM, Faris PM. Closed wound drainage in total hip or total knee replacement. A prospective, randomized study. J Bone Joint Surg Am. 1994;76(1):35–8.

36. Esler CNA, Blakeway C, Fiddian NJ. The use of a closed-suction drain in total knee arthroplasty. J Bone Joint Surg. 2003;85(2):215–7.

37. Muñoz M, Ariza D, Garcerán MJ, Gómez A, Campos A. Benefits of postoperative shed blood reinfusion in patients undergoing unilateral total knee replacement. Arch Orthop Traum Su. 2005;125(6):385–9.

38. Carless P, Moxey A, O'Connell D, Henry D. Autologous transfusion techniques: a systematic review of their efficacy. Transfus Med. 2004;14(2):123–44.

39. Hansen E, Hansen MP. Reasons against the retransfusion of unwashed wound blood. Transfusion. 2004;44(12 Suppl):45S–53.

40. Zamora-Navas P, Collado-Torres F, de la Torre-Solis F. Closed suction drainage after knee arthroplasty. A prospective study of the effectiveness of the operation and of bacterial contamination. Acta Orthop Belg. 1999;65(1):44–7.

41. Greidanus NV, Peterson RC, Masri BA, Garbuz DS. Quality of life outcomes in revision versus primary total knee arthroplasty. J Arthroplasty. 2011;26(4):615–20.

15

Hospital volume and the risk of revision in Oxford unicompartmental knee arthroplasty in the Nordic countries

Mona Badawy[1*], Anne M. Fenstad[2], Christoffer A. Bartz-Johannessen[2], Kari Indrekvam[1,3], Leif I. Havelin[2,3], Otto Robertsson[4,5], Annette W-Dahl[4,5], Antti Eskelinen[6], Keijo Mäkelä[7], Alma B. Pedersen[8,9], Henrik M. Schrøder[10] and Ove Furnes[2,3]

Abstract

Background: High procedure volume and dedication to unicompartmental knee arthroplasty (UKA) has been suggested to improve revision rates. This study aimed to quantify the annual hospital volume effect on revision risk in Oxfordu nicompartmental knee arthroplasty in the Nordic countries.

Methods: 14,496 cases of cemented medial Oxford III UKA were identified in 126 hospitals in the four countries included in the Nordic Arthroplasty Register Association (NARA) database from 2000 to 2012. Hospitals were divided by quartiles into 4 annual procedure volume groups ($\leq$11, 12-23, 24-43 and $\geq$44). The outcome was revision risk after 2 and 10 years calculated using Kaplan Meier method. Multivariate Cox regression analysis was used to assess the Hazard Ratio (HR) of any revision due to specific reasons with 95% confidence intervals (CI).

Results: The implant survival was 80% at 10 years in the volume group $\leq$11 procedures per year compared to 83% in other volume groups. The HR adjusted for age category, sex, year of surgery and nation was 0.87 (95% CI: 0.76-0.99, $p = 0.036$) for the group 12-23 procedures per year, 0.78 (95% CI: 0.68-0.91, $p = 0.002$) for the group 24-43 procedures per year and 0.82 (95% CI: 0.70-0.94, $p = 0.006$) for the group $\geq$44 procedures per year compared to the low volume group. Log-rank test was $p = 0.003$. The risk of revision for unexplained pain was 40-50% higher in the low compared with other volume groups.

Conclusion: Low volume hospitals performing $\leq$11 Oxford III UKAs per year were associated with an increased risk of revision compared to higher volume hospitals, and unexplained pain as revision cause was more common in low volume hospitals.

Keywords: Knee, Osteoarthritis, Arthroplasty, Unicompartmental, Procedure volume, Revision causes

Background

The Oxford unicompartmental knee arthroplasty (UKA) has been investigated in numerous studies due to the deviant results comparing registry results to studies from high volume centers and surgeons. Data from national registries show a significantly higher revision rate for both short and long term results for UKA than for total knee arthroplasty (TKA) [1–5]. Other studies from high-volume Oxford developing centers, however, show excellent long-term results [6, 7]. The existing variability in practice regarding indication and usage of UKA results in low volumes in hospitals using strict criteria [8], and higher volumes in hospitals offering UKA to patients using less strict criteria [9]. The Nordic Arthroplasty Register Association is a collaboration of arthroplasty registers in Sweden, Denmark, Norway and Finland established in 2007. The cooperation has produced a

* Correspondence: mona.badawy@helse-bergen.no
The article is written according to the STROBE guidelines and the RECORD Statement.
[1]Coastal Hospital, 5253 Hagavik, Norway
Full list of author information is available at the end of the article

common defined set of variables agreed upon, enabling analyses of larger statistical material [10]. This is an advantage especially for uncommon methods and procedures, such as the UKA constituting only 11% of the knee arthroplasties in the Nordic countries [11]. The advantage of a registry study for our purpose was the representation of all surgeons in all hospitals in Sweden, Denmark, Finland and Norway resulting in more generalizable findings. The UKA is utilized at similar lower percentage than TKA in the majority of countries with registries worldwide for the treatment of osteoarthritis [2, 12]. The aim of this study was to investigate how the patient risk for revision surgery after Oxford III UKA varied as a function of hospital procedure volume. Adding to the analyses for all causes of revision, the second objective was to assess any differences in the proportion of the specific causes of revision according to volume groups.

Methods

Data sources

We used the NARA database, containing a common defined code set to identify patients undergoing primary cemented medial Oxford III UKA between January 1, 2000 and December 31, 2012 in this population-based register study [11, 13]. Every year all uniform variables from each national register are re-coded according to common definitions and anonymized and then merged into the NARA database. The linkage between primary procedure and subsequent revision or death on individual data is performed in each national register before merged into the NARA database. The first studies focused on differences in patient demographics, surgical methods and implant brands [10, 11, 14]. The main purpose of NARA was the ability to analyze a larger statistical material, which is an advantage especially for uncommon methods and implants. It reflects the current practice in 4 different countries. The knee dataset currently includes 390,525 primary knee arthroplasty operations performed during 1995-2012 [13]. The Oxford UKA was the most commonly registered UKA implant in the NARA.

Study population

Implant brand and type could be a source of confounding in comparison to revision rate according to hospital, and therefore all other brands and types than Oxford III UKA were excluded. Diagnoses other than osteoarthritis (OA) were excluded as inflammatory disease is a contraindication in UKA. The inclusion criteria for this study, to obtain comparable groups for analysis, are shown in the flowchart (Fig. 1). In NARA revision is defined as removal/exchange/addition of one or more implant

component(s) and is linked to the primary procedure by the unique national identification number of the patient.

We identified 4211 (29.0%) Oxford III implants in Denmark in 32 different hospitals: 2218 (15.3%) in Sweden distributed among 18 hospitals, 3910 (27.0%) in Finland in 41 hospitals and 4157 (28.7%) in Norway in 35 hospitals (Table 1). The inclusion of bilateral knee arthroplasty can be a violation of the assumption of independent observations in survival analyses, but studies have shown that the effect is minor regarding statistical precision for survival analysis of knee replacements [15]. In this study, 14% of the patients had bilateral knee arthroplasty.

Exposure

All Oxford III UKA procedures were entered into one of four different annual hospital volume groups. We used quartiles to divide into equal numbered volume groups; ≤11, 12-23, 24-43 and ≥44 procedures per year. Hospitals with inconsistent procedure volume over time may have contributed to different volume groups according to the number of procedures at their hospital in the year of surgery. Thus, for each hospital each year was examined individually. This categorization of the exposure assumes that unspecified hospital-level effects are trumped by a potential volume effect on revision rates. Revision due to any reason as well as specific causes for revision was analysed.

Statistics

Survival analyses were performed with any revision of the implant as endpoint. Kaplan Meier cumulative survival at 2 and 10 years was reported. A 2 year follow-up was chosen to assess early revisions. The follow-up started at the day of primary UKA procedure and ended at the day of first revision, death, emigration or the end of follow-up time (December 31st 2012). The two highest volume groups had shorter follow-up compared to the lower (chi-square test p-value <0.001). Log-rank test was performed, p = 0.003. Differences for categorical variables such as sex, age categories, year of surgery and nations were assessed by Pearson's chi-squared test. Any p-values less than 0.05 were considered significant. To estimate differences in continuous variables the student t-test was used.

The Cox regression model was used to calculate Hazard Ratios (HR) with 95% confidence interval (CI) for the 10 year follow-up period to investigate the association between four hospital procedure volume groups and implant survival time. P-values were presented relative to the lowest volume group (≤ 11). All p-values less than 0.05 were considered to be statistically significant. The Cox model included sex, age category, year of surgery, nation and hospital volume. Death is to be

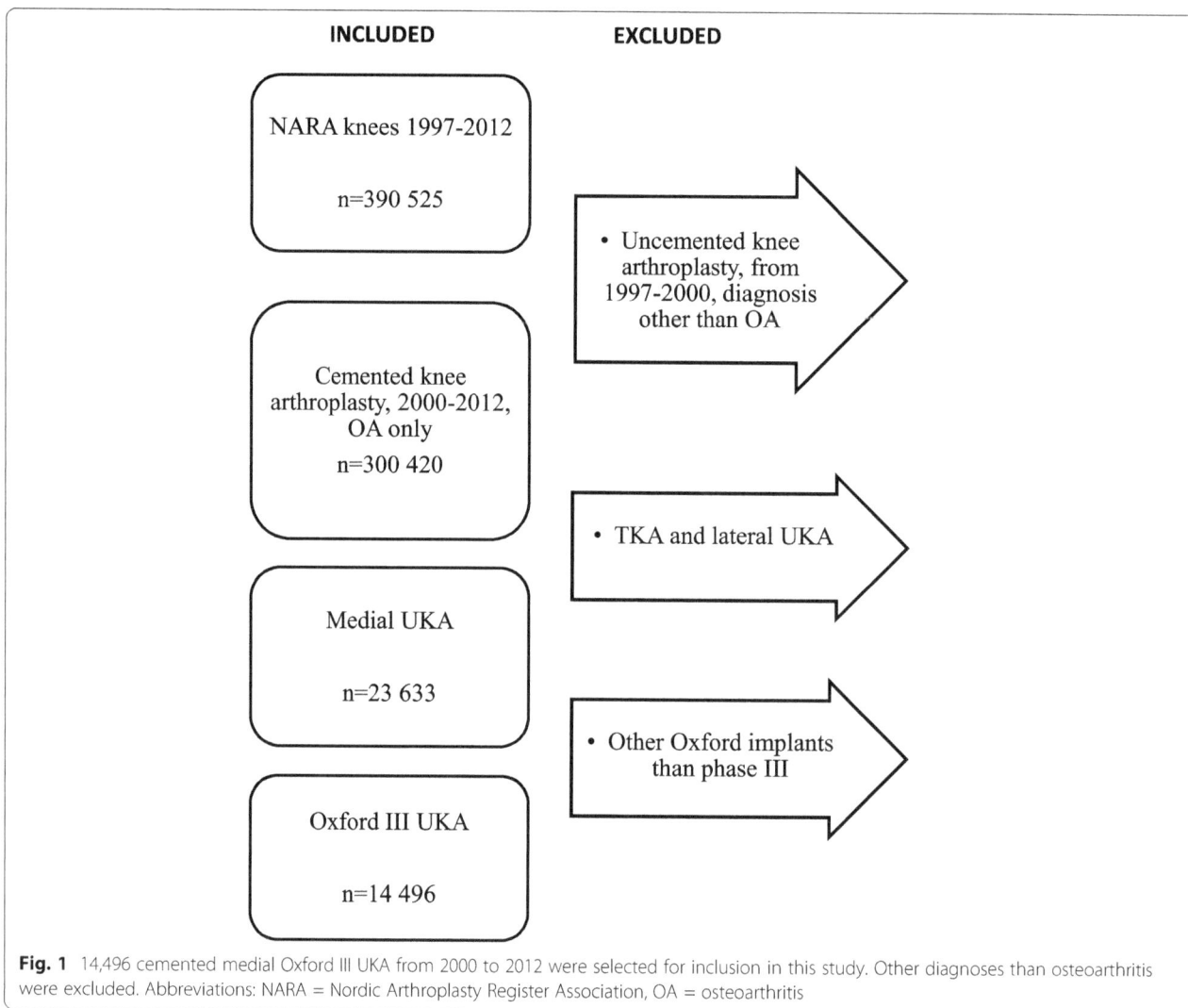

INCLUDED   **EXCLUDED**

NARA knees 1997-2012

n=390 525

• Uncemented knee arthroplasty, from 1997-2000, diagnosis other than OA

Cemented knee arthroplasty, 2000-2012, OA only
n=300 420

• TKA and lateral UKA

Medial UKA

n=23 633

• Other Oxford implants than phase III

Oxford III UKA

n=14 496

Fig. 1 14,496 cemented medial Oxford III UKA from 2000 to 2012 were selected for inclusion in this study. Other diagnoses than osteoarthritis were excluded. Abbreviations: NARA = Nordic Arthroplasty Register Association, OA = osteoarthritis

considered a possible competing risk to revision. We studied the influence of death by performing a competing risk analysis using the statistical software R [16, 17]. The results for the volume groups did not change significantly when accounting for death as a competing risk for revision (Table 2). Cox regression analyses were made for the different confounding variables and are presented in Table 3.

The various reasons for revision were organized hierarchically with infection first and unexplained pain last, as shown in Table 4. Loosening and wear were second in the list and instability and dislocation third. The group 'other reasons' contained new diseases occurring in the joint such as osteoarthritis or osteonecrosis laterally or joint fibrosis with stiffness. Surgical errors such as incorrect sizing of components were also included in this group. When more than one reason was reported, the top reason in the hierarchy was used as endpoint in the analyses. Pain as a cause of revision was used as

endpoint only when pain was the only reason reported. HR with 95% CI was reported for different revision causes with 10 years follow-up. The proportional hazards assumption of the Cox model was tested based on log-minus-log plot and found to be valid. SPSS version 23 and R statistical software package version 3.2.1 were used for the statistical analyses.

Results

126 hospitals performed 14,496 cemented medial Oxford III UKA from 2000 to 2012 in the 4 Nordic countries. Demographics and patient characteristics are shown in Table 1. The median number of procedures performed annually by a hospital was 23 (IQR (inter quartile range) =12-44). The median annual procedure volume per hospital in Denmark was 41 (IQR = 23-61), 27 (IQR = 13-48) in Sweden, 18 (IQR = 9-36) in Finland and 17 (IQR = 10-26) in Norway. The most common annual hospital volume was 1 per year, the second and third

Table 1 Patient and procedure characteristics of 14,496 cemented medial Oxford III unicompartmental knee arthroplasty according to four hospital volume categories with the diagnosis osteoarthritis from 2000 to 2012

	Annual hospital volume groups				
	≤11	12-23	24-43	≥44	
					p-values
No of procedures	3528	3759	3533	3676	
Men %	42	43	44	44	0.17
Age^median^ (range)	62 (28-94)	63 (34-93)	65 (33-94)	65 (33-95)	
Age group n (%)					
<55	731 (21)	652 (17)	501 (14)	540 (15)	<0.001
55-64	1471 (42)	1469 (39)	1199 (34)	1339 (36)	
65-74	946 (27)	1169 (31)	1251 (35)	1240 (34)	
≥75	380 (11)	469 (13)	582 (17)	566 (15)	
Year of surgery					
2000-03	962 (27)	826 (22)	399 (11)	475 (13)	<0.001
2004-06	928 (26)	1061 (28)	562 (16)	1113 (30)	
2007-09	925 (26)	1281 (32)	1349 (38)	900 (25)	
2010-12	713 (20)	654 (18)	1223 (35)	1188 (32)	
Nation n (%)					
Denmark (4211)	558 (16)	615 (16)	1118 (32)	1920 (52)	<0.001
Norway (4157)	1273 (36)	1551 (41)	1147 (33)	186 (5)	
Sweden (2218)	460 (13)	561 (15)	508 (14)	689 (19)	
Finland (3920)	1237 (35)	1032 (28)	760 (21)	881 (24)	

most common annual procedure volume was 2 and 3 per year respectively.

The Kaplan Meier 2 year survival was 95% for the three hospitals groups with annual procedure volume > 11 and 93% for the hospitals performing ≤11 Oxford III UKA per year. The Kaplan Meier estimated survival had dropped to 80% at 10 years follow up with poorest result for the ≤11 per year group (Table 2). The three hospital volume groups of >11 had an estimated survival of 83% at 10 years. The Log-rank test was statistically significant with $p = 0.003$.

In the Cox regression model, the high volume groups (≥44 procedures per year) had a lower risk of any revision during the entire follow-up time of 10 years compared with the lowest volume group (≤ 11 procedures per year) according to adjusted HR = 0.82 (95% CI 0.70-0.94, $p = 0.006$). Similarly, the adjusted HRs were 0.78 (95% CI 0.68-0.91, $p = 0.002$) for the group performing 24-43 procedures per year and 0.87 (95% CI 0.76-0.99, $p = 0.036$) for the group performing 12-23 procedures per year compared to the lowest volume group (Table 2, Fig. 2).

Table 2 Results from survival and Cox regression analyses on hospital volume for 14,496 cemented medial Oxford III unicompartmental knee arthroplasty in NARA 2000-2012

Annual hospital volume groups	Number of procedures	Number of revisions (%)	Number of deaths[a] (%)	K-M 2-year survival (95%CI)	K-M 10-year survival (95%CI)	Cox Regression Unadjusted HR(95%CI) 10 years	p-value	Cox Regression Adjusted RR(95%CI) 10 years	p-value
≤11	3528	481 (13.6)	231 (6.5)	93 (92.4-94.0)	80 (78.0-82.0)	1.0 (ref)		1.0 (ref)	
12-23	3759	429 (11.4)	237 (6.3)	95 (94.1-95.7)	83 (80.8-84.4)	0.85 (0.75-0.97)	0.017	0.87 (0.76-0.99)	0.036
24-43	3533	293 (8.3)	185 (5.2)	95 (94.1-95.7)	83 (80.2-86.2)	0.78 (0.67-0.90)	0.001	0.78 (0.68-0.91)	0.002
≥44	3676	351 (9.5)	227 (6.2)	95 (94.3-95.9)	83 (80.7-85.5)	0.82 (0.72-0.95)	0.006	0.82 (0.70-0.94)	0.006

K-M Kaplan-Meier estimated cumulative survival at 2 and 10 years (%)
HR Hazard Ratio; with adjustment for age category, sex, year of surgery and nation
CI confidence interval
Ref reference
[a]No statistical significant differences in proportion of deaths within the groups, p-value equal to 0.11

Table 3 Cox proportional survival model with Hazard Ratios (HR) adjusted for age, sex, year of surgery and nation as covariates with 95% CI (confidence interval) for all reasons for revision up to 10 years after primary surgery

Variables	No of procedures	HR(95%CI)	p-value
Age group			
55-64	5469	1.0 (ref)	
< 55	2424	1.3 (1.1-1.5)	<0.001
65-74	4606	0.8 (0.7-0.9)	<0.001
≥ 75	1997	0.7 (0.6-0.8)	<0.001
Sex			
Male	6272	1.0 (ref)	
Female	8224	1.0 (0.9-1.1)	0.6
Year of surgery			
2000-03	2662	1.0 (ref)	
2004-06	3664	1.2 (1.0-1.3)	0.04
2007-09	4392	1.2 (1.0-1.4)	0.02
2010-12	3778	1.3 (1.1-1.6)	0.004
Nation			
Sweden	2218	1.0 (ref)	
Denmark	4211	1.4 (1.2-1.7)	<0.001
Norway	4157	1.2 (1.0-1.5)	0.01
Finland	3910	1.2 (1.0-1.4)	0.05

In the multivariable survival model we found inferior results for the youngest age group <55 with Hazard Ratio HR = 1.29 (95% CI 1.13-1.47, p = <0.001) with 55-64 as reference. The ≥75 age group showed better results; HR = 0.65 (95% CI 0.55-0.78, p < 0.001) (Table 3, Table 5). Gender was not found to influence the results. There seems to be a deterioration in results in the more recent

years of surgery (HR = 1.33 (95%CI 1.10-1.62)). Denmark had statistically significant higher relative risk (HR = 1.41 (95%CI 1.19-1.68, p < 0.001)) compared to Sweden as reference. Similarly, Norway had HR = 1.24 (95%CI 1.05-1.47, p = 0.01). Finland had HR = 1.18 (95%CI 1.00-1.39, p = 0.05) (Table 3).

Revision causes

The distribution of revision causes among the 1519 revised cemented medial Oxford III implants from 2000 to 2012—according to hospital volume—is shown in Table 4. We found a difference in the risk of revision for unexplained pain among the volume groups. The volume groups performing >11 Oxford III UKA per year revised 40-50% fewer patients for unexplained pain than the lowest volume hospitals (≤11 per year). The other revision causes did not show any statistically significant differences between the groups (Table 4).

Discussion

In this large population based study based on 14,496 cemented medial Oxford III unicompartmental knee arthroplasty performed in four Scandinavian countries; we showed that high procedure volumes (>11 procedures per year) were associated with a decreased risk for revision.

This study contributes to the knowledge of other previously published results. There are available studies on the impact of procedure volume in UKA, and the common denominator is the Oxford implant since its usage is widespread. The Swedish study from 2001 found that performing less than 23 UKA per year was associated with a higher risk of revision [18], whereas Baker et al. [19] suggested a minimum annual volume of 13. Our previous study from Norway indicated fewer revisions

Table 4 Revisions causes with 10 years follow up. Hazard Ratios with confidence intervals for different hospital volumes, adjusted for sex, age category, year of surgery and nation

Annual hospital volume group	Number of procedures	Number of revisions	Revision causes with adjusted Hazard Ratios (95% confidence interval)					
			Infection	Loosening/Wear	Instability/Dislocation	Unexplained pain	Other reasons	Unknown reasons
		1519	n = 57	n = 545	n = 104	n = 273	n = 498	n = 42
≤11	3528	465	1.0 (ref)	1.0 (ref)	1.0 (ref)	1.0 (ref)	1.0 (ref)	1.0 (ref)
12-23	3759	420	1.02 (0.49-2.16)	1.04 (0.83-1.29)	1.66 (1.00-2.76)	0.54 (0.39-0.75)	0.72 (0.57-0.91)	1.90 (0.83-4.39)
24-43	3533	292	0.92 (0.41-2.02)	0.80 (0.61-1.04)	1.12 (0.61-2.05)	0.64 (0.46-0.89)	0.80 (0.62-1.04)	1.12 (0.44-2.86)
≥44	3676	342	1.20 (0.54-2.64)	0.93 (0.73-1.19)	1.15 (0.58-2.28)	0.56 (0.39-0.80)	0.77 (0.60-0.99)	0.47 (0.14-1.51)
Number of revisions in each volume group:								
≤11		13		157	23	96	168	8
12-23		15		166	43	60	118	18
24-43		13		93	21	61	93	11
≥44		16		129	17	56	119	5

n numbers
ref reference

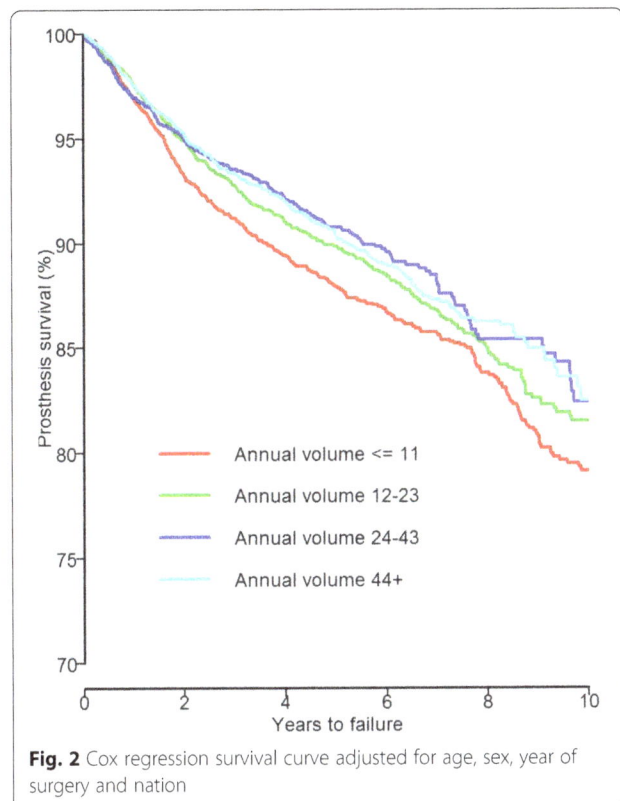

Fig. 2 Cox regression survival curve adjusted for age, sex, year of surgery and nation

studies and results, a threshold value of 11 per year could be considered a conservative value.

Our study included data from 4 different national registers with multiple surgeons and hospitals with varying experience and volume, suggesting high external validity. It reflects the practice in 4 different countries. Due to complete follow up of all patients in the study population with censoring at the time of death, emigration, or at the end of follow up, selection bias is unlikely. Additionally, only patients who received an Oxford III UKA with the diagnosis OA were selected (Fig. 1). We limited the analyses to the latest time period from 2000, excluding older implants and techniques. Using previously described methods of analysing the impact of procedure volume also strengthen the study [20, 22, 24, 25]. The advantage of analyzing each year separately is the reflection of the procedure volume that particular year.

Revision was less likely in older patients compared to the younger in our study. Other studies have shown that young patients experience an increased risk of revision after UKA compared to older patients [21, 26–28]. W-Dahl et al. [29] and Liddle et al. [21] also found that older patients had the greatest benefits and the lowest revision rates. In addition, UKA has been associated with lower rates of morbidity and mortality compared to TKA [30]. Sweden had the best implant survival of all the 4 countries. This could be a result of longer training of Swedish surgeons, starting unicompartmental knee arthroplasty surgery and a knee arthroplasty register before the other Nordic countries, and thereby gaining more experience. Sweden differs from the other nations with less than 50% of the implanted UKAs being Oxford and thus their learning curve could be improved by surgical experience performing other types of UKA. Denmark had inferior results compared to the other countries and contributed to the majority of patients in high volume hospitals (52% in the ≥44 group). We performed sensitivity analysis with and without data from Denmark. The tendency in the results for the volume groups did not change excluding Denmark. Denmark also has poorer results in the low volume groups. The cause of poorer results in Denmark is not possible to verify, but learning curve, threshold for

with an annual caseload of more than 40 [20]. A study from the National Joint Registry of England and Wales (NJR) regarding determinants of revision following UKA supported the importance of experience measured at the unit level as well, and also favoring consultants rather than trainees [21]. A recent study from the NJR recommended surgeons to perform at least 20% of their knee arthroplasties as UKAs to achieve lower rates of revisions [22]. They also found that 81.4% of the surgeons performed less than 10 UKA per year. This corresponds to our findings of extreme skewness with dominance of low-volume performance. Some registers on the other hand recommend the use of fewer UKA due to higher failure rates [23]. Our study from 4 countries suggests a minimum hospital volume per hospital of 11. However, considering the variety of the previously mentioned

Table 5 Results from Kaplan Meier 10 year survival analysis for age as stratification variable according to volume groups with 95% confidence interval

Annual Hospital Volume	Age groups				
	< 55 yrs. $n = 2424$	55-64 $n = 5469$	65-74 $n = 4606$	≥75 $n = 1997$	For all ages (table 2) $n = 14,496$
≤11	74 (69.4-78.2)	79 (76.4-82.4)	82 (78.7-85.9)	89 (84.2-94.2)	80 (78.0-82.0)
12-23	74 (67.3-79.7)	81 (78.1-84.1)	87 (84.4-90.0)	87 (82.0-91.2)	83 (80.8-84.4)
24-43	77 (68.8-84.6)	83 (77.5-87.5)	84 (78.7-88.7)	90 (85.5-93.5)	83 (80.2-86.2)
≥44	79 (69.8-88.2)	81 (77.6-85.2)	84 (79.3-88.5)	90 (86.5-92.9)	83 (80.7-85.5)

n numbers

revision and patient selection could be explanation factors. Theoretically, an increase in inexperienced surgeons implementing a new technique could initially lead to many revisions, but if continued, an expected improvement should occur. This could also explain the deteriorating results in the last time period.

Analyses of specific revision causes revealed a higher risk of revision for unexplained pain in low volume hospitals as compared to higher volume hospitals. We found minor differences for the other revision causes (Table 4). Baker et al. found that while more unicompartmental knee implants than total knee implants were revised for unexplained pain, when these revisions for unexplained pain were discounted, unicompartmental knee arthroplasty still had a significantly greater risk of revision from other reasons than did total knee arthroplasty [31]. However the numbers of revisions in each group were too small to allow making any conclusions regarding the differences between the volume groups.

There has been an on-going discussion regarding the threshold for revision due to unexplained pain [32]. Similarly, the incidence of radiolucent lines at the bone-implant interface [33] could be misinterpreted as loosening by unexperienced Oxford-users, and thereby leading to unnecessary revisions. Nevertheless, in cases with concurrent pain or symptomatology, it could be argued that revision is motivated. These could be explanations to the differences in revision rates, suggesting a lower revision-threshold in low-volume users. However, even the highest volume hospitals could not match the outcomes reported by developers [6, 7, 34] or the results after TKA regarding revision rates [24, 35]. A retrospective independent sample of failures reported to the registers could be one approach to evaluate the indication for revision surgery and identifying critical errors in the primary surgical technique and patient selection. Precise surgical indications for both primary and revision surgery are still debated [8, 22]. Furthermore, whether emphasis should be put on the higher revision rates of UKA compared to TKA or the lower risk of postoperative death and complications comparing UKA to TKA is also important to take into consideration [35].

Limitations to the study may be unmeasured factors such as decision-making regarding pre-operative radiographic changes leading to primary indication for surgery [36]. In addition, information on life style factors and physical activity was not available. The selection of patients considered suitable for UKA surgery is debatable regarding radiographic findings, age and BMI [8, 22]. Only hospital procedure volume was available for analysis in the NARA database, surgeon caseload and experience were not available. Theoretically, a high volume surgeon in a high volume center would gain the best results according to a systematic review regarding surgery volume [37]. However, the volume of a center had an equal if not greater effect on patient outcome than surgeon volume. Categorization of the volume exposure assumes that any (unspecified) hospital-level effects (e.g. the care that patients within a specific hospital receive, independent of volume) are trumped by a potential volume effect on revision rates. The analyses in this study are limited to the cemented medial Oxford III UKA and may limit the generalizability of the results to be valid for other UKA implant types.

Conclusion

Hospitals performing ≤11 Oxford III UKA per year had a higher risk of revision, and were more likely to perform revisions due to unexplained pain.

Abbreviations

CI: Confidence Interval; HR: Hazard Ratio; IQR: Interquartile range; K-M: Kaplan Meier; N: numbers; NARA: Nordic Arthroplasty Register Association; NJR: National Joint Registry of England and Wales; OA: Osteoarthritis; Ref: Reference; TKA: Total Knee Arthroplasty; UKA: Unicompartmental Knee Arthroplasty

Acknowledgements

Not applicable.

Funding

This study was in part funded by Nordforsk grant.

Level of evidence

III, observational registry study.

Authors' contributions

MB, AMF and OF designed the study. MB, AMF, CABJ, LIH, OF, KI, OR, AWD, HS, AP, AE and KM collected the data and edited the manuscript. MB wrote the manuscript and the analyses were done by AMF, CABJ, MB and OF. All authors have read and approved the final manuscript.

Consent for publication

This study was approved through each national registries own ethical process. Patients in Norway give individual written consent to participate. In Finland and Denmark it is mandatory to participate for all hospitalized patients and no consent is required for an approved National medical registry and in Sweden no written consent is needed, but the patient can opt to not participate.

Competing interests

The authors declare that they have no competing interests.

Author details

[1]Coastal Hospital, 5253 Hagavik, Norway. [2]The Norwegian Arthroplasty Register, Department of Orthopaedic Surgery, Haukeland University Hospital,

Bergen, Norway. [3]Department of Clinical Medicine, Institute of Medicine and Dentistry, University of Bergen, Bergen, Norway. [4]The Swedish Knee Arthroplasty Register, Lund, Sweden. [5]Department of Clinical Sciences, Lund University Faculty of Medicine, Orthopedics, Lund, Sweden. [6]The Coxa Hospital for Joint Replacement, Tampere, Finland. [7]Department of Orthopaedics and Traumatology, Turku University Hospital, Turku, Finland. [8]The Danish Knee Arthroplasty Register, Aarhus, Denmark. [9]Department of Clinical Epidemiology, Aarhus University Hospital, Aarhus, Denmark. [10]Department of Orthopaedic surgery, Næstved Hospital, Næstved, Denmark.

References

1. Niinimaki T, Eskelinen A, Makela K, Ohtonen P, Puhto AP, Remes V. Unicompartmental knee arthroplasty survivorship is lower than TKA survivorship: a 27-year Finnish registry study. Clin Orthop Relat Res. 2014; 472:1496–501.
2. Australian Orthopaedic Association National Joint Replacement Registry Annual report. Online source: http://aoanjjr.sahmri.com.
3. Swedish Knee Register Annual Report. Online source: http://www.myknee.se/en.
4. Danish Knee Arthtoplasty Register Annual Report. Online source: http://kea.au.dk/en/ClinicalQuality/.
5. Norwegian Arthroplasty Register Annual Report. Online source: http://www.nrlweb.ihelse.net/eng/.
6. Price AJ, Svard U. A second decade lifetable survival analysis of the Oxford unicompartmental knee arthroplasty. Clin Orthop Relat Res. 2011;469:174–9.
7. Pandit H, Jenkins C, Gill HS, Barker K, Dodd CA, Murray DW. Minimally invasive Oxford phase 3 unicompartmental knee replacement: results of 1000 cases. J Bone Joint Surg Br. 2011;93:198–204.
8. Kozinn SC, Scott R. Unicondylar knee arthroplasty. J Bone Joint Surg Am. 1989;71:145–50.
9. Pandit H, Jenkins C, Gill HS, Smith G, Price AJ, Dodd CA, et al. Unnecessary contraindications for mobile-bearing unicompartmental knee replacement. J Bone Joint Surg Br. 2011;93:622–8.
10. Havelin LI, Robertsson O, Fenstad AM, Overgaard S, Garellick G, Furnes O. A Scandinavian experience of register collaboration: the Nordic Arthroplasty register association (NARA). J Bone Joint Surg Am. 2011;93(Suppl 3):13–9.
11. Robertsson O, Bizjajeva S, Fenstad AM, Furnes O, Lidgren L, Mehnert F, et al. Knee arthroplasty in Denmark, Norway and Sweden. A pilot study from the Nordic Arthroplasty register association. Acta Orthop. 2010;81:82–9.
12. National Joint Registry of England,Wales and Northern Ireland Annual Report. Online source: http://www.njrcentre.org.uk/njrcentre.
13. Nordic Arthroplasty Register Association Report. Online source: http://www.nordicarthroplasty.org.
14. Havelin LI, Fenstad AM, Salomonsson R, Mehnert F, Furnes O, Overgaard S, et al. The Nordic Arthroplasty register association: a unique collaboration between 3 national hip arthroplasty registries with 280,201 THRs. Acta Orthop. 2009;80:393–401.
15. Robertsson O, Ranstam J. No bias of ignored bilaterality when analysing the revision risk of knee prostheses: analysis of a population based sample of 44,590 patients with 55,298 knee prostheses from the national Swedish knee Arthroplasty register. BMC Musculoskelet Disord. 2003;4:1.
16. Ranstam J, Karrholm J, Pulkkinen P, Makela K, Espehaug B, Pedersen AB, et al. Statistical analysis of arthroplasty data. I. Introduction and background. Acta orthop. 2011;82:253–7.
17. Fine JP, Gray RJ. A proportional hazards model for the subdistribution of a competing risk. J Am Stat Assoc. 1999;94:496–509.
18. Robertsson O, Knutson K, Lewold S, Lidgren L. The routine of surgical management reduces failure after unicompartmental knee arthroplasty. J Bone Joint Surg Br. 2001;83:45–9.
19. Baker P, Jameson S, Critchley R, Reed M, Gregg P, Deehan D. Center and surgeon volume influence the revision rate following unicondylar knee replacement: an analysis of 23,400 medial cemented unicondylar knee replacements. J Bone Joint Surg Am. 2013;95:702–9.
20. Badawy M, Espehaug B, Indrekvam K, Havelin LI, Furnes O. Higher revision risk for unicompartmental knee arthroplasty in low-volume hospitals. Acta Orthop. 2014;85:342–7.
21. Liddle AD, Judge A, Pandit H, Murray DW. Determinants of revision and functional outcome following unicompartmental knee replacement. Osteoarthritis Cartilage OARS, Osteoarthritis Res Soc. 2014;22:1241–50.
22. Liddle AD, Pandit H, Judge A, Murray DW. Optimal usage of unicompartmental knee arthroplasty: a study of 41 986 cases from the National Joint Registry for England and Wales. Bone Joint J. 2015;97-b:1506–11.
23. Paxton EW, Inacio MC, Khatod M, Yue EJ, Namba RS. Kaiser Permanente National Total Joint Replacement Registry: aligning operations with information technology. Clin Orthop Relat Res. 2010;468:2646–63.
24. Badawy M, Espehaug B, Indrekvam K, Engesaeter LB, Havelin LI, Furnes O. Influence of hospital volume on revision rate after total knee arthroplasty with cement. J Bone Joint Surg Am. 2013;95:e131.
25. Glassou EN, Hansen TB, Makela K, Havelin LI, Furnes O, Badawy M, et al. Association between hospital procedure volume and risk of revision after total hip arthroplasty: a population-based study within the Nordic Arthroplasty register association database. Osteoarthritis Cartilage OARS, Osteoarthritis Res Soc. 2016;24:419–26.
26. W-Dahl A, Robertsson O, Lidgren L. Surgery for knee osteoarthritis in younger patients. Acta Orthop. 2010;81:161–4.
27. Furnes O, Espehaug B, Lie SA, Vollset SE, Engesaeter LB, Havelin LI. Failure mechanisms after unicompartmental and tricompartmental primary knee replacement with cement. J Bone Joint Surg Am. 2007;89:519–25.
28. Kuipers BM, Kollen BJ, Bots PC, Burger BJ, van Raay JJ, Tulp NJ, et al. Factors associated with reduced early survival in the Oxford phase III medial unicompartment knee replacement. Knee. 2010;17:48–52.
29. W-Dahl A, Robertsson O, Lidgren L, Miller L, Davidson D, Graves S. Unicompartmental knee arthroplasty in patients aged less than 65. Acta Orthop. 2010;81:90–4.
30. Hunt LP, Ben-Shlomo Y, Clark EM, Dieppe P, Judge A, MacGregor AJ, et al. 45-Day mortality after 467,779 knee replacements for osteoarthritis from the National Joint Registry for England and Wales: an observational study. Lancet. 2014;384:1429–36.
31. Baker PN, Petheram T, Avery PJ, Gregg PJ, Deehan DJ. Revision for unexplained pain following unicompartmental and total knee replacement. J Bone Joint Surg Am. 2012;94:e126.
32. Goodfellow JW, O'Connor JJ, Murray DW. A critique of revision rate as an outcome measure: re-interpretation of knee joint registry data. J Bone Joint Surg Br. 2010;92:1628–31.
33. Gulati A, Chau R, Pandit HG, Gray H, Price AJ, Dodd CA, et al. The incidence of physiological radiolucency following Oxford unicompartmental knee replacement and its relationship to outcome. J Bone Joint Surg Br. 2009;91:896–902.
34. Murray DW, Goodfellow JW, O'Connor JJ. The Oxford medial unicompartmental arthroplasty: a ten-year survival study. J Bone Joint Surg Br. 1998;80:983–9.
35. Liddle AD, Judge A, Pandit H, Murray DW. Adverse outcomes after total and unicompartmental knee replacement in 101,330 matched patients: a study of data from the National Joint Registry for England and Wales. Lancet. 2014;384:1437–45.
36. Dowsey MM, Nikpour M, Dieppe P, Choong PF. Associations between pre-operative radiographic changes and outcomes after total knee joint replacement for osteoarthritis. Osteoarthritis Cartilage OARS Osteoarthritis Res Soc. 2012;20:1095–102.
37. Critchley RJ, Baker PN, Deehan DJ. Does surgical volume affect outcome after primary and revision knee arthroplasty? A systematic review of the literature. Knee. 2012;19:513–8.

16

Rotational alignment of femoral component with different methods in total knee arthroplasty

Joon Kyu Lee[1], Sahnghoon Lee[2], Sae Hyung Chun[2], Ki Tae Kim[1] and Myung Chul Lee[2]* 🔟

Abstract

Background: Femoral component rotation (FCR) is one of the most important factors in total knee arthroplasty. In this prospective study, we used three different techniques for FCR and analyzed their accuracy with postoperative axial computed tomography (CT) images. We also evaluated effect of FCR to clinical outcome.

Methods: One hundred sixty-five patients were randomly allocated into three groups. In the measured resection group, FCR was set by externally rotating the axis 3° off the posterior femoral condylar axis. In the tensor group, a gap-tensioning device set at 20 lbf was used. In the block group, spacer blocks of various thicknesses were used. The FCR angle (FCRa) was measured on postoperative axial CT as an angle between the clinical transepicondylar and posterior condylar axes of the femoral component. Outliers were defined as FCRas deviated more than 3° either internally or externally. Postoperative 2 year clinical scores and knee range of motion were checked.

Results: The tensor group had significantly better positioning of the femoral component to the neutral position compared with the measured resection group and the block group (mean FCRa: internal rotation 1.79, 0.43 and 2.63°, respectively, $p < 0.001$). The outliers were also least frequent in the tensor group (35, 16 and 40%, respectively, $p = 0.02$). There were no significant differences in postoperative 2 year clinical results among groups.

Conclusions: Gap technique with a 20-lbf tensor device was the most accurate and precise method for obtaining adequate FCR. Measured resection with 3° external rotation and gap technique with blocks could lead to internal rotation of the femoral component. Postoperative 2 year clinical results were not significantly different among groups with different techniques for FCR.

Keywords: Femoral component rotation, Gap technique, Measured resection technique, Tensor device

Background

Establishing adequate femoral component rotation (FCR) is important in total knee arthroplasty (TKA), and it is widely accepted through many studies. Most surgeons agree that the femoral component should be rotated externally as emphasized by Mochizuki more than 30 years ago [1]. Various patellofemoral complications are observed when the femoral components are rotated internally, such as lateral tilting, subluxation and dislocation of the patella and patellar maltracking [2]. Increased lateral flexion laxity is associated with increased internal rotation of the femoral component and a less favorable clinical outcome [3]. On the contrary, excessive external rotation of the femoral component will increase the medial flexion gap and could lead to symptomatic flexion instability. Combined internal malrotation of the femoral and tibial component is also a significant factor in the development of anterior knee pain after TKA [4]. Patellofemoral

* Correspondence: leemc@snu.ac.kr
[2]Department of Orthopaedic Surgery, Seoul National University Hospital, 101 Daehang-ro, Jongno-gu, Seoul 110-744, Korea
Full list of author information is available at the end of the article

problem, instability, polyethylene wear, osteolysis, aseptic loosening and infection are major causes of early failures in TKA [5].

Two techniques are generally accepted for soft tissue balancing and determining FCR, which are measured resection and gap techniques [6, 7]. An external rotation of 3° off the posterior femoral condylar axis is considered to be satisfactory and generally accepted in the measured resection technique [8, 9]. However, several other methods have been proposed in an effort to increase its accuracy. Many studies have reported that the transepicondylar axis is more reliable in a typical varus knee with medial tibiofemoral arthritis [10–13]. Two methods are used to determine the flexion gap and femoral component position in axial plane in the gap technique. The tensor device is commonly used to achieve symmetric gap. It is still unclear how much force is appropriate for distraction using the tensor device, and surgeons usually determine the device tension through their experience [14, 15]. Alternatively, gap blocks of various thickness can be used to perform the gap technique.

The primary purpose of this study was to find whether different methods may result in different outcomes in FCR accuracy and outlier frequency. The secondary purpose was to identify the effect of FCR to the clinical outcome. The hypotheses were that there would be significant differences in FCR accuracy among techniques and FCR would affect clinical outcome significantly. We prospectively performed TKAs with three different methods and analyzed its FCR accuracy by measuring the degree of FCR to the clinical transepicondylar axis (cTEA) on the postoperative axial computed tomography (CT) images. Postoperative 2 year clinical scores and knee range of motion were evaluated to check the effect of FCR to the clinical outcome.

Methods

Consecutive patients, who were scheduled to undergo primary TKAs, were enrolled prospectively between June 2011 and August 2012. In 132 patients, TKAs were performed on 189 knees during the enrollment period of this study. Patients with a diagnosis other than primary osteoarthritis or valgus deformity of the knee and those who refused to participate were excluded. After written informed consents were obtained, 168 knees in 119 patients were assigned to one of the three groups. Block randomization using sealed envelopes was carried out in the operation room. CT scans were performed approximately 3 months after surgery, and 15 knees in 12 patients were lost to follow-up because these patients did not undergo CT scanning. Consequently, 153 knees in 107 patients were analyzed in this study (Fig. 1).

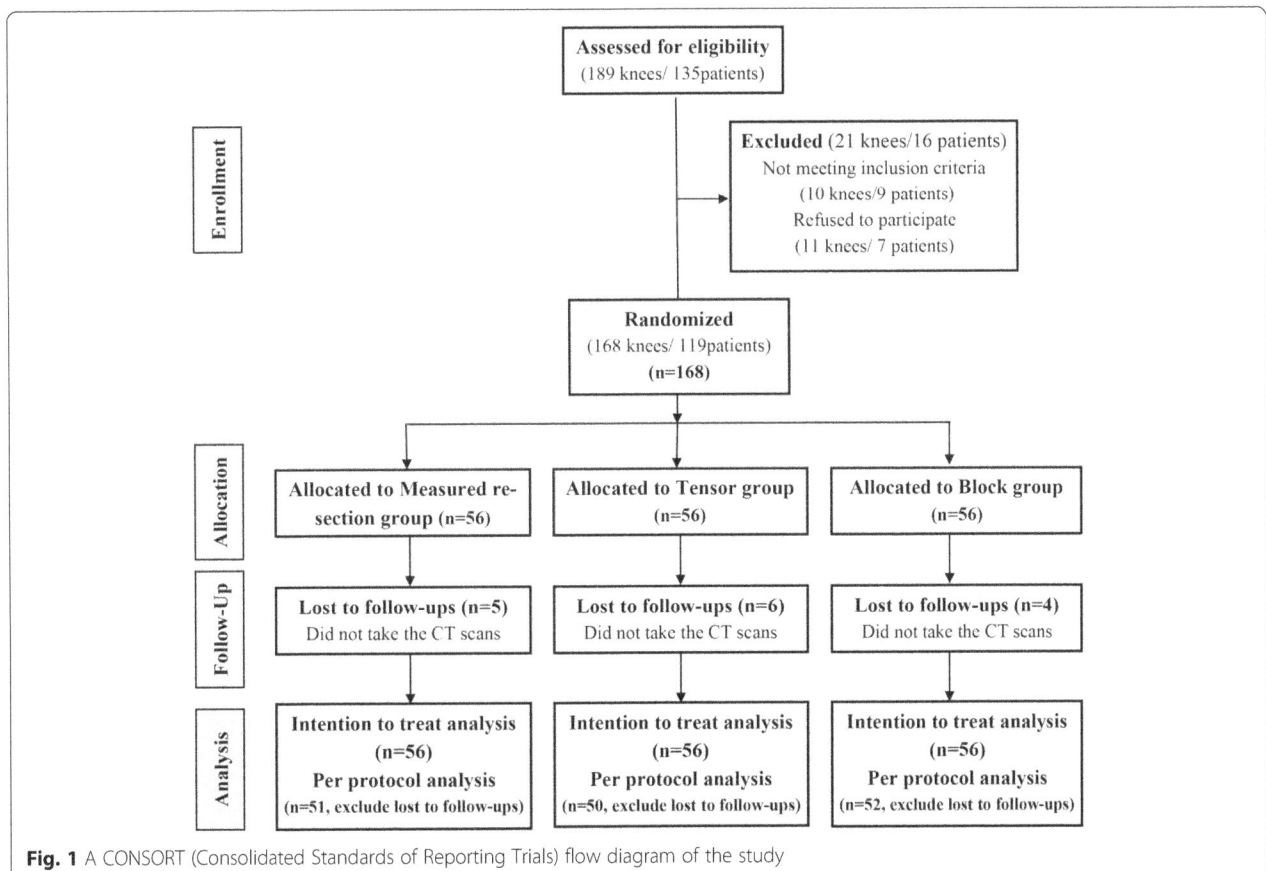

Fig. 1 A CONSORT (Consolidated Standards of Reporting Trials) flow diagram of the study

No inter-group differences were evident in preoperative demographics and clinical status (Table 1).

All surgical procedures were performed by a single experienced surgeon (*). We used the P.F.C Sigma RP-F (DePuy Orthopaedics, Leeds, United Kingdom), Buechel-Pappas TKA system (Endotec, Orlando, Florida, USA) and Low Contact Stress TKA system (DePuy, Warsaw, IN, USA) for the measured resection, tensor and block groups, respectively. A medial parapatellar arthrotomy was used, and both cruciate ligaments were resected. In the measured resection group, we resected the distal femur and proximal tibia and subsequently determined the FCR using the sizing guide instrument. The FCR axis was set by externally rotating the axis 3° off the posterior femoral condylar axis. In the tensor group, we cut the proximal tibia, then used the tensor device to determine component rotation in which the joint distraction force was set at 20 lbf (89 N) (Fig. 2a). After that, we resected the anterior and posterior femur, and then, the distal femur. In the block group, the procedure was the same as that in the tensor group, but instead of using the tensor device, gap blocks with 10, 12.5, 15 and 17.5-mm thicknesses were used (Fig. 2b). Most patellae were resurfaced. However, normal-shaped patellae with thickness less than 20 mm or relatively good cartilage status (International Cartilage Repair Society grade 0 or 1) were retained selectively. All prostheses were fixed with cement.

Using CT scans (Siemens Somatom; Siemens Medical Solutions, Malvern, PA, USA), 1-mm thickness axial images were obtained. We measured the angle between the cTEA and the posterior condylar axis (PCA) of the femoral component (FCR angle, FCRa) using the OnDemand3D program (CyberMed, Seoul, Korea) (Fig. 3).

We calculated the mean value of the FCRa and the frequency of outlier, which was defined as the deviation of more than 3° either internally or externally, in each group [6, 16]. Clinical effect of the FCR was evaluated with clinical scores (Knee society scores, Hospital for special surgery score and WOMAC score) and knee range of motion at 2 years postoperatively.

Statistical analysis

A priori sample size analysis using G*Power program version 3.1.2 showed that 50 cases per group were required to detect a statistical difference in the component rotation among three groups with a 1° precision, ($\alpha = 0.05$, $\beta = 0.8$). The results were evaluated only in the per-protocol analyses after excluding patients lost to follow-ups rather than applying an intention-to-treat protocol. The Kolmogorov-Smirnov test was used to check the data for normality in continuous variables. The inter-group differences were determined using mixed model for adjustment of auto-correlation and Pearson's chi-square test with posthoc tests for continuous and categorical variables, respectively. All statistical analyses were performed using two-tailed test, and significance was accepted for p value of <0.05. Two of authors (* and *) measured the FCRa on axial CT images twice, with an interval of 2 weeks between measurements. The intra- and interobserver reliabilities in measurements were verified by measuring agreement with kappa statistics [17].

Table 1 Comparison of pre-operative demographics and clinical status among the groups

	Measured resection (n = 51)	Tensor (n = 50)	Block (n = 52)	p-value
Gender (M/F)	2/49	1/49	2/50	0.828[a]
Age[c] (year)	68.6 (55–81)	70.8 (56–86)	69.3 (56–78)	0.178[b]
Body mass index[c] (kg/m^2)	26.6 (20.8–33.7)	25.6 (20.7–31.2)	25.8 (20.2–33.3)	0.169[b]
Involved knee (Rt./Lt.)	27/24	21/29	25/27	0.545[a]
Range of knee motion[c] (degree)				
Flexion contracture	9.4 (0–25)	8.8 (0–30)	8.8 (0–20)	0.859[b]
Further flexion	124.7 (100–150)	125.9 (90–150)	125.5 (40–150)	0.937[b]
Total range of motion	115.3 (80–145)	117.1 (60–145)	116.7 (35–145)	0.889[b]
Tibiofemoral angle (degree)	Varus 4.5 (varus 24 - valgus 7)	Varus 2.8 (varus 19 - valgus 6)	Varus 2.9 (varus 18 - valgus 7)	0.225[b]
KS score[c] (points)				
Knee	48.6 (19–90)	45.1 (6–74)	46.6 (24–71)	0.259[b]
Function	42.7 (0–86)	39.7 (0–71)	39.4 (2–71)	0.163[b]
HSS score (points)	62.2 (38–84)	60.9 (27–82)	61.9 (43–78)	0.802[b]
WOMAC score (points)	52.8 (19–96)	58.3 (17–96)	55.8 (17–91)	0.094[b]

Abbreviations: *KS* Knee Society, *HSS* Hospital for Special Surgery, *WOMAC* Western Ontario and McMaster Universities Osteoarthritis Index (LK 3.1 version)
[a]Chi-square test
[b]Mixed model for adjustment of auto-correlation
[c]The values are given as the mean and the range in parenthesis

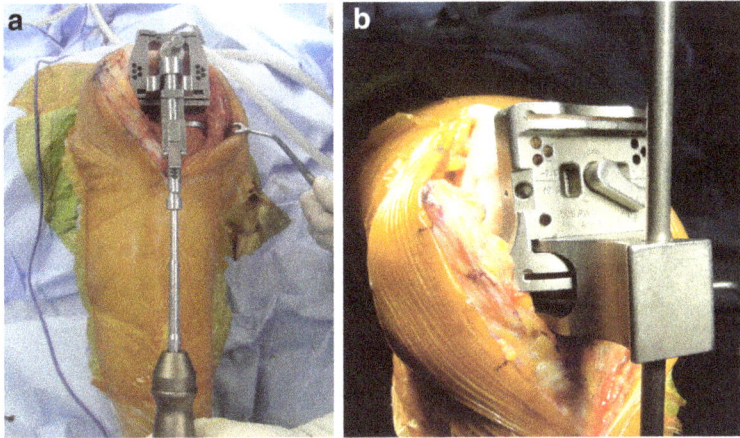

Fig. 2 Devices used during the surgery to set femoral component rotation: **a** the tensor device set by 20 lbf which was used in the tensor group, **b** the gap block which was used in the block group

Results

The mean FCRa was $-1.79° \pm 2.25°$, $-0.43° \pm 2.36°$, and $-2.63° \pm 2.50°$ in the measured resection, tensor and block groups ('-' means internal rotation of the femoral component), respectively. The tensor group had significantly better positioning of the femoral component to the neutral position compared with the measured resection and block groups ($p < 0.001$).

The outliers were also least frequent in the tensor group (35, 16 and 40% in the measured resection, tensor and block groups, respectively, $p = 0.02$). The measured resection group and the block group showed internally rotated positioning of the femoral component, and no significant difference was found between the two groups. The outlier cases were also similar between the two groups (Table 2).

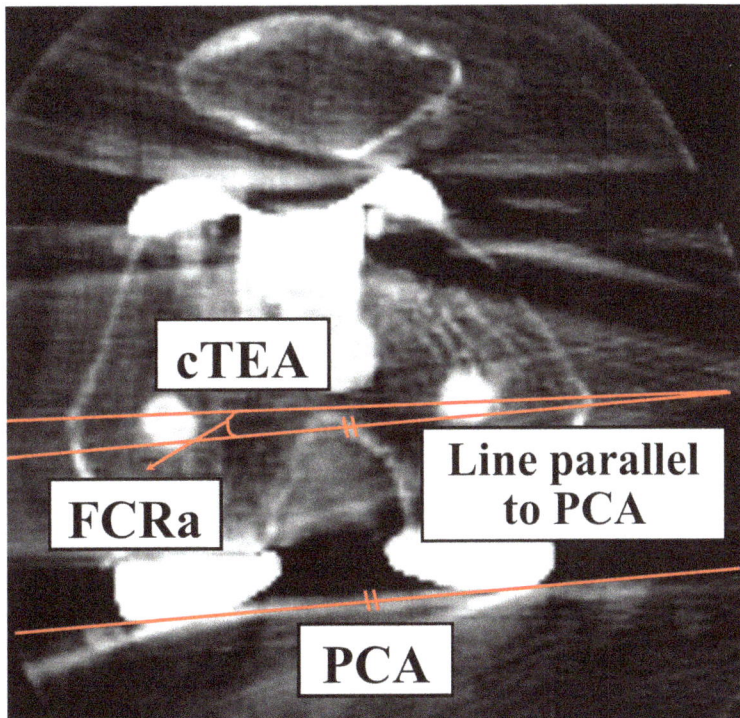

Fig. 3 Angle on the axial CT image manipulated with use of the OnDemand3D program (Cybermed) to measure femoral component rotation (Tensor group). cTEA, clinical transepicondylar axis; PCA, posterior condylar axis; FCRa, Femoral component rotation angle, the angle between cTEA and PCA of the femoral component

Table 2 Comparison of the femoral component rotation

		Measured resection ($n = 51$)	Tensor ($n = 50$)	Block ($n = 52$)	p-value
Femoral component rotation[c,d] (degree)	Mean	−1.79	−0.43	−2.63	0.0001[a]
	Range	−6.9 ~ 3.4	−5.5 ~ 6.1	−10.8 ~ 1.5	
	95% confidence interval	−2.43 ~ −1.16	−1.10 ~ 0.24	−3.32 ~ −1.93	
Outlier[e]	Total	18 (35%)	8 (16%)	21 (40%)	0.020[b]
	>3° IR	16	5	21	
	>3° ER	2	3	0	

Comparison between Measured resection group and Tensor group; p-value 0.0063[a] Comparison between Tensor group and Block group; p-value <0.0001[a]
Comparison between Measured resection group and Block group; p-value 0.0691[a]
Femoral component rotation: angle between clinical transepicondylar axis and posterior condylar axis of femoral component
Outlier: Femoral component rotation with more than 3° of external rotation or internal rotation
Abbreviations: *IR* internal rotation, *ER* external rotation
[a]Mixed model for adjustment of auto-correlation
[b]Chi-square test
[c]Subgroup analysis of femoral component rotation angle among groups
[d]+ : external rotation, − : internal rotation
[e]The values are given as the number of cases with percentage in parenthesis

There were no significant differences in postoperative 2 year clinical results among groups, although the tensor group had slightly better results compared to two other groups (Table 3).

All kappa values >0.8 confirmed substantial intra- and interobserver reliabilities of the FCRa measurements.

Discussion

We showed that there are differences in the accuracy of FCR in TKA based on the technique used in this study. Gap technique with tensor device of 20 lbf showed the most accurate and precise results. The measured resection technique with 3° external rotation and gap technique with spacer blocks showed a tendency of internal rotation in FCR. Postoperative 2 year clinical results were not significantly different among groups with different techniques for FCR.

Gap technique with the 89 N tensor device was the most accurate and precise method in obtaining the adequate FCR, but the ideal amount of tension has still not been determined. Asano et al. reported that the mean

soft tissue tension was 126.8 N and 120.7 N in extension and flexion, respectively, in 77 knees. They concluded that 80–160 N was the appropriate tension, and tension in that range did not affect postoperative range of motion [14]. In their other report, the mean soft tissue tension in extension was 91.7 N in 64 knees, and the range of distribution was also very wide (approximately 55–175 N, not exactly revealed in the article, only revealed in the graph) [18]. Yoshino et al. reported that 86.1 N and 97.1 N in patellar eversion and reset, respectively, were the appropriate tensions in 25 PS-TKAs [15]. Lee et al. chose loads of 35 N for distraction force in their study [6] and Hanada et al. chose loads of 50 N for their study [7]. We used the 89 N tensor device in our study, and this value is similar to that documented in the above-mentioned reports.

In the measured resection group, 3° external rotation off the PCA was set based on previous reports [8, 9]. However, the FCRa was inconsistent and the percentage of outlier cases was high because of the variations in the extent of the posterior condylar erosion and position of the bony landmarks of each patient. Fehring et al. also

Table 3 Comparison of postoperative clinical scores and knee range of motion among the groups

	Measured resection ($n = 45$)	Tensor ($n = 48$)	Block ($n = 49$)	p-value
Range of knee motion[b] (degree)	127.7 (90–145)	128.0 (100–145)	125.9 (95–145)	0.400[a]
KS score[b] (points)				
Knee	95.2 (84–100)	96.2 (84–100)	95.9 (89–100)	0.783[a]
Function	85.3 (61–100)	85.0 (64–100)	83.4 (61–100)	0.760[a]
HSS score (points)	91.7 (82–99)	92.0 (84–99)	91.8 (84–98)	0.899[a]
WOMAC score (points)	12.1 (1–24)	11.4 (1–27)	11.9 (2–27)	0.831[a]

Abbreviations: *KS* Knee Society, *HSS* Hospital for Special Surgery, *WOMAC* Western Ontario and McMaster Universities Osteoarthritis Index (LK 3.1 version)
[a]Mixed model for adjustment of auto-correlation
[b]The values are given as the mean and the range in parenthesis

reported higher rotational errors of at least 3° when FCR was determined by bony landmarks compared with the tension gap technique [16].

Several technical issues have been identified with the block placement method, which may be the cause of unsatisfactory implant placements. First, gap block could easily be rotated internally during the insertion or inevitably causes the femur to rotate externally because of the medial tightness in the varus knee, which applies to most of the participants in this study. This might have led to the internal rotation of femoral components in the block group. Second, the true tension of each participant might be underestimated. For example, if the true gap width of a patient is between 10 and 12.5 mm, it is evaluated uniformly as 10 mm because a thicker gap block cannot be inserted. Therefore, the block technique has a greater chance of inaccuracy. Some reports using gap block also introduced similar results although the causes were not explained clearly, that is, internal rotation of the femoral component [19].

The best reference for the FCR is still in debate. Several bony landmarks of the distal femur were proposed as the reference, including the PCA, cTEA, surgical transepicondylar axis (sTEA) and antero-posterior axis (Whiteside's line). Fehring and Laskin found that the result was inferior to that of tensioned gap technique when the PCA was used as reference [16, 20]. Griffin also reported that the posterior condyles were potentially unreliable references [21]. Arima stated that Whiteside's line was a reliable landmark in a valgus knee, and Whiteside reported that a better clinical outcome was observed in the group using Whiteside's line as a reference compared with that using the PCA as a reference in a valgus knee [22, 23]. On the other hand, Nagamine's study revealed that the PCA was more reliable than Whiteside's line in knees with medial tibiofemoral arthritis [24]. Victor also reported that Whiteside's line was least consistent on his CT-based kinematic study using cadavers [25]. Several studies concluded that the transepicondylar axis was more reliable than other landmarks in a typical varus knee with medial tibiofemoral arthritis. However, there are two transepicondylar axes (cTEA and sTEA), and several authors did not clearly state which of the two used in their studies [26–29]. Which of the two references is more appropriate and reproducible is unclear and there are several conflicting studies on this [28, 30, 31]. Based on our experience, we chose cTEA as a reference in this study.

This study has several limitations. First, the prosthesis and the instrument sets used for each group were different from one another. Although we think the type of prosthesis and instrument would not affect the FCRa significantly, different instruments could lead to different accuracy and precision. Second, because we chose the best cut image in axial CT with 1 mm thickness for measurement of FCRa rather subjectively, it could have not been the exact image to evaluate the FCRa of the case. However, we made it clear that axial CT cut was the best available image for FCRa measurement for the case. Third, the concept of FCR alignment in this study was based on mechanical alignment after TKA; meanwhile, there are several reports that patient-specific kinematic alignment is more important and more related to clinical outcome after TKA [32]. However, the focus of this study was to find the best method that can align the femoral component to the cTEA which the authors chose as the FCR reference based on literature reviews and personal experience. Fourth, surgeon errors could possibly occur with these three different techniques, due to each one having their own technical difficulties. Fifth, because this study was a single surgeon series, it is possible that the implementation of these three techniques could be different with different surgeons and the results could change if different surgeons were included in the study. However, this could also be an asset to this study that surgeon bias could be eliminated from the evaluation. And lastly, postoperative clinical evaluations were performed with 2-year postoperative data with less patients. Since the FCR could be a major factor to the long-term survival of the implant, longer follow-up clinical evaluations should be performed.

Conclusions

Although there are both good and bad points in techniques for determining FCRs, the gap technique with the 20-lbf tensor device was the most accurate and precise method in obtaining adequate FCR. Measured resection with 3° external rotation and gap technique with blocks could lead to internal rotation of the femoral component. Postoperative 2 year clinical results were not significantly different among groups with different techniques for FCR.

Abbreviations
CT: Computed tomography; cTEA: Clinical transepicondylar axis; FCR: Femoral component rotation; FCRa: Femoral component rotation angle; PCA: Posterior condylar axis; sTEA: Surgical transepicondylar axis; TKA: Total knee arthroplasty

Acknowledgement
The authors thank Medical Research Collaborating Center of Seoul National University Hospital for support in the statistical analysis

Funding
There was no external funding for this study.

Authors' contributions
JKL collected the data, performed the measurement and analysis, participated in the study design and drafted the manuscript. SL participated in the study design, supervised the analysis and helped to draft the manuscript. SHC

collected the data, performed the measurement. KTK helped to draft the manuscript and review the manuscript. MCL designed the study, supervised the whole study process and helped to draft and review the manuscript. All authors read and approved the final manuscript.

Competing interests

The authors declare that they have no competing interests.

Consent for publication

Not applicable.

Author details

[1]Department of Orthopaedic Surgery, Hallym University Sacred Heart Hospital, 22 Gwanpyeong-ro, 170beon-gil, Dongan-gu, Anyang-si, Gyeonggi-do 431-796, Korea. [2]Department of Orthopaedic Surgery, Seoul National University Hospital, 101 Daehang-ro, Jongno-gu, Seoul 110-744, Korea.

References

1. Mochizuki RM, Schurman DJ. Patellar complications following total knee arthroplasty. J Bone Joint Surg Am. 1979;61(6A):879–83.
2. Berger RA, Crossett LS, Jacobs JJ, Rubash HE. Malrotation causing patellofemoral complications after total knee arthroplasty. Clin Orthop Relat Res. 1998;356:144–53.
3. Romero J, Stahelin T, Binkert C, Pfirrmann C, Hodler J, Kessler O. The clinical consequences of flexion gap asymmetry in total knee arthroplasty. J Arthroplasty. 2007;22(2):235_40.
4. Barrack RL, Schrader T, Bertot AJ, Wolfe MW, Myers L. Component rotation and anterior knee pain after total knee arthroplasty. Clin Orthop Relat Res. 2001;392:46–55.
5. Fehring TK, Odum S, Griffin WL, Mason JB, Nadaud M. Early failures in total knee arthroplasty. Clin Orthop Relat Res. 2001;392:315–8.
6. Lee DH, Padhy D, Park JH, Jeong WK, Park JH, Han SB. The impact of a rectangular or trapezoidal flexion gap on the femoral component rotation in TKA. Knee Surg Sports Traumatol Arthrosc. 2011;19(7):1141_7.
7. Hanada H, Whiteside LA, Steiger J, Dyer P, Naito M. Bone landmarks are more reliable than tensioned gaps in TKA component alignment. Clin Orthop Relat Res. 2007;462:137–42.
8. Figgie 3rd HE, Goldberg VM, Heiple KG, Moller 3rd HS, Gordon NH. The influence of tibial-patellofemoral location on function of the knee in patients with the posterior stabilized condylar knee prosthesis. J Bone Joint Surg Am. 1986;68(7):1035–40.
9. Rhoads DD, Noble PC, Reuben JD, Tullos HS. The effect of femoral component position on the kinematics of total knee arthroplasty. Clin Orthop Relat Res. 1993;286:122–9.
10. Berger RA, Rubash HE, Seel MJ, Thompson WH, Crossett LS. Determining the rotational alignment of the femoral component in total knee arthroplasty using the epicondylar axis. Clin Orthop Relat Res. 1993;286:40_7.
11. Churchill DL, Incavo SJ, Johnson CC, Beynnon BD. The transepicondylar axis approximates the optimal flexion axis of the knee. Clin Orthop Relat Res. 1998;356:111–8.
12. Miller MC, Berger RA, Petrella AJ, Karmas A, Rubash HE. Optimizing femoral component rotation in total knee arthroplasty. Clin Orthop Relat Res. 2001;392:38–45.
13. Poilvache PL, Insall JN, Scuderi GR, Font-Rodriguez DE. Rotational landmarks and sizing of the distal femur in total knee arthroplasty. Clin Orthop Relat Res. 1996;331:35–46.
14. Asano H, Hoshino A, Wilton TJ. Soft-tissue tension total knee arthroplasty. J Arthroplasty. 2004;19(5):558–61.
15. Yoshino N, Watanabe N, Watanabe Y, Fukuda Y, Takai S. Measurement of joint gap load in patella everted and reset position during total knee arthroplasty. Knee Surg Sports Traumatol Arthrosc. 2009;17(5):484–90.
16. Fehring TK. Rotational malalignment of the femoral component in total knee arthroplasty. Clin Orthop Relat Res. 2000;380:72–9.
17. Viera AJ, Garrett JM. Understanding interobserver agreement: the kappa statistic. Fam Med. 2005;37(5):360–3.
18. Asano H, Muneta T, Sekiya I. Soft tissue tension in extension in total knee arthroplasty affects postoperative knee extension and stability. Knee Surg Sports Traumatol Arthrosc. 2008;16(11):999–1003.
19. Boldt JG, Stiehl JB, Munzinger U, Beverland D, Keblish PA. Femoral component rotation in mobile-bearing total knee arthroplasty. Knee. 2006;13(4):284–9.
20. Laskin RS. Flexion space configuration in total knee arthroplasty. J Arthroplasty. 1995;10(5):657–60.
21. Griffin FM, Insall JN, Scuderi GR. The posterior condylar angle in osteoarthritic knees. J Arthroplasty. 1998;13(7):812–5.
22. Arima J, Whiteside LA, McCarthy DS, White SE. Femoral rotational alignment, based on the anteroposterior axis, in total knee arthroplasty in a valgus knee. A technical note. J Bone Joint Surg Am. 1995;77(9):1331–4.
23. Whiteside LA, Arima J. The anteroposterior axis for femoral rotational alignment in valgus total knee arthroplasty. Clin Orthop Relat Res. 1995;321:168–72.
24. Nagamine R, Miura H, Inoue Y, Urabe K, Matsuda S, Okamoto Y, Nishizawa M, Iwamoto Y. Reliability of the anteroposterior axis and the posterior condylar axis for determining rotational alignment of the femoral component in total knee arthroplasty. J Orthop Sci. 1998;3(4):194–8.
25. Victor J, Van Doninck D, Labey L, Van Glabbeek F, Parizel P, Bellemans J. A common reference frame for describing rotation of the distal femur: a ct-based kinematic study using cadavers. J Bone Joint Surg (Br). 2009;91(5):683–90.
26. Jenny JY, Boeri C. Low reproducibility of the intra-operative measurement of the transepicondylar axis during total knee replacement. Acta Orthop Scand. 2004;75(1):74–7.
27. Jerosch J, Peuker E, Philipps B, Filler T. Interindividual reproducibility in perioperative rotational alignment of femoral components in knee prosthetic surgery using the transepicondylar axis. Knee Surg Sports Traumatol Arthrosc. 2002;10(3):194–7.
28. Mantas JP, Bloebaum RD, Skedros JG, Hofmann AA. Implications of reference axes used for rotational alignment of the femoral component in primary and revision knee arthroplasty. J Arthroplasty. 1992;7(4):531–5.
29. Olcott CW, Scott RD. The Ranawat Award. Femoral component rotation during total knee arthroplasty. Clin Orthop Relat Res. 1999;367:39–42.
30. Akagi M, Matsusue Y, Mata T, Asada Y, Horiguchi M, Iida H, Nakamura T. Effect of rotational alignment on patellar tracking in total knee arthroplasty. Clin Orthop Relat Res. 1999;366:155–63.
31. Yoshino N, Takai S, Ohtsuki Y, Hirasawa Y. Computed tomography measurement of the surgical and clinical transepicondylar axis of the distal femur in osteoarthritic knees. J Arthroplasty. 2001;16(4):493–7.
32. Dossett HG, Estrada NA, Swartz GJ, LeFevre GW, Kwasman BG. A randomised controlled trial of kinematically and mechanically aligned total knee replacements: two-year clinical results. Bone Joint J. 2014;96-B(7):907–13.

17

A new classification of TKA periprosthetic femur fractures considering the implant type

Johannes K. M. Fakler[1*†], Cathleen Pönick[1†], Melanie Edel[1,2], Robert Möbius[1,2], Alexander Giselher Brand[1], Andreas Roth[1], Christoph Josten[1,2] and Dirk Zajonz[1,2] (iD)

Abstract

Background: The treatment aims of periprosthetic fractures (PPF) of the distal femur are a gentle stabilization, an early load-bearing capacity and a rapid postoperative mobilization of the affected patients. For the therapy planning of PPF a standardized classification is necessary which leads to a clear and safe therapy recommendation. Despite different established classifications, there is none that includes the types of prosthesis used in the assessment. For this purpose, the objective of this work is to create a new more extensive fracture and implant-related classification of periprosthetic fractures of the distal femur based on available classifications which allows distinct therapeutic recommendations.

Methods: In a retrospective analysis all patients who were treated in the University Hospital Leipzig from 2010 to 2016 due to a distal femur fracture with total knee arthroplasty (TKA) were established. To create an implant-associated classification the cases were discussed in a panel of experienced orthopaedists and well-practiced traumatologists with a great knowledge in the field of endoprosthetics and fracture care. In this context, two experienced surgeons classified 55 consecutive fractures according to Su et al., Lewis and Rorabeck and by the new created classification. In this regard, the interobserver reliability was determined for two independent raters in terms of Cohen Kappa.

Results: On the basis of the most widely recognized classifications of Su et al. as well as Lewis and Rorabeck, we established an implant-dependent classification for PPF of the distal femur. In accordance with the two stated classifications four fracture types were created and defined. Moreover, the four most frequent prosthesis types were integrated. Finally, a new classification with 16 subtypes was generated based on four types of fracture and four types of prosthesis. Considering all cases the presented implant-associated classification ($\kappa = 0.74$) showed a considerably higher interobserver reliability compared to the other classifications of Su et al. ($\kappa = 0.39$) as well as Lewis and Rorabeck ($\kappa = 0.31$). Excluding the cases which were only assessable by the new classification, it still shows a higher interobserver reliability ($\kappa = 0.70$) than the other ones ($\kappa = 0.63$ or $\kappa = 0.45$).

Conclusions: The new classification system for PPF of the distal femur following TKA considers fracture location and implant type. It is easy to use, shows agood interobserver reliability and allows conclusions to be drawn on treatment recommendations. Moreover, further studies on the evaluation of the classification are necessary and planned.

Keywords: Implant-dependent classification, Periprosthetic fractures, Distal femur, Total knee arthroplasty

* Correspondence: Johannes.Fakler@medizin.uni-leipzig.de
†Equal contributors
[1]Department of Orthopaedic Surgery, Traumatology and Plastic Surgery, University Hospital Leipzig, Liebigstrasse 20, D-04103 Leipzig, Germany
Full list of author information is available at the end of the article

Background

The increased number of performed TKAs combined with longer implant survival and consecutive biomechanical changes of the adjacent bone is associated with a growing number of late complications [1]. The number of revisions after total knee arthroplasty increased by 40%, whereas total hip arthroplasty (THA) revisions increased by only 23% between 2006 and 2010 in the Nationwide Inpatient Sample (NIS) of the USA. During the same period both the primary TKA and the primary THA increased by only 31% [2, 3]. The most frequent reason for revisions in knee endoprosthetics is aseptic loosening due to osteolysis [2, 4]. Polyethylene abrasion is discussed as a main cause of osteolysis with a resulting implant loosening [5, 6]. Besides endoprosthetic loosening, reduced bone quality through osteoporosis and physical impairment of geriatric patients with a tendency to fall are related to an increased periprosthetic fracture risk [7, 8]. The incidence of PPF in knee prostheses varies between 0.6% and 5.5% in current literature [9–11]. For most of geriatric pre-disabled people PPF have serious consequences. With the duration of immobilization the risk for nosocomial infections, thromboses and embolisms rises and thus the mortality increases [12, 13]. In this context, conservative therapy does not serve as clinical standard due to its low efficiency which is based on often longer persisting or not guaranteed bony healing [14]. In a large meta-analysis the failure rates were partially indicated as very high with up to 50%. Especially the non-union rates vary between 1.5% and 29%, whereas the corresponding revision rates range from 4.6 to 40% [15]. Treatment aims are a gentle stabilization, an early load-bearing capacity and a rapid postoperative mobilization of the affected patients. In addition to a well-founded understanding of the possibilities of treating these fractures, which require a case-adapted and individualized therapy in principal, a clear procedure is needed. Therefore, a standardized classification of PPF, that allows distinct and safe therapy recommendations, is helpful for creating such a specific therapy concept. The first classification of supracondylar femoral fractures in knee endoprostheses dates from 1967 by Neer and colleagues [16]. It only considers the dislocation and is rarely used today. In 1991, DiGioia and Rubash extended this classification for bone quality, fracture orientation and extent of dislocation [16, 17]. Nevertheless, just like Neer it is only used in rare cases. In contrast, a widely accepted classification with therapeutic recommendations was presented by Lewis and Rorabeck in 1997. Here, the degree of dislocation and the stability of the prosthesis play a decisive role [18]. Currently, one of the most common used and newest classifications of PPF of the knee is described by Su et al. in 2003. The three types of this classification are based on

a simple anatomical assignment: **type I:** fractures are proximal to the femoral component, **type II:** fracture starts at the proximal border of the femoral component and extends proximally, **type III:** all fracture parts are below the proximal border of the anterior prosthesis shield [19]. However, none of these classifications includes the various types of endoprosthesis in their assessment. In recent years, the importance of endoprosthesis revision has steadily increased and complex revision systems are widespread in the current patient population. The differently constructed systems with individual specifications have a significant influence on the surgical supply of the occurred PPF [2, 3]. In particular, technical developments for the medical treatment of periprosthetic fractures in revision systems have become established. The successful clinical usage of different investigations such as retrograde intramedullary nails with angular stable locking options, plate osteosynthesis with multidirectional locking options or polyaxial locking compression plates (LCP) as well as attachment plates has also often been described in the literature [20–24]. Based on the increase of different types of prosthesis with an accumulation of revision systems and the development of new care strategies it is necessary to create a novel more extensive classification with a clear reference to the implant.

The intention of this work is to generate a new fracture and implant-related classification of periprosthetic TKA fractures of the femur on the basis of available classifications and through a retrospective analysis of specific patients from the University Hospital Leipzig. Moreover, it is intended to accomplish a classification from which clear therapeutic recommendations can be derived.

Methods

Prior to the start of the investigation, the local university's ethics committee was consulted and after examination a positive vote was issued. The vote-number of the audit authority is 044/14032016. The written, informed consent was obtained from all study participants, including their consent for publication of the results. By means of a retrospective analysis all patients who were treated due to a femur fracture in the University Hospital Leipzig from 2010 to 2016 were identified (1468 patients). Subsequently, all people with a periprosthetic fracture of the femur were determined (178 patients). Excluding all femur fractures with THA, 55 TKAs with PPF of the distal femur could be recorded.

All available data were obtained from the patient documentation system which contains archived records and electronic files in IS-H SAP (Siemens AG Healthcare Sector, Erlangen, Germany), radiological findings as well as images from SIENET MagicWeb/ACOM (Siemens AG

Healthcare Sector, Erlangen, Germany), among other things. Based on this, we examined each fracture localization and configuration. Furthermore, the descriptions of the fractures which were noted in the operational report were analyzed. In this context, fracture size, bone quality, stability of the prosthesis and type of care were documented. The cases were discussed in a panel of four senior orthopaedic surgeons experienced in adult reconstruction and orthopaedic trauma surgery and with a great knowledge in the field of endoprosthetics as well as fracture care. Within the scope of this case discussion, a classification together with therapeutic recommendations were derived and formulated.

Implant-dependent classification of periprosthetic fractures of the distal femur

Based on the most widely recognized classifications of Su et al. as well as Lewis and Rorabeck, we have established an implant-dependent classification for periprosthetic fractures of the distal femur relating to the most common types of prosthesis [18, 19]. In this context four fracture types (I – IV) were created and defined relevant to the already mentioned classifications.

- Type I: Fracture is distant from the TKA (proximal of the femoral component) referring to Su type I
- Type II: Fracture starts at the level of the proximal border of TKA and extends proximally referring to Su type II
- Type III: All fracture parts are below the proximal prosthesis border referring to Su type III
- Type IV: Supracondylar fracture with prosthetic loosening referring to Lewis and Rorabeck type III

In addition, the most frequent prosthesis types (A - D) were taken into account and summarized in four groups which are defined as follows:

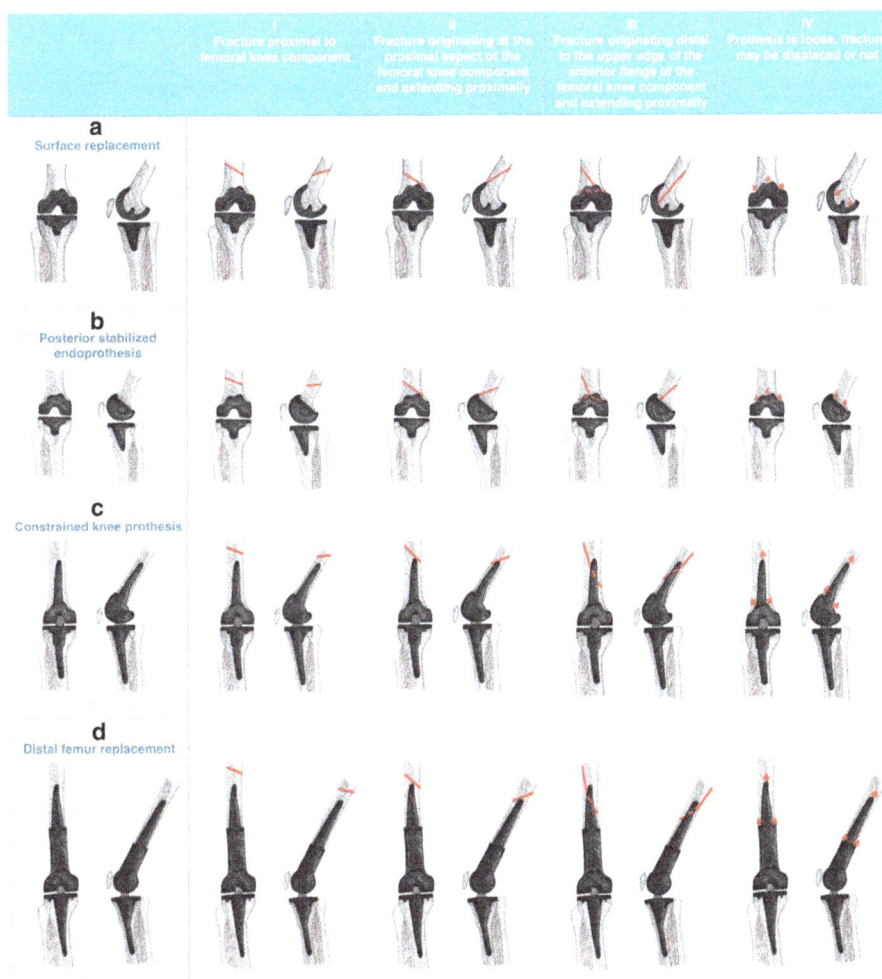

Fig. 1 Schematic representation of the implant-dependent classification for periprosthetic fractures of the distal femur **a**: Unconstrained bikondylär TKA, **b**: posterior stabilized TKA, **c**: constrained (rotating-hinge) TKA, **d**: Distal femoral replacement. I-III: Location and expansion of fracture, IV: fracture with implant loosening. Red line depicts fracture line

Table 1 Treatment recommendations in gradation with respect to the classification of the fracture

	I	II	III	IV
A	Locking plate, retrograde nail, (antegrade nail)	Locking plate, retrograde nail,	Locking plate, revision arthroplasty (constraint endoprosthesis, eventually distal femoral replacement)	Revision arthroplasty (constraint endoprosthesis, eventually distal femoral replacement)
B	Locking plate, antegrade nail	Locking plate, revision arthroplasty (distal femoral replacement, eventually constraint endoprosthesis)	revision arthroplasty (distal femoral replacement)	revision arthroplasty (distal femoral replacement)
C	Locking plate (polyaxial, attachment plates), revision arthroplasty (distal femoral replacement)	Locking plate (polyaxial, attachment plates), revision arthroplasty (distal femoral replacement)	revision arthroplasty (distal femoral replacement)	revision arthroplasty (distal femoral replacement)
D	Locking plate (polyaxial, attachment plates), revision arthroplasty (distal femoral replacement)	revision arthroplasty (distal femoral replacement), Locking plate (polyaxial, attachment plates),	revision arthroplasty (distal femoral replacement)	revision arthroplasty (distal femoral replacement)

- Type A: bicondylar uncoupled endoprosthesis (surface replacement)
- Type B: Semi-constraint bicondylar sledges prosthesis (posterior stabilized)
- Type C: Constraint prosthesis with intramedullary anchoring
- Type D: Distal femur replacement

Finally, a classification with 16 subtypes was made based on four types of fracture and four groups of prostheses. A schematic representation of the new implant-dependent classification of periprosthetic fractures of the distal femur is shown in Fig. 1.

Classification-related therapeutic recommendations

For the purpose of creating classification-related therapeutic recommendations all relevant cases were assessed with regard to the new classification and appropriate treatment recommendations were derived. These recommendations are based on the expertise of the experts and the analysis of current literature. The recommendations were formulated in first, second, and third line therapy. A corresponding overview is given in Table 1.

Finally, two senior orthopaedic surgeons classified independently the conventional X-ray images of the chosen fractures (n = 55) according to Su et al., Lewis and Rorabeck plus the new classification [18, 19]. With regard to the different classifications, the interobserver reliability was determined for two independent raters

pursuant to Cohen Kappa [25]. On this occasion, Kappa was defined by Landis and Koch as follows: $\kappa < 0$ poor agreement, $\kappa = 0$–0.20 slight, $\kappa = 0.21$–0.40 fair, $\kappa = 0.41$–0.60 moderate, $\kappa = 0.61$–0.80 substantial, $\kappa = 0.81$–1.00 (almost) perfect [26].

Results

The interobserver reliability for two independent raters of the three classifications (Su et al., Rorabeck et al. and implant-associated classification) is presented in Table 2. Since implant group C and D are not clearly defined by the classifications of Su et al. as well as Lewis and Rorabeck, they are excluded from the investigation. Therefore, only 41 cases were taken into account, whereas the implant-related classification could be applied in all 55 cases ($\kappa = 0.74$). As a result, the new classification showed the highest interobserver reliability ($\kappa = 0.70$). While Su et al. got similar results ($\kappa = 0.63$), just a moderate agreement could be verified by Lewis and Rorabeck ($\kappa = 0.45$).

Discussion

Periprosthetic fractures in patient's TKA show an incidence of 0.3–5.5% and after revision surgery even up to 6% [9, 10]. However, data of most studies are of reduced significance due to their small number of cases. By means of a meta-analysis of Probst and colleagues, including 55 studies with 1370 patients in total, an average number of 25 patients was obtained [27]. Despite the rarity, the

Table 2 Interobserver reliability of all classifications (Su et al., Lewis and Rorabeck, new implant-related classification) according to Cohen Kappa for two independent testers with: $\kappa < 0$ poor agreement, $\kappa = 0$–0.20 slight, $\kappa = 0.21$–0.40 fair, $\kappa = 0.41$–0.60 moderate, $\kappa = 0.61$–0.80 substantial, $\kappa = 0.81$–1.00 (almost) perfect

interobserver reliability (Kappa)	Su et al. classification	Lewis & Rorabeck classification	new implant-associated classification
without exclusion ($n = 55$)	0.388 (fair)	0.309 (fair)	0.743 (substantial)
with exclusion ($n = 41$)	0.633 (substantial)	0.445 (moderate)	0.696 (substantial)

Exclusion is based on implant typ C and D, which are only defined by the new classification

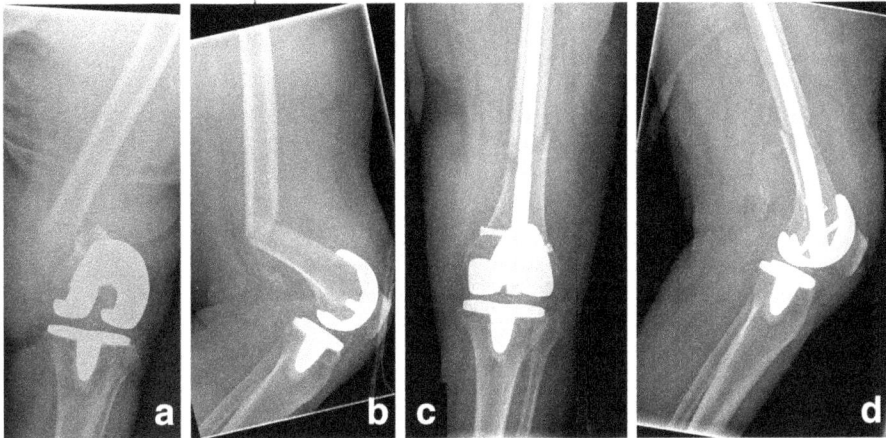

Fig. 2 X-ray images of a 92-year-old woman with a periprosthetic fracture of the left femur after cruciate retaining (CR) bicondylar TKA (type A I); **a**: anterior-posterior and **b**: lateral radiation path with representation of the fracture before supply; **c**: anterior-posterior and **d**: lateral radiation path after reconstruction and supply by retrograde nail osteosynthesis

incidence increases with the raise in primary knee and relevant revision endoprosthetics [2, 3]. Moreover, these are serious diagnoses, which should be treated in centers with experienced orthopaedists and traumatologists. In general, the treatment of periprosthetic fractures requires an optimal combination of endoprosthetics and fracture care [9, 12, 17]. The aim in this is to restore the limb's original functional capability for achieving a rapid recovery of mobility and to avoid complications like bedrest of the often multimorbid patients. For this purpose and to ensure a safe treatment, a clear acute care concept with an individually adapted treatment is indispensable. For the treatment of distal thigh fractures good and clear guidelines already exist [28–30]. In this context, the classifiable treatment is established and well evaluated, too [24, 31, 32]. There are also many different classifications for the treatment of periprosthetic distal femoral fractures with clear therapeutic deductions [16, 18, 19, 33, 34]. A meta-analysis of Ebraheim and colleagues, containing 41 articles with 448 fractures, revealed Rorabeck type II as the most common fracture. Standard treatments for these types of fracture are locked plating and intra-medullary nailing with similar healing rates of 87% and 84%, respectively [35]. However, despite intensive literature research, we were unable to find a classification which also refers to the type of prosthesis in addition to the fracture configuration. Although some classifications involve the loosening of the femoral component, no clear statements are made about the type of prosthesis [18]. Moreover, the range of prosthesis types has expanded considerably due to the increasing number of endoprosthesis replacements. Thus, it appears that an establishment of a

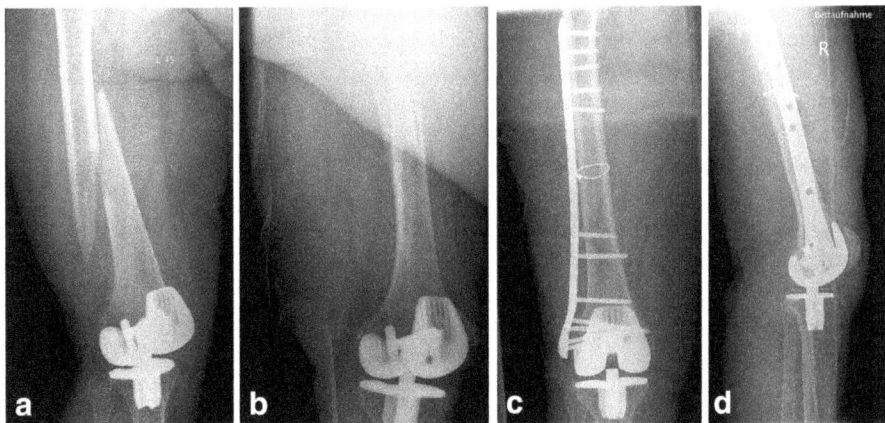

Fig. 3 X-ray images of an 84-year-old woman with a periprosthetic fracture of the right femur with posterior stabilized (PS) TKA (type B I); **a**: anterior-posterior and **b**: lateral radiation path with representation of the fracture before supply; **c**: anterior-posterior and **d**: lateral radiation path after reconstruction and supply by plate osteosynthesis. The insertions of the distal screws were complicated by the box

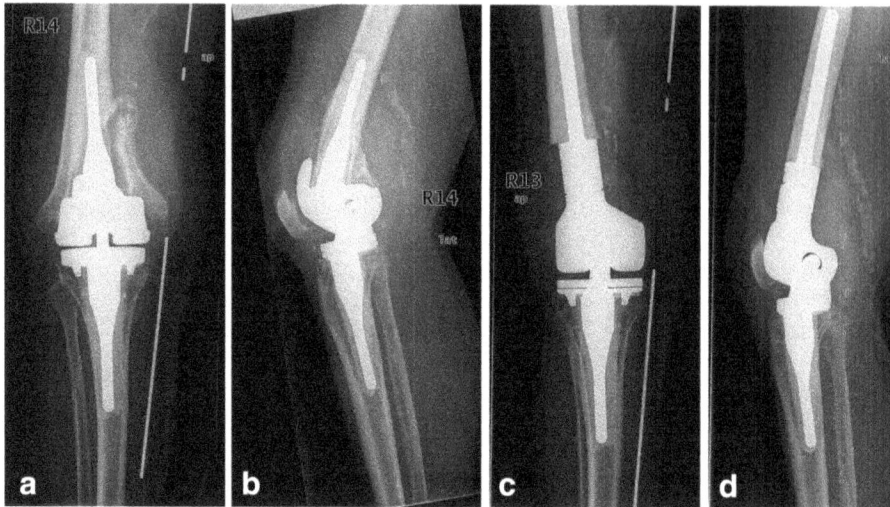

Fig. 4 X-ray images of a 77-year-old woman with a periprosthetic fracture of the right femur with loose constrained TKA and intramedullary stem (type C IV); **a**: anterior-posterior and **b**: lateral radiation path with representation of the fracture before supply; **c**: anterior-posterior and **d**: lateral radiation path after implantation of a modular TKA

classification, which relates in particular to the prosthesis properties, is necessary. For this purpose, the presented implant-dependent classification for periprosthetic fractures of the distal femur involves both the fracture localization and orientation according to Su et al. as well as the loosening of the implant relating to Lewis and Rorabeck [18, 19]. Based on this, these specifications combined with the four prosthesis types are grouped into 16 subtypes (Fig. 1). Due to the independent evaluation of two experienced orthopaedic surgeons, we were able to prove that the presented implant-associated classification shows a higher interobserver reliability compared to the classifications of Su et al. or Lewis and Rorabeck, respectively (Table 2). A major advantage of the new classification is the inclusion of the implant types C and D, which are not defined by the other ones [18, 19]. The classification of loosening is generally problematic, because of their limited detectability using conventional X-ray imaging. Most inconsistencies of our investigators were based on this fact. For this purpose, the intraoperative findings are always essential.

As already shown, therapy is a patient-specific process which presupposes a high level of expertise and experience. Therefore, a dogmatic therapy recommendation is not always effective. Type A I fracture, for example, shows that an absolute recommendation for intramedullary nails is only possible to a limited extent. On the one hand, different types of prosthesis, varying in depth of their intercondylar boxes, exist. Thus, prostheses with a widely dorsally drawn box complicate the choice of the correct nail's point of intersection. On the other hand, there are prosthetic designs with a smaller intercondylar

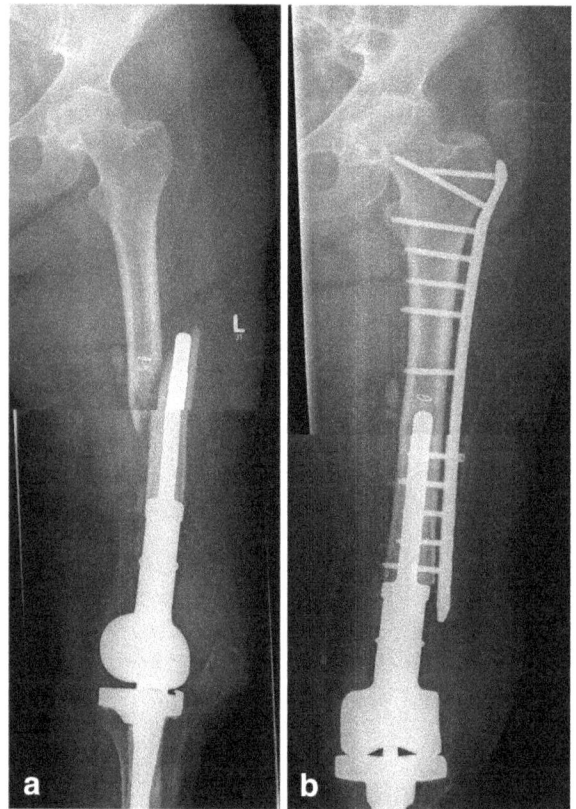

Fig. 5 X-ray images of an 82-year-old woman with a periprosthetic fracture of the/left femur with distal femoral replacement; (Type D II) **a**: anterior-posterior radiation path with representation of the fracture before supply; **b**: anterior-posterior radiation path after reconstruction and supply by plate osteosynthesis

distance of the femoral component than the nail diameter [36]. In these cases, retrograde intramedullary nailing of periprosthetic fractures of the distal femur is not or only partly feasible. Furthermore, more than 40° deficit in knee flexion may be an obstacle for the insertion of a nail [37]. Additionally, a cemented anchoring of the femoral component can make the insertion or locking of the nail more difficult or impossible. Here, an angle stable plate osteosynthesis is more useful (Fig. 2). In type B fractures (posterior stabilized TKA) a retrograde nail osteosynthesis is impossible in most systems because of the closed design of the box. However, there also exist PS-systems in which retrograde nailing is feasible due to the open box (NexGen or Persona by Zimmer). Nevertheless, on the basis of the box the entry point can also lead to difficulties in these systems. Special nails for osteosynthesis with TKAs can simplify this problem. Especially in typ C II and III fractures, which extend far distally, osteosynthesis with plates is complex. In this context, the insertion of the distal screws is hampered by the box's configuration in particular (Fig. 3). In these cases and in case of loosening (type IV fractures), only an implant revision often remains as ultima ratio (Fig. 4). If modular endoprostheses fail a revision is frequently indicated as well. Here, the only available treatment is a larger modular mega-endoprosthesis. In order to preserve remaining bone stock an osteosynthesis should be aspired (Fig. 5). These few examples already show the complexity of PPF's operative care, which can also be only partially covered by the new classification. There still remains a single case decision which depends on additional multiple factors, such as bone structure (osteoporosis), cementation, stature of the patient, surgeon's experience, etc. [38, 39]. The presented classification is just intended to ease the decision-making process, which must be adapted to each individual case.

A further aim of our working group is to evaluate the classification by means of retrospective investigations followed by prospective ones.

Conclusions

We present an implant-dependent classification for periprosthetic fractures of the distal femur. Based on the widespread and established classifications according to Su et al. as well as Lewis and Rorabeck we created a more detailed one. In favour of a better categorization the four classic prosthesis types are additionally included. Thus, fractures can not only be classified by their anatomical assignment but in combination with the existing prosthesis. Therefore, clear treatment recommendations can be easier derived from the presented 16 subtypes, taking the individual situation into account.

Further studies on the evaluation of the classification are necessary and planned.

Abbreviations
LCP: Locking compression plates; NIS: Nationwide Inpatient Sample; PPF: Periprosthetic fractures; THA: Total hip arthroplasty; TKA: Total knee arthroplasty

Acknowledgements
We acknowledge the support of the German Research Foundation (DFG) and the University Hospital Leipzig within the program of Open Access Publishing. We would also like to thank Prof. Th. Kahn, Department of Diagnostic and Interventional Radiology, for providing the radiographs.

Funding
This study was funded by the German Research Foundation (DFG) and the University Hospital Leipzig within the program of Open Access Publishing. The funding body had no impact on the design of the study, collection, analysis and interpretation of data as well as writing the manuscript.

Authors' contributions
JF initiated the work and is the head of the expert team. CP has carried out the data collection and presentation. She also has contributed significantly to the preparation of the manuscript. DZ was part of the expert team and a major contributor in writing the manuscript. ME gave statistical support, endorsed the drafting of the article and revised it critically. AB helped with data collection. MG, CJ, AR and JF were mainly responsible for the treatment of the patients as well as members of the expert group. All authors read and approved the final manuscript.

Consent for publication
Not applicable.

Competing interests
JKMF is a member of the Editorial Board of BMC Musculoskeletal Disorders. The other authors declare no competing interests.

Author details
[1]Department of Orthopaedic Surgery, Traumatology and Plastic Surgery, University Hospital Leipzig, Liebigstrasse 20, D-04103 Leipzig, Germany. [2]ZESBO – Center for Research on Musculoskeletal Systems, University of Leipzig, Semmelweisstrasse 14, D-04103 Leipzig, Germany.

References
1. Cholewinski P, Putman S, Vasseur L, Migaud H, Duhamel A, Behal H, Pasquier G. Long-term outcomes of primary constrained condylar knee arthroplasty. Orthop Traumatol Surg Res. 2015;101:449–54. doi:10.1016/j.otsr.2015.01.020.
2. Bozic KJ, Kamath AF, Ong K, Lau E, Kurtz S, Chan V, et al. Comparative epidemiology of revision arthroplasty: failed THA poses greater clinical and economic burdens than failed TKA. Clin Orthop Relat Res. 2015;473:2131–8. doi:10.1007/s11999-014-4078-8.

3. Bozic KJ, Kurtz SM, Lau E, Ong K, Chiu V, Vail TP, et al. The epidemiology of revision total knee arthroplasty in the United States. Clin Orthop Relat Res. 2010;468:45–51. doi:10.1007/s11999-009-0945-0.

4. Cherian JJ, Jauregui JJ, Banerjee S, Pierce T, Mont MA. What host factors affect aseptic loosening after THA and TKA? Clin Orthop Relat Res. 2015;473: 2700–9. doi:10.1007/s11999-015-4220-2.

5. Gonzalez MH, Mekhail AO. The failed total knee arthroplasty: evaluation and etiology. J Am Acad Orthop Surg. 2004;12:436–46.

6. Lonner JH, Siliski JM, Scott RD. Prodromes of failure in total knee arthroplasty. J Arthroplast. 1999;14:488–92.

7. Chang CB, Kim TK, Kang YG, Seong SC, Kang S-B. Prevalence of osteoporosis in female patients with advanced knee osteoarthritis undergoing total knee arthroplasty. J Korean Med Sci. 2014;29:1425–31. doi:10.3346/jkms.2014.29.10.1425.

8. Smith JW, Marcus RL, Peters CL, Pelt CE, Tracy BL, LaStayo PC. Muscle force steadiness in older adults before and after total knee arthroplasty. J Arthroplast. 2014;29:1143–8. doi:10.1016/j.arth.2013.11.023.

9. Gruner A, Hockertz T, Reilmann H. Periprosthetic fractures: classification, management, therapy. Unfallchirurg. 2004;107:35–49.

10. Wick M, Muller EJ, Kutscha-Lissberg F, Hopf F, Muhr G. Periprosthetic supracondylar femoral fractures: LISS or retrograde intramedullary nailing? Problems with the use of minimally invasive technique. Unfallchirurg. 2004;107:181–8. doi:10.1007/s00113-003-0723-5.

11. Culp RW, Schmidt RG, Hanks G, Mak A, Esterhai JL. JR, Heppenstall RB. Supracondylar fracture of the femur following prosthetic knee arthroplasty. Clin Orthop Relat Res. 1987:212–22.

12. Agarwal S, Sharma RK, Jain JK. Periprosthetic fractures after total knee arthroplasty. J Orthop Surg (Hong Kong). 2014;22:24–9.

13. Gavaskar AS, Tummala NC, Subramanian M. The outcome and complications of the locked plating management for the periprosthetic distal femur fractures after a total knee arthroplasty. Clin Orthop Surg. 2013;5:124–8. doi:10.4055/cios.2013.5.2.124.

14. Tomas T, Nachtnebl L, Otiepka P. Distal femoral periprosthetic fractures: classification and therapy. Acta Chir Orthop Traumatol Cechoslov. 2010;77:194–202.

15. Hagel A, Siekmann H, Delank K-S. Periprosthetic femoral fracture - an interdisciplinary challenge. Dtsch Arztebl Int. 2014;111:658–64. doi:10.3238/arztebl.2014.0658.

16. Neer CS2, Grantham SA, Shelton ML. Supracondylar fracture of the adult femur. A study of one hundred and ten cases. J Bone Joint Surg Am 1967; 49:591–613.

17. DiGioia AM3, Rubash HE. Periprosthetic fractures of the femur after total knee arthroplasty. A literature review and treatment algorithm. Clin Orthop Relat Res 1991:135–142.

18. Rorabeck CH, Angliss RD, Lewis PL. Fractures of the femur, tibia, and patella after total knee arthroplasty: decision making and principles of management. Instr Course Lect. 1998;47:449–58.

19. Su H, Aharonoff GB, Hiebert R, Zuckerman JD, Koval KJ. In-hospital mortality after femoral neck fracture: do internal fixation and hemiarthroplasty differ? Am J Orthop (Belle Mead NJ). 2003;32:151–5.

20. Smith WR, Stoneback JW, Morgan SJ, Stahel PF. Is immediate weight bearing safe for periprosthetic distal femur fractures treated by locked plating? A feasibility study in 52 consecutive patients. Patient Saf Surg. 2016;10:26. doi:10.1186/s13037-016-0114-9.

21. Kammerlander C, Kates SL, Wagner M, Roth T, Blauth M. Minimally invasive periprosthetic plate osteosynthesis using the locking attachment plate. Oper Orthop Traumatol. 2013;25:398–408, 410. doi:10.1007/s00064-011-0091-1.

22. Wahnert D, Schliemann B, Raschke MJ, Kosters C. Treatment of periprosthetic fractures: new concepts in operative treatment. Orthopade. 2014;43:306–13. doi:10.1007/s00132-013-2165-2.

23. Fakler JKM, Hepp P, Marquass B, von Dercks N, Josten CI. Distal femoral replacement an adequate therapeutic option after complex fractures of the distal femur? Z Orthop Unfall. 2013;151:173–9. doi:10.1055/s-0032-1328424.

24. Agrawal A, Kiyawat V. Complex AO type C3 distal femur fractures: results after fixation with a lateral locked plate using modified swashbuckler approach. Indian J Orthop. 2017;51:18–27. doi:10.4103/0019-5413.197516.

25. Cohen J. Weighted kappa: nominal scale agreement with provision for scaled disagreement or partial credit. Psychol Bull. 1968;70:213–20.

26. Landis JR, Koch GG. The measurement of observer agreement for categorical data. Biometrics. 1977;33:159–74.

27. Probst A, Schneider T, Hankemeier S, Brug E. The prosthesis nail – a new stable fixation device for periprosthetic fractures and critical fractures of the proximal femur. Unfallchirurg. 2003;106:722–31. doi:10.1007/s00113-003-0621-x.

28. Vandenbussche E, LeBaron M, Ehlinger M, Flecher X, Pietu G. Blade-plate fixation for distal femoral fractures: a case-control study. Orthop Traumatol Surg Res. 2014;100:555–60. doi:10.1016/j.otsr.2014.06.006.

29. Toro G, Calabro G, Toro A, de SA, Iolascon G. Locking plate fixation of distal femoral fractures is a challenging technique: a retrospective review. Clin Cases Miner Bone Metab. 2015;12:55–8. doi:10.11138/ccmbm/2015.12.3s.054.

30. Griffin XL, Parsons N, Zbaeda MM, McArthur J. Interventions for treating fractures of the distal femur in adults. Cochrane Database Syst Rev. 2015: CD010606. doi:10.1002/14651858.CD010606.pub2.

31. Weight M, Collinge C. Early results of the less invasive stabilization system for mechanically unstable fractures of the distal femur (AO/OTA types A2, A3, C2, and C3). J Orthop Trauma. 2004;18:503–8.

32. Hutson JJ. JR, Zych GA. Treatment of comminuted intraarticular distal femur fractures with limited internal and external tensioned wire fixation. J Orthop Trauma. 2000;14:405–13.

33. Backstein D, Safir O, Gross A. Periprosthetic fractures of the knee. J Arthroplast. 2007;22:45–9. doi:10.1016/j.arth.2006.12.054.

34. Tabutin J, Cambas P-M, Vogt F. Tibial diaphysis fractures below a total knee prosthesis. Rev Chir Orthop Reparatrice Appar Mot. 2007;93:389–94.

35. Ebraheim NA, Kelley LH, Liu X, Thomas IS, Steiner RB, Liu J. Periprosthetic distal femur fracture after Total knee arthroplasty: a systematic review. Orthop Surg. 2015;7:297–305. doi:10.1111/os.12199.

36. Biber R, Bail HJ. Retrograde intramedullary nailing for periprosthetic fractures of the distal femur. Oper Orthop Traumatol. 2014;26:438–54. doi:10.1007/s00064-014-0303-6.

37. Thompson SM, Lindisfarne EAO, Bradley N, Solan M. Periprosthetic supracondylar femoral fractures above a total knee replacement: compatibility for fixation with a retrograde intramedullary nail. J Arthroplast. 2014;29:1639–41. doi:10.1016/j.arth.2013.07.027.

38. Beris AE, Lykissas MG, Sioros V, Mavrodontidis AN, Korompilias AV. Femoral periprosthetic fracture in osteoporotic bone after a total knee replacement: treatment with Ilizarov external fixation. J Arthroplast. 2010;25:1168.e9–12. doi:10.1016/j.arth.2009.10.009.

39. Solarino G, Vicenti G, Moretti L, Abate A, Spinarelli A, Moretti B. Interprosthetic femoral fractures-a challenge of treatment. A systematic review of the literature. Injury. 2014;45:362–8. doi:10.1016/j.injury.2013.09.028.

18

Cytokine and neuropeptide levels are associated with pain relief in patients with chronically painful total knee arthroplasty

Jasvinder A. Singh[1,2,3,4*], Siamak Noorbaloochi[6,7] and Keith L. Knutson[5]

Abstract

Background: There are few studies with an assessment of the levels of cytokines or neuropeptides as correlates of pain and pain relief in patients with painful joint diseases. Our objective was to assess whether improvements from baseline to 2-months in serum cytokine, chemokine and substance P levels were associated with clinically meaningful pain relief at 2-months post-injection in patients with painful total knee arthroplasty (TKA).

Methods: Using data from randomized trial of 60 TKAs, we assessed the association of change in cytokine/chemokine/Substance P levels with primary study outcome, clinically important improvement in Western Ontario McMaster Osteoarthritis Index (WOMAC) pain subscale at 2-months post-injection using Student's t-tests and Spearman's correlation coefficient (non-parametric). Patients were categorized as pain responders (20-point reduction or more on 0-100 WOMAC pain) vs. pain non-responders. Sensitivity analysis used 0–10 daytime pain numeric rating scale (NRS) instead of WOMAC pain subscale.

Results: In a pilot study, compared to non-responders ($n = 23$) on WOMAC pain scale at 2-months, pain responders ($n = 12$) had significantly greater increase in serum levels of IL-7, IL-10, IL-12, eotaxin, interferon gamma and TNF-α from baseline to 2-months post-injection ($p < 0.05$ for all). Change in several cytokine/chemokine and substance P levels from pre-injection to 2-month follow-up correlated significantly with change in WOMAC pain with correlation coefficients ranging −0.37 to −0.51: IL-2, IL-7, IL-8, IL-9, IL-16, IL-12p, GCSF, IFN gamma, IP-10, MCP, MIP1b, TNF-α and VEGF ($n = 35$). Sensitivity analysis showed that substance P decreased significantly more from baseline to 2-months in the pain responders (0.54 ± 0.53; $n = 10$) than in the pain non-responders (0.48 ± 1.18; $n = 9$; $p = 0.023$) and that this change in serum substance P correlated significantly with change in daytime NRS pain, correlation coefficient was 0.53 ($p = 0.021$; $n = 19$). Findings should be interpreted with caution, since cytokine analyses were performed for a sub-group of the entire trial population.

Conclusion: Serum cytokine, chemokine and Substance P levels correlated with pain response in patients with painful TKA after an intra-articular injection in a randomized trial.

Keywords: Cytokine, Substance P, Pain, Primary total knee arthroplasty, TKA

* Correspondence: Jasvinder.md@gmail.com
[1]Medicine Service, VA Medical Center, 700 19th St S, Birmingham, AL 35233, USA
[2]Department of Medicine at School of Medicine, University of Alabama at Birmingham Faculty Office Tower, 805B, 510 20th Street S, Birmingham, AL 35294, USA
Full list of author information is available at the end of the article

Background

Total knee arthroplasty (TKA) is one of the most successful procedures performed in patients with end-stage osteoarthritis (OA) and other arthritides with refractory pain [1]. While most patients report improved pain and function outcomes after TKA, persistent pain is reported by 6.5% or more patients post-TKA [2].

The role that cytokines and neurotransmitters play in joint pain is of great interest and has been the focus of recent research [3]. In an animal model of OA, cytokine levels were higher in OA joints, which were reduced by treatment with coenzyme Q-10 that also led to significant pain relief [4]. TNF-α levels were associated with WOMAC pain scores in patients with OA [5]. Joint fluid substance P (SP) levels in knee joints were elevated in painful knee joints with OA [6] and in preoperative joint fluid in those with greater pain relief after knee arthroplasty [6]. Studies showed that higher levels of cytokines such as interleukin-8 (IL-8), IL-6 and tumor necrosis factor-alpha (TNF-α) were associated with implant loosening in patients with joint arthroplasty [7, 8]. To our knowledge, there are limited or no data regarding the role of cytokines in pain severity in patients with painful TKA or relief with interventions.

We examined the data from a randomized trial of patients with persistently painful TKA [9] to test the hypotheses whether in patients with painful TKA, change (baseline to 2-months) in serum cytokine, chemokine and substance P (neuropeptide) levels was associated with clinically meaningful pain relief at 2-months post-injection. We also assessed whether baseline to 2-month change in cytokine/chemokine/substance P level correlated with change in pain severity from baseline to 2 months.

Methods

Clinical trial population

We used the data from patients enrolled in a previously published 6-month, 2-arm, parallel group, blinded placebo-controlled randomized trial (NCT00403273), details provided elsewhere [9]. Briefly, 60 TKAs were randomized in 1:1 to single intra-articular injection of active (onabotulinum toxin A) vs. placebo (saline) to assess its short-term anti-nociceptive efficacy. The research pharmacist prepared computerized randomization with permuted blocks of four patients each and prepared the treatment and placebo syringes using a strict standardized protocol. Both placebo and onabotulinum toxin A injections were transparent and could not be differentiated. In this triple-blind study, patients, investigators (PI, blinded investigators performing assessments, research associates) and the statistician were blinded (all analyses were completed and tables finalized before the pharmacist revealed the designation for group 1 vs. group 2). The PI injected the affected TKA joint using the standardized medial or lateral approach [10, 11]. This study was adequately

powered with 19 patients/group were needed for 80% power and 24 patients/group for 90% power (assuming 25% loss to follow-up), to detect a difference of 43% in proportion of patients reporting a clinically meaningful improvement in pain, based on previously published studies [12, 13].

Primary outcome assessment was at 2-months. A protocol modification to collect blood specimens to understand the mechanism of pain relief in patients with persistently painful TKA was made around the mid-point of patient recruitment upon receipt of federal funds, which provided resources to perform these assays, which were not available previously [9]. The Institutional Review Board (IRB) at the Minneapolis VA approved the study.

Serum cytokine and neuropeptide assays

Specimens were drawn both at baseline pre-injection and 2-month post-injection. We performed the serum cytokine assay using the BioRad human 27-plex cytokine panel (Cat # 171-A11127, Bio-Rad, San Diego CA; Table 1; http://www.bio-rad.com/en-jp/sku/m500kcaf0y-bio-plex-pro-human-cytokine-27-plex-assay). 100 μl of Bio-Plex assay buffer was added to each well of a Multiscreen MABVN 1.2 μm microfiltration plate followed by the addition of 50 μl of the multiplex bead preparation. Following washing of the beads with the addition of 100 μl of wash buffer, 50 μl of the samples or the standards was added to each well and incubated with shaking for 30 min at room temperature. Standard curves were generated with a mixture of 27 cytokine standards and eight serial dilutions ranging from 0 to 32,000 picogram/ml. The plate was then washed three times followed by incubation of each well in 25 μl of pre-mixed detection antibodies for 30 min with shaking. The plate was further washed and 50 μl of streptavidin solution were added to each well and incubated for 10 min at room temperature with shaking. The beads were given a final washing and re-suspended in 125 μl of Bio-Plex assay buffer. Cytokine

Table 1 Components of the 27-cytokine panel

Interleukins (IL): IL-1 beta, IL-1 alpha, IL-2, IL-4, IL-5, IL-6, IL-7, IL-8, IL-9, IL-10, IL-12 (p70), IL-13, IL-15, IL-17

Basic fibroblast growth factor (FGF)

Eotaxin

granulocyte colony stimulating factor (G-CSF), granulocyte macrophage colony stimulating factor (GM-CSF)

Interferon gamma (IFN- γ), Interferon gamma-induced protein 10 (IP-10)

Monocyte chemoattractant protein-1 (MCP-1)

Macrophage Inflammatory Protein-1 alpha (MIP-1α), MIP-1 beta (MIP-1β)

Platelet-derived growth factor (PDGF)

Regulated upon Activation, Normal T cell Expressed and presumably Secreted (RANTES)

Tumor necrosis factor-alpha (TNF-α)

Vascular endothelial growth factor (VEGF)

levels in the sera were quantitated by analyzing 100 μl of each well on a Bio-Plex using Bio-Plex Manager software version 4.0.

Serum neuropeptide assay included enzyme linked immunoassays for Substance P (SP), (R&D Systems, Minneapolis, MN; https://www.rndsystems.com/products/substance-p-parameter-assay-kit_kge007#product-details), which was performed as per manufacturer's instructions in a standard fashion. Samples, standards and controls were placed in a 96 well plate pre-coated with a polyclonal antibody. Primary antibody (for SP) solution and SP conjugated to horseradish peroxidase, were added to the wells and the plate was incubated overnight at 4° Celsius. After washing, substrate solution was added to the wells, incubated for 30 min, at room temp, in the dark and stop solution was added. The optical density of wells was determined using a micro plate reader set to 450 nm, with a reference wavelength of 570 nm.

Statistical analyses

Change in serum cytokine, chemokine and Substance P levels were calculated as baseline minus 2-month levels for each patient, where specimen was available. We decided a priori not to impute any values. We defined clinically important improvement in pain as the following: WOMAC pain scale as 20-point absolute improvement or more (range 0–100; higher = more pain; main analysis); or 2-point reduction or more in index TKA daytime numeric rating scale (NRS) pain severity on 0–10 scale (higher = more pain) at 2-month post-injection (sensitivity analysis), as previously published [14]. Patients were categorized as pain responder (achieved clinically important improvement in WOMAC pain) vs. pain non-responders (did not achieve this clinically improvement in WOMAC pain). We used student's t-tests to compare the mean change in cytokine chemokine and Substance P levels baseline to 2-months post-injection between pain responders and non-responders. We assessed non-parametric Spearman's correlation between cytokine/neurotransmitter level change from baseline to 2-months and the decrease in WOMAC pain (main analysis) or 0–10 daytime pain numeric rating scale (NRS; sensitivity analyses), baseline to 2-months, to account for non-normal distributions.

Results

Patients in the randomized trial had a mean age of 67 years, 84% were male and 96% were Caucasian. The mean duration of TKA pain was 4.5 years (SD, 4.8) and 75% were primary TKAs.

Compared to non-responders ($n = 23$) on WOMAC pain scale at 2-months, pain responders ($n = 12$) had significantly greater increase in serum levels of IL-7, IL-10, IL-12 (p70), eotaxin, IFN- γ and TNF-α from baseline to 2-months post-injection ($p < 0.05$ for all; Table 2). Several

other cytokines showed a non-significant trend by pain-responder status ($p ≤0.32$; Table 2). In sensitivity analysis in a smaller set of patients, who reported daytime NRS pain on 0–10 scale, serum substance P decreased significantly more in the pain responders (0.54 ± 0.53; $n = 10$) than in the pain non-responders (0.48 ± 1.18; $n = 9$; $p = 0.023$) 2-months post-injection.

Change in several cytokine and chemokine levels from pre-injection to 2-month follow-up correlated significantly with change in WOMAC pain with correlation coefficients ranging –0.37 to –0.51: IL-2, IL-7, IL-8, IL-9, IL-16, IL-12 (p70), GCSF, IFN- γ, IP-10, MCP, MIP1b, TNF-α and VEGF ($n = 35$; Table 3). In sensitivity analysis, we additionally noted a change in serum substance P from pre-injection to 2-month follow-up correlated significantly with change in daytime NRS pain, correlation coefficient was 0.53 ($p = 0.021$; $n = 19$).

Discussion

In this ancillary pilot study, we assessed whether changes in serum levels of cytokines, chemokines and Substance P from baseline to 2-month post-injection were associated with clinically meaningful pain relief at 2-month post-injection. We performed a mechanistic study and used data from our randomized study of intra-articular injection for painful TKA [9]. In many patients, the pain improvement lasted through the 6-month follow-up period, indicating that the joint pain relief was somewhat durable [9]. We found that several cytokine levels, including IL-7, IL-10, IL-12 (p70), eotaxin, IFN- γ and TNF-α, changed significantly more in WOMAC pain responders compared to pain non-responders (responders defined as those with pain decrement of 20 points or more on 0-100 scale). Correlation analyses identified additional cytokines with moderate correlations with WOMAC pain scores (baseline to 2-month change in cytokine level with baseline to 2-month change in WOMAC pain) in addition to these, including IL-2, IL-8, IL-9, IL-16, GCSF, IP-10, MCP, MIP1b and VEGF. In sensitivity analysis using a smaller dataset, serum substance P level reduction was greater in pain responders using the 0–10 daytime NRS pain than pain non-responders (pain decrement of two points or more o 0–10 scale). The direction and magnitude were similar to the responder analysis by WOMAC pain, however, standard deviations were larger in WOMAC pain analysis, leading to the difference in substance P levels being non-significant ($p = 0.32$) in the main analysis, but significant in sensitivity analysis ($p = 0.023$). This is a hypothesis-generating study and therefore, these findings need to be replicated in future studies.

The traditional view of cytokines/chemokines being either anti- or pro-inflammatory [15] has been challenged [16], since they can serve either role depending on the condition and the body organ. Higher levels of pro-

Table 2 Association of change in serum cytokine and neurotransmitter levels from baseline to 2-months with pain responder status on WOMAC pain at 2-month post-injection in painful TKA

	WOMAC Pain Responder*	N	Mean Change (FU-Baseline)	Std. Deviation	Std. Error Mean	P-value
Interleukin (IL)-7	No	23	0.084	0.91	0.19	**0.01**
	Yes	12	1.07	1.17	0.34	
IL-10	No	23	8.51	20.90	4.36	**0.01**
	Yes	12	27.72	21.56	6.22	
IL-12 p70	No	23	3.36	8.17	1.70	**0.004**
	Yes	12	12.91	9.60	2.77	
Eotaxin	No	23	−2.03	13.92	2.90	**0.046**
	Yes	12	7.85	12.28	3.54	
Interferon gamma (IFN-γ)	No	23	−1.24	23.18	4.83	**0.03**
	Yes	12	15.61	13.35	3.85	
Tumor necrosis factor-alpha (TNF-α)	No	23	4.46	21.32	4.44	**0.03**
	Yes	12	22.22	24.65	7.12	
IL-4	No	23	−0.02	0.16	0.03	0.12
	Yes	12	0.06	0.12	0.03	
IL-6	No	23	−15.90	275.66	57.48	0.09
	Yes	12	137.35	182.09	52.56	
IL-13	No	23	4.90	13.25	2.76	0.15
	Yes	12	12.18	14.87	4.29	
IL-15	No	23	0.31	11.87	2.47	0.09
	Yes	12	7.36	10.52	3.038	
Macrophage Inflammatory Protein-1 beta (mip1b)	No	23	5.55	91.43	19.06	0.16
	Yes	12	53.35	96.39	27.82	
Substance P	No	14	0.08	1.11	0.298	0.32
	Yes	5	−0.46	0.61	0.273	

Only those associations that either had a significant p-value or a p-value <0.33 are listed; The levels of other cytokine did not differ significantly between pain responders and pain non-responders (IL-1 beta, IL-1 alpha, IL-2, IL-5, IL-8, IL-9, IL-17, Basic FGF, G-CSF, GM-CSF, IP-10, MCP-1, MIP-1 alpha, PDGF, RANTES, and VEGF). Significant p-values <0.05 are in bold

Positive changes mean that at the 2-month follow-up time, the levels were higher than the baseline and a negative sign means follow-up levels were lower

WOMAC Pain Responder* is defined as reduction in WOMAC pain subscale of 20 or more 0–100 scale

inflammatory cytokines have been linked to pain [17–20]. On the other hand, change in pro- and anti-inflammatory cytokines with treatment in other pain conditions do not map precisely to their associations with pain condition at baseline [21–24]. Studies that have investigated the potential mechanisms of joint pain relief in intervention studies are lacking. Such studies can provide insights into mechanisms of action of an intervention, and discover mediators of joint pain relief in patients with OA. Our study begins to fill this knowledge gap by providing data among patients with painful joint arthroplasty.

Other recent uncontrolled studies have documented a potential role of cytokines, chemokines and Substance P in the failure of total joint replacement. In a recent study, both IL-1 beta and IL-2 levels were significantly lower ($p < 0.025$) in 10 patients with stable, painless, well-functioning, cemented total knee or hip arthroplasties (TKA/THA) than patients with aseptically loosened, painful, arthroplasties [25]. Genetic variants of pro-inflammatory cytokines TNF-alpha and IL-6 were associated with susceptibility to severe osteolysis after THA, a condition that is associated with increasing pain and functional limitation [7]. Compared to OA, aseptic loosening of TKA was associated with up-regulated expression of several cytokines including IL-8 and MMP9 and low levels of inflammatory cytokines [8].

In patients undergoing revision surgery for painful primary hip arthroplasty, nerve fibers with positive immunostaining to Substance P were found in bone-prosthesis interface membranes [26]. Joint fluid Substance P levels were elevated in painful knee joints with osteoarthritis that underwent TKA, but not in normal/asymptomatic contralateral knees [6]. Significantly greater pain relief after knee arthroplasty was seen in patients with an

Table 3 Non-parametric correlation of change in serum cytokine and neurotransmitter levels from baseline to 2-months with change in WOMAC pain at 2-month post-injection in painful TKA, showing statistically significant associations

Baseline to 2-month change in serum levels*	Spearman's correlation coefficient	P-value
IL2	−0.37	0.03
IL7	−0.42	0.01
IL8	−0.51	**0.002**
IL9	−0.50	**0.002**
IL16	−0.48	**0.004**
IL12p70	−0.56	**<0.001**
GCSF	−0.34	0.04
IFN gamma	−0.48	**0.003**
IP10	−0.38	0.02
MCP	−0.35	0.03
MIP1b	−0.49	**0.003**
TNF-alpha	−0.42	0.01
VEGF	−0.38	0.02

*Data from 35 patients were available
Only those cytokines that had a significant p-value <0.05 are listed in bold; other cytokines were not significantly associated with change in WOMAC pain at 2-month post-TKA

elevated preoperative joint fluid Substance P level compared to patients with normal Substance P levels [6]. In an animal model of OA, MMP-13, IL-1b, IL-6 and IL-15 were up-regulated in OA joints and the levels were reduced by treatment with coenzyme Q-10 that led to significant pain relief [4]. In a study of 47 OA patients, TNF-alpha levels were associated with WOMAC pain and overall scores [5]. Thus, cytokine levels have been correlated with OA and arthroplasty joint pain in observational studies. Our study provides evidence showing that a change in cytokine levels correlated with pain relief in patients with painful TKA in a clinical trial who had a clinically meaningful pain relief after an intra-articular injection.

Our study findings must be interpreted considering study limitations. The sample size for this ancillary study was small. A protocol modification was made to the main study on receipt of federal funding that allowed us to collect specimens and perform analyses, and therefore these analyses were performed on a subset of the main trial, since almost 40% of the study cohort had already been enrolled in the study. Therefore, we likely missed several important findings due to type II error. Subsequent studies should enroll a larger number of patients to explore this important aspect of treatment for patients with painful arthroplasty. We examined the patients in the pain responder vs. non-responder categories, as specified a priori in our analytic plan. Since our hypothesis was to assess the cytokine, chemokine and neuropeptide mediators of joint pain relief in painful arthroplasty, we limited our

analyses by whether patient was or was not a responder by clinically meaningful pain relief at 2-months post-injection. We adopted this approach rather than comparing Botulinum toxin group vs. placebo group, since we only had samples on half of the study participants in the RCT and both groups of patients with samples consisted of a mix of pain responders and non-responders, leading to an inadequate sample size for this comparison. We believe that the associations we noted are unlikely to be drug-specific, since responders included patients from both intervention and control arms. This analysis addressed our main objective to better understand the mechanism of pain improvement in patients who have had a failed TKA, and are undergoing a medical treatment to improve pain. Study strengths include the randomized, blinded study design, use of paired samples and focus on a condition that has significant public health impact. The presence of significant associations, even under the stringent categorization (responders/non-responders), with the current sample size, supports our underlying theoretical framework that cytokine, chemokine and substance P level changes after an intra-articular injection might be associated with pain relief.

Conclusions

In conclusion, our exploratory study shows that patients who experience pain relief after an intra-articular injection have a different pattern of change in serum cytokine/chemokine levels than patients without pain relief. Our study identifies several cytokines that might play a role in relief of joint pain with local therapies. Our study has generated interesting hypotheses of mechanisms of pain relief in patients with painful TKA. Future studies need to confirm our findings in patients with painful arthroplasty, with similar intra-articular interventions, but also other dissimilar interventions, since pain pathways/mechanisms may be similar.

Abbreviations
NRS: Numeric rating scale; OA: Osteoarthritis; TKA: Total knee arthroplasty; WOMAC: Western Ontario and McMaster Universities Osteoarthritis Index

Acknowledgements
None.

Funding
This study was supported by the resources and use of facilities at Birmingham and Minneapolis Veterans Affairs medical centers and the NIH CTSA award 1 KL2 RR024151-01 (Mayo Clinic Center for Clinical and Translational Research). JAS is supported by the resources and the use of facilities at the VA Medical Center at Birmingham, Alabama, USA.

Authors' contributions
JAS designed the study, developed study protocol, collected data, reviewed data analyses and wrote the first draft of the paper. SN performed the data analyses. KK supervised all cytokine and other assays. All authors revised the manuscript, read, and approved the final manuscript.

Authors' information

JAS is the co-chair of the special Interest group assessing the outcome measures in arthroplasty and has served as expert/lead on task forces for the specialty societies and the US FDA. Other authors have no other relevant information

Each author certifies that his or her institution has approved the human protocol for this investigation and that all investigations were conducted in conformity with ethical principles of research.

"The views expressed in this article are those of the authors and do not necessarily reflect the position or policy of the Department of Veterans Affairs or the United States government."

Competing interests

JAS has received research grants from Takeda and Savient and consultant fees from Savient, Takeda, Regeneron, Merz, Bioiberica, Crealta and Allergan pharmaceuticals, WebMD, UBM LLC and the American College of Rheumatology. JAS serves as the principal investigator for an investigator-initiated study funded by Horizon pharmaceuticals through a grant to DINORA, Inc., a 501 (c)(3) entity. JAS is a member of the executive of OMERACT, an organization that develops outcome measures in rheumatology and receives arms-length funding from 36 companies; a member of the American College of Rheumatology's (ACR) Annual Meeting Planning Committee (AMPC); Chair of the ACR Meet-the-Professor, Workshop and Study Group Subcommittee; and a member of the Veterans Affairs Rheumatology Field Advisory Committee. Other authors have no relevant disclosures. None of the authors have any non-financial disclosures.

Author details

[1]Medicine Service, VA Medical Center, 700 19th St S, Birmingham, AL 35233, USA. [2]Department of Medicine at School of Medicine, University of Alabama at Birmingham Faculty Office Tower, 805B, 510 20th Street S, Birmingham, AL 35294, USA. [3]Division of Epidemiology at School of Public Health, University of Alabama at Birmingham, 1720 Second Ave. South, Birmingham, AL 35294-0022, USA. [4]Department of Orthopedic Surgery, Mayo Clinic College of Medicine, 200 1st St SW, Rochester, MN 55905, USA. [5]Department of Immunology, Mayo Clinic College of Medicine, 200 1st St SW, Rochester, MN 55905, USA. [6]Center for chronic disease Outcomes Research, Minneapolis Veterans Affairs Health are System Center, Minneapolis, MN 55121, USA. [7]Department of Medicine, University of Minnesota, 401 East River Parkway, Minneapolis, MN 55455, USA.

References

1. Singh JA, Vessely MB, Harmsen WS, Schleck CD, Melton 3rd LJ, Kurland RL, Berry DJ. A population-based study of trends in the use of total hip and total knee arthroplasty, 1969-2008. Mayo Clin Proc. 2010;85(10):898–904.

2. Singh JA, Gabriel S, Lewallen D. The impact of gender, age, and preoperative pain severity on pain after TKA. Clin Orthop Relat Res. 2008; 466(11):2717–23.

3. Miller RE, Miller RJ, Malfait AM. Osteoarthritis joint pain: The cytokine connection. Cytokine. 2014;70(2):185–93.

4. Lee J, Hong YS, Jeong JH, Yang EJ, Jhun JY, Park MK, Jung YO, Min JK, Kim HY, Park SH, et al. Coenzyme Q10 ameliorates pain and cartilage degradation in a rat model of osteoarthritis by regulating nitric oxide and inflammatory cytokines. PLoS One. 2013;8(7):e69362.

5. Orita S, Koshi T, Mitsuka T, Miyagi M, Inoue G, Arai G, Ishikawa T, Hanaoka E, Yamashita K, Yamashita M, et al. Associations between proinflammatory cytokines in the synovial fluid and radiographic grading and pain-related scores in 47 consecutive patients with osteoarthritis of the knee. BMC Musculoskelet Disord. 2011;12:144.

6. Pritchett JW. Substance P level in synovial fluid may predict pain relief after knee replacement. J Bone Joint Surg (Br). 1997;79(1):114–6.

7. Gallo J, Mrazek F, Petrek M. Variation in cytokine genes can contribute to severity of acetabular osteolysis and risk for revision in patients with ABG 1 total hip arthroplasty: a genetic association study. BMC Med Genet. 2009;10:109.

8. Tomankova T, Kriegova E, Fillerova R, Luzna P, Ehrmann J, Gallo J. Comparison of periprosthetic tissues in knee and hip joints: differential expression of CCL3 and DC-STAMP in total knee and hip arthroplasty and similar cytokine profiles in primary knee and hip osteoarthritis. Osteoarthritis Cartilage. 2014;22(11):1851–60.

9. Singh JA, Mahowald ML, Noorbaloochi S. Intraarticular botulinum toxin A for refractory painful total knee arthroplasty: a randomized controlled trial. J Rheumatol. 2010;37(11):2377–86.

10. Courtney P, Doherty M. Joint aspiration and injection. Best Pract Res Clin Rheumatol. 2005;19(3):345–69.

11. Lopes RV, Furtado RN, Parmigiani L, Rosenfeld A, Fernandes AR, Natour J. Accuracy of intra-articular injections in peripheral joints performed blindly in patients with rheumatoid arthritis. Rheumatology (Oxford). 2008;47(12):1792–4.

12. Bellamy N, Bell MJ, Goldsmith CH, Pericak D, Walker V, Raynauld JP, Torrance GW, Tugwell P, Polisson R. The effectiveness of hylan G-F 20 in patients with knee osteoarthritis: an application of two sets of response criteria developed by the OARSI and one set developed by OMERACT-OARSI. Osteoarthritis Cartilage. 2005;13(2):104–10.

13. Singh J, Mahowald M, Krug H, Gioe T, Santos E, Schmidt R. Intra-articular Botulinum Toxin A for Painful Total Knee Arthroplasty (TKA). Arthritis Rheum. 2006;54(9; Supp):S541–542.

14. Farrar JT, Portenoy RK, Berlin JA, Kinman JL, Strom BL. Defining the clinically important difference in pain outcome measures. Pain. 2000;88(3):287–94.

15. Opal SM, DePalo VA. Anti-inflammatory cytokines. Chest. 2000;117(4):1162–72.

16. Cavaillon JM. Pro- versus anti-inflammatory cytokines: myth or reality. Cell Mol Biol (Noisy-le-grand). 2001;47(4):695–702.

17. Alexander RB, Ponniah S, Hasday J, Hebel JR. Elevated levels of proinflammatory cytokines in the semen of patients with chronic prostatitis/chronic pelvic pain syndrome. Urology. 1998;52(5):744–9.

18. Hu C, Yang H, Zhao Y, Chen X, Dong Y, Li L, Dong Y, Cui J, Zhu T, Zheng P, et al. The role of inflammatory cytokines and ERK1/2 signaling in chronic prostatitis/chronic pelvic pain syndrome with related mental health disorders. Sci Rep. 2016;6:28608.

19. Jiang YH, Peng CH, Liu HT, Kuo HC. Increased pro-inflammatory cytokines, C-reactive protein and nerve growth factor expressions in serum of patients with interstitial cystitis/bladder pain syndrome. PLoS One. 2013;8(10):e76779.

20. Kiguchi N, Kobayashi Y, Kishioka S. Chemokines and cytokines in neuroinflammation leading to neuropathic pain. Curr Opin Pharmacol. 2012;12(1):55–61.

21. Bushehri A, Chow E, Zhang L, Azad A, Vuong S, Pasetka M, Zhou M, Hird A, Dennis K, McDonald R, et al. Urinary cytokines/chemokines pattern in patients with painful bone metastases undergoing external beam radiotherapy experiencing pain flare. Ann Palliat Med. 2016;5(2):107–15.

22. Degenhardt BF, Johnson JC, Fossum C, Andicochea CT, Stuart MK. Changes in Cytokines, Sensory Tests, and Self-Reported Pain Levels After Manual Treatment of Low Back Pain. Clin Spine Surg. 2016. [Epub ahead of print]. doi:10.1097/BSD.0000000000000231.

23. Johnston IN, Milligan ED, Wieseler-Frank J, Frank MG, Zapata V, Campisi J, Langer S, Martin D, Green P, Fleshner M, et al. A role for proinflammatory cytokines and fractalkine in analgesia, tolerance, and subsequent pain facilitation induced by chronic intrathecal morphine. J Neurosci. 2004;24(33):7353–65.

24. Kraychete DC, Sakata RK, Issy AM, Bacellar O, Jesus RS, Carvalho EM. Proinflammatory cytokines in patients with neuropathic pain treated with Tramadol. Rev Bras Anestesiol. 2009;59(3):297–303.

25. Chadha HS, Wooley PH, Sud S, Fitzgerald Jr RH. Cellular proliferation and cytokine responses to polymethylmethacrylate particles in patients with a cemented total joint arthroplasty. Inflamm Res. 1995;44(4):145–51.

26. Ahmed M, Bergstrom J, Lundblad H, Gillespie WJ, Kreicbergs A. Sensory nerves in the interface membrane of aseptic loose hip prostheses. J Bone Joint Surg (Br). 1998;80(1):151–5.

19

How do orthopaedic surgeons inform their patients before knee arthroplasty surgery?

Aamir Mahdi[1,2]* (iD), Maria Hälleberg Nyman[3] and Per Wretenberg[1,2]

Abstract

Background: Total knee arthroplasty (TKA) is a successful and common procedure. However, 6–28% of patients are dissatisfied postoperatively. The provision of preoperative patient information, inquiring about patients' expectations, and taking a psychiatric history are essential parts of both preoperative evaluation and postoperative outcome. The aim of this study was to investigate how orthopaedic knee surgeons in Sweden inform their patients before surgery.

Methods: A questionnaire was distributed to all knee surgeons performing TKA in Sweden. Responses were received from 60 of the 65 orthopaedic departments performing TKA in Sweden (92%), covering 219 of the approximately 311 knee surgeons at the 65 departments (70%). The answers were analysed with descriptive statistics. A content analysis of the surgeons' opinions was also performed using a thematic method.

Results: In terms of information provision, 58% of the surgeons always gave written information while 92% informed orally. Only 44% always asked about the patient's expectations, and only 42% always informed patients about the 20% dissatisfaction rate after TKA. Additionally, 24% never operated on mild indication of arthrosis, 20% always took a psychiatric history, and half never or seldom consulted a psychiatrist. However, all the knee surgeons believed in a psychiatric impact on TKA outcome. Qualitative analysis revealed five common causes of patient dissatisfaction, which in descending frequency were: patients' expectations, choice of patients to operate on, surgical factors, combinations of factors, and insufficient information provision to patients.

Conclusions: Knee surgeons in Sweden have considerable awareness of the importance of preoperative patient information, the impact of patient expectations, and psychiatric illness. However, they need to improve their preoperative routines when it comes to providing written information, asking about the patient's expectations, and psychiatric assessment.

Keywords: Expectation, Postoperative outcome, Preoperative information, Psychiatric history, TKA

Background

Total knee arthroplasty (TKA) is a common procedure with generally good results. By 2030, the annual number of TKA operations performed in the USA is expected to have reached 3.48 million, an increase of 673% from the figures for 2005 [1]. The most recent annual report from the Swedish knee arthroplasty register shows a similar trend, with an increase from 70 to 140 TKA procedures per 100,000 inhabitants between 2000 and 2015 [2]. However, despite advances in design and technique, there are still patients who are not satisfied after this procedure. Previous studies have shown many reasons for dissatisfaction [3–24], for example early- and late postoperative complications, unfulfilled expectations, anxiety and depression. Further, earlier studies have shown a correlation between dissatisfaction and mechanical [5, 14] and/or psychological factors [16]. In Sweden, the risk of

* Correspondence: aamir.mahdi@oru.se
[1]Department of Orthopaedics, Örebro County, Sweden
[2]Faculty of Medicine and Health, School of Medical Sciences, Örebro University, Örebro, Sweden
Full list of author information is available at the end of the article

dissatisfaction after knee arthroplasty is about 8% in the absence of complications [22, 23].

Patient dissatisfaction contradicts the aim of TKA surgery in improving patient's quality of life [10, 25–27]. It implies a burden for both patients and health care professionals [28–32]. Most of the previous studies conducted to address the problem of dissatisfaction and to analyse the preventable factors in order to decrease this rate. [6, 10, 12, 15, 25, 26, 33–38]

Orthopaedic surgeons may have different ways of dealing with how patients are informed preoperatively, as well as different opinions about the importance of preoperative information in relation to postoperative outcome. Preoperative information includes a general written and verbal information, patient expectations, information about the 20%-non-satisfaction's rate and psychiatric history. A previous study showed a discordance between surgeon and patient satisfaction after knee arthroplasty surgery [39]. Moreover, a qualitative study by Conrades et al. showed a relationship between how the TKA patient was informed preoperatively and how much they trusted the department [40].

When it comes to reducing the risk for patient dissatisfaction, we know the importance of a qualified preoperative information according to the patient's needs and selection of the right patient for surgery [12, 18, 40–44], but we do not know the extent of the problem in Sweden in terms of the surgeon's attitude to the information, patient selection, and the surgeon's opinion about patient dissatisfaction. There are few studies which describe orthopaedic surgeons' attitudes toward giving information to patients. The aim of this study was therefore to investigate how TKA surgeons in Sweden inform their patients preoperatively, and what kind of information they give. This will lead to strategies and possibly changing protocols to improve the knee surgeon's attitude in preoperative patient's information. In turn, it will possibly decrease the dissatisfactions rate in Sweden.

Methods

Design

We conducted a cross-sectional descriptive study including qualitative and quantitative data collection.

Methods and analyses

A study-specific questionnaire was distributed in paper form to all 65 TKA clinics in Sweden in May 2016. A list of all orthopaedic clinics performing TKA was obtained from the Swedish knee registry. A reminder letter was sent in October 2016 to increase the response rate. For each department, the questionnaire was sent to the orthopaedic surgeon locally responsible for registration of TKAs in the Swedish Knee Arthroplasty Register, who then distributed the questionnaire to all orthopaedic surgeons who performed TKA at that department. Knee departments in Sweden are located in either state-funded university hospitals, regional hospitals, small hospitals, or private clinics.

The initial response rate was 55%, but the reminder letter increased this to 92% (60 clinics) (Appendix 1). The five orthopaedic clinics that failed to return the questionnaire were located in a university hospital ($n = 1$) and local hospitals ($n = 4$). Of the approximately 311 knee arthroplasty surgeons in Sweden, 219 answered the questionnaire. Thus, about 70% of the surgeons who regularly perform TKA surgery in Sweden answered the questionnaire. The reasons of 30% non-response were the surgeon's unwilling and uninterestingness according to orthopaedic chief managers. This rate was not related to the kind of hospital (University hospital, county council hospital or local hospital).

The sixteen-item questionnaire was designed by the researchers with the aim of investigating how information was given to and discussed with patients before surgery. The first fourteen questions covered written and oral information, patients' expectations, surgery on mild indication, and patients' psychiatric history. The choice of questions was based on evidence from the literature that these factors can have an impact on outcome [4, 9, 12, 13, 16, 19, 20, 32, 42–45]. A five-point Likert scale was used, with response alternatives of always, often, sometimes, seldom, and never after a discussion with a statistician (Appendix 2).

The final two questions were concerned with what the surgeons believed were the most common reasons for dissatisfaction after TKA, and were answered in the form of free text. These two questions were analysed qualitatively with a quantitative component. The text was coded inductively and grouped into five main categories based on 262 responses, and then analysed with a method based on thematic qualitative analysis [46, 47]. Initial coding was performed by the first author(AM). Then, the second author(MH) checked the quality of the coding and changes were made until consensus was reached. To facilitate thematic analysis, responses on the two-free text items were uploaded into Version 11 of the NVivo software package (Boston, MA, USA).

There was no previous validated questionnaire which cover all the items that we intended to study. The questionnaire was written in Swedish by the major supervisor and the main researcher. The co-supervisor

How do orthopaedic surgeons inform their patients before knee arthroplasty...

143

made then several changes on the language and the construct. It sent then to two independent orthopaedic surgeons to study the construct of the questionnaire. Further changes were made to the final version of the questionnaire. No comments have been received from the ethical board committee or knee orthopaedic surgeons if something in the questionnaire were ambiguous or not-understandable.

Statistical analysis

The statistical data analysis was divided into two parts:

1. **General analysis:** The data were described in terms of frequencies of answers. Duration of experience was not taken into consideration.
2. **Specific analysis:** The surgeons were divided into subgroups classified in terms of years of experience, volume of primary TKA/revision surgeries per year, and percentage of work done on knees. For statistical purposes, orthopaedic surgeons who performed 75% of their work on knees were grouped with those working solely on knees. Subgroup analysis was performed to see if there were differences between the groups (Table 1).

Data were analysed as frequencies of each answer (always, often, sometimes, seldom, and never). More specifically, subgroup data analysis was performed to see if there were any statistically significant differences (Table 1). The chi-square test was used to compare multiple categorical groups. Version 24 of the SPSS software package (IBM, SPSS Inc., Chicago, Illinois, USA) was used for the quantitative data analysis.

Results

Descriptive statistics

Only 8% of orthopaedic surgeons in Sweden worked solely on TKA surgery. In terms of experience, 43% had 5–15 years of experience in knee arthroplasty, 47% performed 22–50 primary TKA procedures per year, and more than 50% performed revision arthroplasty of varying degrees of complexity (Table 1). The results are presented below in terms of the nine main questions. Those represented question 1,2,7,8,9,10,11,13 and 14. The answers of question 12 were presented together with question 13. Question 3,4,5 and 6 were dealt with knee surgeons experiences (Table 1, Appendix 2). The answer of question 15 and 16 were analysed qualitatively (Appendix 2).

Written information

The results showed that 58% of the knee surgeons always gave written information to their patients,

Table 1 Characteristics of Swedish knee surgeons ($N = 219$)

Variable	Orthopaedic knee surgeon ($N = 219$)
Experience, n (%)	
< 5 years	32 (15)
5–15 years	95 (43)
15–30 years	80 (37)
> 30 years	11 (5)
Missing	1 (0.5)
[a]Knee specialist, n (%)	
100% Knee specialist	18 (8)
50% knee specialist	81 (37)
25% Knee specialist	120 (55)
Primary TKA/year, n (%)	
< 22	33 (15)
22–50	103 (47)
50–100	54 (25)
> 100	24 (11)
Missing	5 (2)
Revision TKA/year, n (%)	
No revision	98 (45)
< 5 revisions	54 (25)
> 5 revisions	65 (29)
Missing	2 (1)

The table shows the classification of knee surgeons according to the years of experience, the percentages of daily clinical work with knee joint, the volume of primary TKA performed by every surgeon per year and the volume of revision knee replacement surgery performed by every surgeon per year
[a]Percentage of daily clinical work with knee joint

while 18% never gave written information (Table 2). The highest percentages of written information were given by surgeons with more than 30 years of experience (64%), who performed more than 100 primary TKA procedures per year (71%), who performed more than 5 revisions per year (60%), and who worked solely on knees (67%). However, there was no statistically significant differences between the groups (Table 3).

Surgeons who said they never gave written information had the following characteristics: 15–30 years of experience (23%), performed fewer than 22 primary TKA procedures per year (27%), did not perform any knee revisions (21%), and spent 25% of their time as knee surgeons (23%) (Table 4).

Oral information

Almost all knee surgeons informed their patients orally about the procedure. Oral information included indications, contraindications of surgery, benefits, risks,

Table 2 Knee surgeons' measures regarding preoperative patient information

Variable	Orthopaedic knee surgeon (N = 219)
Written information, n (%)	
Always	127 (58)
Often	24 (11)
Sometimes	7 (3.2)
Seldom	19 (9)
Never	40 (18)
Oral information, n (%)	
Always	202 (92)
Often	16 (7)
Sometimes	1 (1)
Seldom	0 (0)
Never	0 (0)
Patient expectation, n (%)	
Always	97 (44)
Often	78 (36)
Sometimes	32 (15)
Seldom	9 (4)
Never	3 (1)
Dissatisfaction rate, n (%)	
Always	91 (42)
Often	76 (35)
Sometimes	27 (12)
Seldom	15 (7)
Never	9 (4)
Mild indications, n (%)	
Always	2 (1)
Often	12 (6)
Sometimes	54 (25)
Seldom	98 (45)
Never	52 (24)
Psychiatric consultation, n (%)	
Always	21 (10)
Often	38 (17)
Sometimes	45 (21)
Seldom	75 (35)
Never	38 (17)
Impact of psychiatric disorder, n (%)	
Always	63 (29)
Often	119 (54)
Sometimes	34 (16)
Seldom	3 (1)

Table 2 Knee surgeons' measures regarding preoperative patient information *(Continued)*

Variable	Orthopaedic knee surgeon (N = 219)
Never	0 (0)
Psychiatric history, n (%)	
Always	42 (19)
Often	83 (38)
Sometimes	59 (27)
Seldom	28 (13)
Never	7 (3)
Psychiatric questionnaire, n (%)	
No	213 (97)
Yes	2 (1)
EQ-5D	3 (1)
HADS	1 (1)

The table shows the numbers and percentages of all knee surgeons regarding the given preoperative patient's information

expected results, and prognosis. In terms of consistency, 92% always informed their patients, 7% often informed their patients, and 1% sometimes informed their patients (Table 2).

Further classification of surgeons into subgroups did not show any statistically significant differences. The highest proportions of surgeons informing their patients orally were seen in surgeons with 15–30 years of experience (94%), performing 22–50 primary TKA procedures per year (95%), performing no revisions (94%), and conducting 50% of their work on knees (95%) (Table 3).

While experienced knee surgeons did not report the highest frequency of providing oral information, the percentage who did provide oral information was still high and there were no statistically significant differences between the groups. The lowest frequencies of giving oral information were in surgeons who "sometimes" informed patients verbally as follows: < 5 years of experience (3%), 50–100 primary TKA procedures per year (2%), < 5 revisions per year (1%), and conducting 50% of their work on knees (1%) (Table 4).

Expectations

There was an unequal distribution of orthopaedic surgeons asking about the patient's expectations: 44% always asked, 35% often asked, 14% sometimes asked, and the remaining 5% never or seldom asked (Table 2).

Table 3 The sub groups of knee surgeons who gave the highest preoperative information ($N = 219$)

Characteristics of knee surgeons:	Years of experience	P-value*	TKA volume per year	P-value*	Knee revision per year	P-value*	Knee specialist	P-value*
Preoperative measures:								
Written information	> 30	0.72	> 100	0.25	> 5	0.31	100%	0.24
Oral information	15–30	0.39	22–50	0.50	0	0.33	50%	0.32
Expectations	> 30	0.22	> 100	0.51	0	0.19	50%	0.08
Dissatisfaction rate	> 30	0.69	> 100	0.17	< 5	0.47	50%	0.79
Surgery on mild indication	> 30	0.89	< 22	0.70	< 5	0.04	25%	0.77
Psychiatric history	< 5	0.09	> 100	0.59	< 5	0.70	50%	0.94
Psychiatric consultation	> 30	0.03	22–50	0.07	0	0.31	25%	0.07
Psychiatric impact	< 5	0.14	22–50	0.36	0	0.18	50%	0.38

The table shows the highest preoperative given information according to different groups of knee surgeons that were described in Table 1
*Chi ^{2} test

In terms of subgroups, 82% of surgeons with more than 30 years of experience, 54% of surgeons who performed more than 100 primary TKA procedures per year, 47% of surgeons who did not perform revisions, and 47% of surgeons who conducted 50% of their work on knees "always" asked about patient expectations. However, the differences again were not statistically significant (Table 3). The lowest results were among the following, who "never" asked about expectations: < 5 years of experience (3%), 50–100 TKA procedures per year (4%), < 5 revisions per year (4%), and specialising 100% in knees (6%) (Table 4).

Informing patients about the 20% dissatisfaction rate after TKA surgery

Only 42% of surgeons always informed patients about the risk of dissatisfaction; 35% often provided this information while approximately 10% never or seldom

informed patients (Table 2). Surgeons who informed patients frequently had the following characteristics: > 30 years of experience (37%), > 100 primary TKA procedures per year, < 5 knee revisions per year (52%), and conducting 50% of their work on knees (49%) (Table 3). The lowest results were found among the following categories: < 5 years of experience (6%), > 100 primary TKA procedures per year (8%), no knee revisions (6%), and specialising 100% in knees (6%) (Table 4).

Surgery on mild indications

Only 24% of the surgeons never operated on mild indication, though an additional 45% seldom proceeded with surgery in these cases. However, the proportion of surgeons who sometimes, often, or always operated despite a suspicious indication was still high, at 31% (Table 2).

Table 4 The sub groups of knee surgeons who gave the least preoperative information ($N = 219$)

Characteristics of knee surgeons:	Years of experience	P-value*	TKA volume per year	P-value*	Knee revisions per year	P-value*	Knee specialist	P-value*
Preoperative measures:								
Written information	15–30	0.72	< 22	0.25	0	0.31	25%	0.24
Oral information	< 5	0.39	50–100	0.50	< 5	0.33	50%	0.32
Expectations	< 5	0.22	50–100	0.51	< 5	0.19	100%	0.08
Dissatisfaction rate	< 5	0.69	> 100	0.17	0	0.47	100%	0.79
Surgery on mild indication	< 5	0.89	50–100	0.70	< 5	0.04	50%	0.77
Psychiatric history	> 30	0.09	50–100	0.59	> 5	0.70	100%	0.94
Psychiatric consultation	< 5	0.03	50–100	0.07	0	0.31	100%	0.07
Psychiatric impact	15–30	0.14	> 100	0.36	> 5	0.18	50%	0.38

This table shows the lowest preoperative given information according to different groups of knee surgeons that were described in Table 1
*Chi ^{2} -test

The most appropriate answer on this issue is "seldom" [30, 45]. Orthopaedic surgeons who provided those answers had the following characteristics: > 30 years of experience (55%), < 22 TKA procedures per year (55%), < 5 revisions per year (57%, $p = 0.04$), and conducting 25% of work on knees (45%) (Table 3). Surgeons who gave the answer of "always" operating on mild indication had the following characteristics: < 5 years of experience, 50–100 primary TKA procedures per year (4%), < 5 revisions per year (2%) and conducting 50% of their work on knees (1%) (Table 4).

Psychiatric consultation

Despite the known impact of psychiatric illness on TKA outcome, only one in ten of the surgeons always consulted a psychiatric unit; 17% did this often and a fifth did it sometimes (Table 2).

Stratifying the surgeons into four groups showed that surgeons who mostly answer "always" had the following criteria: > 30 years of experience (18%, $p = 0.03$), 22–50 primary TKA procedures per year (15%), no revisions (12%), and spending 25% of their time on knees (13%). The only subgroup with a statistically significant difference was the group with more than 30 years of experience. Knee surgeons who never consulted a psychiatrist had the following characteristics: < 5 years of experience (25%), 50–100 primary TKA procedures per year (22%), no revisions (24%), and specialising 100% in knees (Table 4).

Impact of psychiatric problems on outcome

A total of 29% of the surgeons believed that psychiatric problems always had a negative impact on outcome after TKA, 54% believed there was often an impact, and 16% believed there was sometimes an impact. Although 2% answered "rarely" to this question, there were no surgeons who answered "never" (Table 2).

The knee surgeons who believed that there was always a relationship had the following profile: < 5 years of experience (41%), 22–50 primary TKA procedures per year (34%), no revisions (34%), and conducting 50% of their work on knees (Table 3). Knee surgeons who believed that TKA outcome was seldom related to psychiatric problems had the following characteristics: 15–30 years of experience (3%), > 100 primary TKA procedures per year (4%), > 5 revisions per year (3%), and conducting 50% of their work on knees (Table 4).

Psychiatric history

Only a few of the surgeons used a psychiatric evaluation questionnaire (3%) (Table 2), and only 20% always took a psychiatric history. Forty percent often took a psychiatric history, and 16% rarely or never used this kind of evaluation (Table 2).

Surgeons who always took a psychiatric history had the following characteristics: < 5 years of experience (28%), > 100 primary TKA procedures per year (25%), < 5 revisions per year (26%), and conducting 50% of their work on knees (22%). The differences were not statistically significant (Table 3). Surgeons who never or seldom took a psychiatric history belonged to the following groups: > 30 years of experience (18%), 50–100 primary TKA procedures per year (20%), > 5 revisions per year (20%), and specialising 100% in knees (17%) (Table 4).

Psychological or mechanical reasons for dissatisfaction

One third of the surgeons believed that psychological factors were a reason for patient dissatisfaction, a quarter believed that mechanical factors played the biggest role, and another quarter believed that combinations of factors were behind this (Table 5).

Thematic analysis: Reasons for dissatisfaction after knee surgery

Five categories emerged in the thematic analysis, and are discussed below in descending order of their frequency of being mentioned.

Patient expectations

Almost half of the surgeons (122/262) stated that patients' expectations were a predictive factor of bad outcome. They described these expectations as too great, unrealistic, high, wrong, and unreasonable.

Choice of patients to operate on

The second most common reason for dissatisfaction was the choice of patients to operate on. A considerable number of surgeons (72/262) related bad outcome to patient selection. Their statements included mentions of bad preoperative physical and psychological

Table 5 TKA surgeon's opinion about the general cause of dissatisfaction ($N = 219$)

Variables, n (%)	Surgeon's opinion
Psychological/expectations	66 (30)
Mechanical/soft tissue	56 (26)
Combination	59 (27)
Unknown	14 (6)
Miscellaneous	8 (4)
Missing	16 (7)

The table shows what knee surgeons thought in general as the main cause of patient's non-satisfaction after primary total knee arthroplasty plan, inadequate motivation for postoperative training, multiple previous surgeries, surgery in early stages of arthrosis, mild complaint, obesity, low pain threshold, anxiety, depression, wrong indication, co-morbidities, poor preoperative range of motion, and insufficient rehabilitation.

Surgical factors

The third factor was related to surgery. Many of the orthopaedic surgeons (41/262) mentioned surgery-related factors as a cause of dissatisfaction after TKA, including unskilled/inexperienced surgeon, insufficient surgical performance, mechanical issues, poor implant positioning, no implant better than the natural knee, scar tissue, instability, swelling, soft tissue envelope, ligament balance, and patella.

Combination of factors

A few of the surgeons (18/262) stated that poor outcome was determined by a combination of factors. This was the fourth common cause mentioned by the surgeons.

Insufficient information

The fifth and least commonly-mentioned factor that determined the poor outcome was patient information. Very few of the surgeons (9/262) mentioned this as an important factor, and none named it as a sole factor; it was mainly grouped with patient expectations.

Discussion

The Swedish orthopaedic surgeons in the present study described preoperative patient expectations as an important issue in predicting outcome after TKA surgery. However, this descriptive study revealed deficiencies among many TKA surgeons in supplying preoperative information. The discussion below aims to outline the extent of this problem among knee surgeons in Sweden.

All knee surgeons provided some kind of information to their patients preoperatively. However, only 58% of knee surgeons always provided written information, though 92% always informed their patients verbally. Preoperative information included information about indications, contraindications, surgical procedure, risks and benefits, outcome, and prognosis. Preoperative written and oral information has been shown to reduce postoperative pain and thereby enhance postoperative outcome [40, 41, 48], and a qualitative study on TKA patients showed that patients who were well informed preoperatively trusted their health care providers [40]. However, an earlier study showed that preoperative information

about anatomy and patho-anatomy had a limited effect on pain management, while information about pain was more effective [42]. Furthermore, it is of utmost importance that the patients understand the information given. A recent study found that patients with low health literacy had impaired postoperative recovery and lower postoperative quality of life [49].

Written information in the form of booklets has been shown to have a positive effect on outcome after TKA [48]. Another study pointed out the importance of providing both verbal and written information together in order to facilitate postoperative pain control [41]. Consequently, the preoperative provision of written information to all TKA patients could offer a way to increase the satisfaction rate.

In terms of asking about patients' expectations, only 44% of the surgeons always discussed this important issue with their patients. An earlier study showed that TKA surgery failed to meet the patients' expectations when it came to kneeling, squatting, and stair climbing, and in particular that the fulfilment of expectations was highly correlated with satisfaction [43]. Tilbury et al. came to a similar conclusion, emphasizing the importance of preoperative information and education due to the substantial number of TKA patients with unfulfilled expectations [44]. It is very important for the surgeon to ask about the patient's expectations, and make it clear to them which activities might be difficult to perform after the surgery. A study revealed that only young, strong patients who did not have a problem with ascending or descending stairs preoperatively were likely to be able to use stairs postoperatively without a problem [32]. Expectations of improvement in this functional ability may thus contribute to patients' feeling disappointed after surgery, and so impelling knee surgeons to ask their patients about expectations may decrease the rate of dissatisfaction due to unfulfilled expectations. Patient's expectations on the outcome of the TKA are not only based on the information given by the knee surgeons, but rather from discussions with other people like friends, family and from information in media [50].

It is not known whether information about dissatisfaction rate affects outcome after TKA. Earlier research revealed that up to 20% of TKA patients were disappointed with their results [3, 4, 19, 22] .We therefore suggest that informing patients about the dissatisfaction rate before surgery is of importance, as it could increase their awareness of the expected success rate. Further research is needed to create an individualized risk prediction's tool.

Only 42% of surgeons in our study always discussed the success rate after TKA surgery, and 10% never discussed this with their patients. Previous studies have shown that the severity of osteoarthritis correlates with satisfaction rate. Schnurr et al. found that patients suffering from mild or moderate osteoarthritis were at risk of dissatisfaction after TKA, and recommended that patients should be told about this [45]. Another study showed a similarly high dissatisfaction rate among people with mild osteoarthritis changes, and also revealed a high prevalence of chronic non-orthopaedic conditions among these patients, including anxiety/depression, fibromyalgia, low back pain, and prior brain injury [13].

Our Swedish data showed a high percentage (31%; 68/219) of knee surgeons who sometimes, often or always operated on painful knees with mild radiological osteoarthritis in patients with anxiety/depression. Previous medical history is fundamental in preoperative evaluation. Nonetheless, medical and psychiatric illnesses are equally important, and should always be included in preoperative judgment. In recent years, there has been more recognition of the impact of psychological factors on joint prosthesis outcome. Many studies show a negative relationship between depression/anxiety and prosthesis outcome [3, 4, 6, 9, 12, 13, 16, 17]. However, only 20% of the surgeons in our study always took a psychiatric history, and 10% never or rarely enquired about psychiatric problems. Earlier research has shown that the rate of depression is 10–13% among the arthroplasty population, and that depression is correlated with an increased risk of poor outcome after surgery [8, 9]. Thus, awareness of this patient category needs to be increased, at least among Swedish knee surgeons.

Many studies recommend preoperative evaluation and management of psychiatric problems to mitigate postoperative complaints, thereby decreasing dissatisfaction rate after TKA [3, 8, 11, 15, 17, 18, 24, 51, 52]. In our survey, only 10% of orthopaedic surgeons always consulted a psychiatrist when they suspected a psychiatric problem, and 16% never or rarely did this. Moreover, only 3% of the surgeons used preoperative psychiatric questionnaires. With the support of the above-mentioned literature, the use of this kind of questionnaire can detect patients with a psychiatric disorder. There are no systematic protocols yet in Sweden to refer patients with psychiatric diseases for a professional psychiatric evaluation before TKA surgery. We recommend to build up such systems which we consider as important as referral for physical evaluation before surgery.

The knee surgeon's responses were consistent with literature considering their believes about the causes of dissatisfaction. This was regarded patients' expectations [12, 20, 32, 43, 44, 53], the choice of patient to operate on [3, 7, 13, 15, 18, 45, 52, 54–56], surgery related factors [21, 57, 58], combination of factors [10] and poor provision of information [12, 40, 44, 48, 59].

One limitation of this study is its descriptive design; However, the study does reveal the extent of the knee surgeons who do not provide a sufficient preoperative patient information in Sweden, which may be similar in other countries. Descriptive studies are ranked low in the hierarchy of evidence [60], but the strength of this survey is that it is unique in describing for the first time Swedish knee surgeons' attitude to preoperative information. In addition, the qualitative analysis of surgeons' beliefs shows how surgeons think about dissatisfaction after TKA patients in Sweden. Another weakness is the absence of psychometric analysis of the questionnaire. The questionnaire was constructed by the researchers with the aim of investigating the attitudes of knee surgeons, as there was no validated questionnaire which could answer the aim of the study. Many differences between the groups were statistically non-significant because of multi-categorical comparison between the groups. When we condensed these categories, the differences became statistically significant, however without clinical importance. The high response rate added more strength to this study.

Another limitation of the study is that it only evaluated frequency of information provision, which does not tell us anything about the quality of this information, which may also be important and influence patients' expectations and satisfaction [35, 40–42, 48, 59, 61]. Moreover, the surgeon's believes and attitude that showed by the study may not represent the actual daily behavior of knee surgeons.

Conclusions

The findings in this survey show that Swedish knee surgeons are aware of factors which predict poor outcome after knee arthroplasty surgery, and that they take these factors into consideration when verbally informing patients preoperatively. On the other hand, more effort is needed in improving written information, analysis of preoperative patient expectations, taking a psychiatric history, consulting a psychiatrist, and not operating on mild indications. Many studies support the negative effect of these factors on outcome. Changing the attitudes of knee surgeons towards preoperative care might decrease dissatisfaction rate. This survey may serve as background for future research regarding preoperative patient selection, surgeon attitudes, and satisfaction rate.

Appendix 1

Table 6 Swedish hospitals which participated in the survey. SPSS statistical program

No.	Hospital	Knee surgeons (total no.)	percent	Knee surgeons (answered)
1.	Akademiska Uppsala	8	2.8	2
2.	Aleris Motala	4	1.4	3
3.	Alingsås	5	1.7	4
4.	Blekinge	7	2.4	7
5.	Bollnäs	3	1.0	2
6.	Capio Movement/Halms.	5	1.7	2
7.	Carlanderska	2	0.7	2
8.	Danderyd	6	2.1	6
9.	Eksjö-Nässjö-Högla	4	1.4	4
10.	Elisabeth/Uppsala	1	0.3	1
11.	Enköping	6	2.1	6
12.	Falun	6	2.1	2
13.	Gävle	6	2.1	6
14.	Halmstad	7	2.4	3
15.	Helsingborg	5	1.7	1
16.	Huddinge	7	2.4	1
17.	Hudiksvall	3	1.0	1
18.	Hässleholm	3	1.0	2
19.	Kalmar	3	1.0	3
20.	Karlskoga	5	1.7	5
21.	Karlstad	5	1.7	3
22.	Karolinska /Solna	4	1.4	4
23.	Kungsälv	4	1.4	4
24.	Lidköping	5	1.7	3
25.	Lindesberg	6	2.1	6
26.	Ljungby	5	1.7	3
27.	Lycksele	2	0.7	2
28.	Mora	6	2.1	1
29.	Mälar/Eskilstuna	8	2.8	7
30.	Nacka Aleris	3	1,0	3
31.	Norrtälje	3	1.0	3
32.	Nyköping	4	1.4	2
33.	Orthocenter/Göteborg	3	1.0	3
34.	Orthocenter/Löwenstr	4	1.4	4
35.	Ortopediska huset	4	1.4	3
36.	Oskarshamn	3	1.0	3
37.	Piteå/Sunderby	6	2.1	5
38.	Ryhov/Jönköping	3	1.0	1
39.	Sahlgrenska/Mölndal	12	4.2	10
40.	Skellefteå	4	1.4	4
41.	Skene/Södra Älvsborgs	5	1.7	5
42.	Skövde	3	1.0	3
43.	Sollefteå	2	0.7	2

Table 6 Swedish hospitals which participated in the survey. SPSS statistical program *(Continued)*

No.	Hospital	Knee surgeons (total no.)	percent	Knee surgeons (answered)
44.	St. Görans	4	1.4	4
45.	Sundsvall	2	0.7	2
46.	SUS(Lund/Malmö)	16	5.6	10
47.	Södertälje	5	1.7	5
48.	Södersjukhuset	9	3.1	8
49.	Torsby	4	1.4	2
50.	Uddevalla	5	1.7	2
51.	USÖ/Örebro	3	1.0	3
52.	Varberg	5	1.7	5
53.	Vrinnevis/Norrköping	4	1.4	4
54.	Värnamo	4	1.4	4
55.	Västervik	3	1.0	3
56.	Västerås	5	1.7	2
57.	Växjö	7	2.4	7
58.	Ängelholm	3	1.0	3
59.	Örnsköldsvik	3	1.0	3
60.	Östersund	5	1.7	5
		287	100	219

The table shows the numbers and names of participating hospitals. It shows also the total number of knee surgeons who are working in each hospital and the number of knee surgeons who participated in the survey

Appendix 2

Table 7 The questions answered by knee surgeons in the survey

No.	Question text
1	Do you use **written** information with clear text about risks, complications and benefits of TKA surgery?
2	Do you use **oral** information with clear text about risks, complications and benefits of TKA surgery?
3	How many years do you work with Knee arthroplasty?
4	How many primary TKA do you operate per year?
5	How many knee revision arthroplasty do you operate per year?
6	The percentage of working with knee surgery: a. 100% knee specialist b. 75% c. 50% D. 25%
7	Do you ask patients about their **expectations**?
8	Do you inform patient that about 20% of patients are not satisfied after TKA surgery despite the absence of obvious explanation?
9	If you get a patient with severe knee pain, mild radiological arthrosis, large desire to be operated and the patient has anxiety/depression. How often do you proceed with surgery?
10	Do you enquire routinely about psychiatric history?
11	If you realize that patient suffering from depression/anxiety, do you consult psychiatrist before proceeding with surgery?
12	Do you use a psychiatric enquiry sheet for evaluation of psychiatric problems?
13	If you use a psychiatric enquiry which reveal depression or anxiety, do you control that patient received firstly psychiatric treatment
14	Do you think that psychiatric problem play some role in the results?
15	Many of dissatisfied patients describe a pain. What do you think generally the most important reason to the pain if we excluded radiating pain
16	What do you think about the single most important reason that patient is dissatisfied after TKA

The table shows the English translated version of the questionnaire which was sent to the Swedish knee surgeons

Abbreviations

SPSS: Statistical Package for the Social Sciences; TKA: Total knee arthroplasty

Acknowledgements

We wish to thank Ole Brus Clinical Epidemiology and Biostatistics, School of Medical Sciences, Örebro University, Örebro, Sweden) for statistical advice and help with the SPSS software package. We are also grateful to all the surgeons who answered the study questionnaire.

Funding

This study was funded by the Örebro Research Committee, Sweden, and the Orthopaedic Department, Karlskoga Hospital, Sweden. No external funding or benefits were received. The funders had no role in the design and conduct of the study; collection, management, analysis, and interpretation of the data; preparation, review, or approval of the manuscript; and decision to submit the manuscript for publication.

Authors' contributions

AM created the study protocol and design, collected the data, performed the analysis, and wrote the manuscript. MHN and PW contributed to the study design, the analysis, and revision of the manuscript. All authors read and approved the final manuscript.

Consent for publication

Not applicable.

Competing interests

The authors declare that they have no competing interests.

Author details

Department of Orthopaedics, Örebro County, Sweden. ²Faculty of Medicine and Health, School of Medical Sciences, Örebro University, Örebro, Sweden. ³Faculty of Medicine and Health, School of Health Sciences, Örebro University, Örebro, Sweden.

References

1. Kurtz S, Ong K, Lau E, Mowat F, Halpern M. Projections of primary and revision hip and knee arthroplasty in the United States from 2005 to 2030. J Bone Joint Surg Am. 2007;89(4):780–5.
2. Skar: the swedish knee arthroplasty register – Annu Rep 2016 – PART I. In., vol. 2016, 2016 edn: The swedish knee arthroplasty register – Annu Rep 2016 – Part I; 2016: 15.
3. Ali A, Lindstrand A, Sundberg M, Flivik G. Preoperative anxiety and depression correlate with dissatisfaction after Total knee arthroplasty: a prospective longitudinal cohort study of 186 patients, with 4-year follow-up. J Arthroplast. 2017;32(3):767–70.
4. Ayers DC, Franklin PD, Trief PM, Ploutz-Snyder R, Freund D. Psychological attributes of preoperative total joint replacement patients: implications for optimal physical outcome. J Arthroplasty. 2004;19(7 Suppl 2):125–30.
5. Berger RA, Crossett LS, Jacobs JJ, Rubash HE. Malrotation causing patellofemoral complications after total knee arthroplasty. Clin Orthop Relat Res. 1998;356:144–53.
6. Bletterman AN, de Geest-Vrolijk ME, Vriezekolk JE, Nijhuis-van der Sanden MW, van Meeteren NL, Hoogeboom TJ. Preoperative psychosocial factors predicting patient's functional recovery after total knee or total hip arthroplasty: a systematic review. Clin Rehabil. 2017;32(4):512–25.
7. Bozic KJ, Lau E, Ong K, Chan V, Kurtz S, Vail TP, Rubash HE, Berry DJ. Risk factors for early revision after primary TKA in Medicare patients. Clin Orthop Relat Res. 2014;472(1):232–7.
8. Browne JA, Sandberg BF, D'Apuzzo MR, Novicoff WM. Depression is associated with early postoperative outcomes following total joint arthroplasty: a nationwide database study. J Arthroplast. 2014;29(3):481–3.
9. Gandhi R, Zywiel MG, Mahomed NN, Perruccio AV: Depression and the overall burden of painful joints: an examination among individuals undergoing hip and knee replacement for osteoarthritis. Arthritis 2015, 2015:327161.
10. Gibon E, Goodman MJ, Goodman SB. Patient satisfaction after Total knee arthroplasty: A Realistic or Imaginary Goal? Orthop Clin North Am. 2017; 48(4):421–31.
11. Gold HT, Slover JD, Joo L, Bosco J, Iorio R, Oh C. Association of Depression with 90-day hospital readmission after Total joint arthroplasty. J Arthroplast. 2016;31(11):2385–8.
12. Greene KA, Harwin SF. Maximizing patient satisfaction and functional results after total knee arthroplasty. J Knee Surg. 2011;24(1):19–24.
13. Jacobs CA, Christensen CP, Karthikeyan T. Chronic non-orthopedic conditions more common in patients with less severe degenerative changes that have elected to undergo Total knee arthroplasty. J Arthroplast. 2015;30(7):1146–9.
14. Jeffery RS, Morris RW, Denham RA. Coronal alignment after total knee replacement. J Bone Joint Surg Br. 1991;73(5):709–14.
15. Judge A, Arden NK, Cooper C, Kassim Javaid M, Carr AJ, Field RE, Dieppe PA. Predictors of outcomes of total knee replacement surgery. Rheumatology (Oxford). 2012;51(10):1804–13.
16. Khatib Y, Madan A, Naylor JM, Harris IA. Do psychological factors predict poor outcome in patients undergoing TKA? A systematic review. Clin Orthop Relat Res. 2015;473(8):2630–8.
17. Klement MR, Nickel BT, Penrose CT, Bala A, Green CL, Wellman SS, Bolognesi MP, Seyler TM. Psychiatric disorders increase complication rate after primary total knee arthroplasty. Knee. 2016;23(5):883–6.
18. Lingard EA, Katz JN, Wright EA, Sledge CB: Predicting the outcome of total knee arthroplasty. J Bone Joint Surg Am 2004, 86-a(10):2179–2186.
19. Lostak J, Gallo J, Zapletalova J. Patient satisfaction after Total knee arthroplasty. Analysis of pre-operative and Peri-operative parameters influencing results in 826 patients. Acta Chir Orthop Traumatol Cechoslov. 2016;83(2):94–101.
20. Nilsdotter AK, Toksvig-Larsen S, Roos EM. Knee arthroplasty: are patients' expectations fulfilled? A prospective study of pain and function in 102 patients with 5-year follow-up. Acta Orthop. 2009;80(1):55–61.
21. Norton EC, Garfinkel SA, McQuay LJ, Heck DA, Wright JG, Dittus R, Lubitz RM. The effect of hospital volume on the in-hospital complication rate in knee replacement patients. Health Serv Res. 1998;33(5 Pt 1):1191–210.
22. Robertsson O, Dunbar M, Pehrsson T, Knutson K, Lidgren L. Patient satisfaction after knee arthroplasty: a report on 27,372 knees operated on between 1981 and 1995 in Sweden. Acta Orthop Scand. 2000;71(3):262–7.
23. Robertsson O, Dunbar MJ. Patient satisfaction compared with general health and disease-specific questionnaires in knee arthroplasty patients. J Arthroplast. 2001;16(4):476–82.
24. Santaguida PL, Hawker GA, Hudak PL, Glazier R, Mahomed NN, Kreder HJ, Coyte PC, Wright JG. Patient characteristics affecting the prognosis of total hip and knee joint arthroplasty: a systematic review. Can J Surg. 2008;51(6): 428–36.
25. Ali A, Sundberg M, Robertsson O, Dahlberg LE, Thorstensson CA, Redlund-Johnell I, Kristiansson I, Lindstrand A. Dissatisfied patients after total knee arthroplasty: a registry study involving 114 patients with 8–13 years of followup. Acta Orthop. 2014;85(3):229–33.
26. Clement ND, Bardgett M, Weir D, Holland J, Deehan DJ. Increased symptoms of stiffness 1 year after total knee arthroplasty are associated with a worse functional outcome and lower rate of patient satisfaction. Knee Surg Sports Traumatol Arthrosc. 2018. Online ISSN1433-7347.
27. Dailiana ZH, Papakostidou I, Varitimidis S, Liaropoulos L, Zintzaras E, Karachalios T, Michelinakis E, Malizos KN. Patient-reported quality of life after primary major joint arthroplasty: a prospective comparison of hip and knee arthroplasty. BMC Musculoskelet Disord. 2015;16:366.
28. Kievit AJ, van Geenen RC, Kuijer PP, Pahlplatz TM, Blankevoort L, Schafroth MU. Total knee arthroplasty and the unforeseen impact on return to work: a cross-sectional multicenter survey. J Arthroplast. 2014;29(6):1163–8.
29. Van Onsem S, Verstraete M, Dhont S, Zwaenepoel B, Van Der Straeten C, Victor J. Improved walking distance and range of motion predict patient satisfaction after TKA. Knee Surg Sports Traumatol Arthrosc. 2018.
30. Verra WC, Witteveen KQ, Maier AB, Gademan MG, van der Linden HM, Nelissen RG. The reason why orthopaedic surgeons perform total knee

replacement: results of a randomised study using case vignettes. Knee Surg Sports Traumatol Arthrosc. 2016;24(8):2697–703.

31. Weinberg DB, Gittell JH, Lusenhop RW, Kautz CM, Wright J. Beyond our walls: impact of patient and provider coordination across the continuum on outcomes for surgical patients. Health Serv Res. 2007;42(1 Pt 1):7–24.

32. Zeni JA Jr, Snyder-Mackler L. Preoperative predictors of persistent impairments during stair ascent and descent after total knee arthroplasty. J Bone Joint Surg Am. 2010;92(5):1130–6.

33. Bethge M, Kohler L, Kiel J, Thren K, Gutenbrunner C. Sports activity following joint arthroplasty: experiences and expectations of elderly patients--findings from a qualitative content analysis of guided interviews. Rehabilitation (Stuttg). 2015;54(4):233–9.

34. Brander VA, Stulberg SD, Adams AD, Harden RN, Bruehl S, Stanos SP, Houle T. Predicting total knee replacement pain: a prospective, observational study. Clin Orthop Relat Res. 2003;416:27–36.

35. Clement ND, Bardgett M, Weir D, Holland J, Gerrand C, Deehan DJ. The rate and predictors of patient satisfaction after total knee arthroplasty are influenced by the focus of the question. Bone Joint J. 2018;100-b(6):740–8.

36. Clode NJ, Perry MA, Wulff L. Does physiotherapy prehabilitation improve pre-surgical outcomes and influence patient expectations prior to knee and hip joint arthroplasty? Int J Orthop Trauma Nurs. 2018;30:14–9.

37. Filbay SR, Judge A, Delmestri A, Arden NK: Evaluating Patients' expectations from a novel patient-centered perspective predicts knee arthroplasty outcome. J Arthroplast 2018, 33(7):2146–2152.e2144.

38. Indications for Total Knee Arthroplasty and Choice of Prosthesis [http://www.med.or.jp/english/pdf/2001_04/153_158.pdf].

39. Harris IA, Harris AM, Naylor JM, Adie S, Mittal R, Dao AT. Discordance between patient and surgeon satisfaction after total joint arthroplasty. J Arthroplast. 2013;28(5):722–7.

40. Conradsen S, Gjerseth MM, Kvangarsnes M. Patients' experiences from an education programme ahead of orthopaedic surgery - a qualitative study. J Clin Nurs. 2016;25(19–20):2798–806.

41. Andersson V, Otterstrom-Rydberg E, Karlsson AK. The importance of written and verbal information on pain treatment for patients undergoing surgical interventions. Pain Manag Nurs. 2015;16(5):634–41.

42. Louw A, Diener I, Butler DS, Puentedura EJ. Preoperative education addressing postoperative pain in total joint arthroplasty: review of content and educational delivery methods. Physiother Theory Pract. 2013;29(3):175–94.

43. Scott CE, Bugler KE, Clement ND, MacDonald D, Howie CR, Biant LC. Patient expectations of arthroplasty of the hip and knee. J Bone Joint Surg Br. 2012; 94(7):974–81.

44. Tilbury C, Haanstra TM, Leichtenberg CS, Verdegaal SH, Ostelo RW, de Vet HC, Nelissen RG, Vliet Vlieland TP. Unfulfilled expectations after Total hip and knee arthroplasty surgery: there is a need for better preoperative patient information and education. J Arthroplast. 2016;31(10):2139–45.

45. Schnurr C, Jarrous M, Gudden I, Eysel P, Konig DP. Pre-operative arthritis severity as a predictor for total knee arthroplasty patients' satisfaction. Int Orthop. 2013;37(7):1257–61.

46. Boyatzis RE. Transforming qualitative information, thematic analysis and code development, vol. 1. London, New Delhi: International educational and profissional publisher, thousands oaks; 1998.

47. Braun V, Clarke V. What can "thematic analysis" offer health and wellbeing researchers? Int J Qual Stud Health Well-being. 2014;9:26152.

48. Eschalier B, Descamps S, Pereira B, Vaillant-Roussel H, Girard G, Boisgard S, Coudeyre E. Randomized blinded trial of standardized written patient information before total knee arthroplasty. PLoS One. 2017;12(7):e0178358.

49. Halleberg Nyman M, Nilsson U, Dahlberg K, Jaensson M. Association between functional health literacy and postoperative recovery, health care contacts, and health-related quality of life among patients undergoing day surgery: secondary analysis of a randomized clinical trial. JAMA Surg. 2018.

50. Meneghini RM, Russo GS, Lieberman JR. Modern perceptions and expectations regarding total knee arthroplasty. J Knee Surg. 2014;27(2):93–7.

51. Rasouli MR, Menendez ME, Sayadipour A, Purtill JJ, Parvizi J. Direct cost and complications associated with Total joint arthroplasty in patients with preoperative anxiety and depression. J Arthroplast. 2016;31(2):533–6.

52. Schwartz FH, Lange J. Factors that affect outcome following Total joint arthroplasty: a review of the recent literature. Curr Rev Musculoskelet Med. 2017.

53. Dowsey MM, Scott A, Nelson EA, Li J, Sundararajan V, Nikpour M, Choong PF. Using discrete choice experiments as a decision aid in total knee arthroplasty: study protocol for a randomised controlled trial. Trials. 2016; 17(1):416.

54. Pagnotta G, Rich E, Eckardt P, Lavin P, Burriesci R. The effect of a rapid rehabilitation program on patients undergoing unilateral Total knee arthroplasty. Orthop Nurs. 2017;36(2):112–21.

55. Fernandes L, Roos EM, Overgaard S, Villadsen A, Sogaard R. Supervised neuromuscular exercise prior to hip and knee replacement: 12-month clinical effect and cost-utility analysis alongside a randomised controlled trial. BMC Musculoskelet Disord. 2017;18(1):5.

56. Vavro M, Ziakova E, Gazdikova K, Farkasova D. Does standard post-operative rehabilitation have its place after total knee replacement? Bratisl Lek Listy. 2016;117(10):605–8.

57. Liddle AD, Pandit H, Judge A, Murray DW. Effect of surgical caseload on revision rate following Total and Unicompartmental knee replacement. J Bone Joint Surg Am. 2016;98(1):1–8.

58. Wilson S, Marx RG, Pan TJ, Lyman S. Meaningful thresholds for the volume-outcome relationship in Total knee arthroplasty. J Bone Joint Surg Am. 2016;98(20):1683–90.

59. Majid N, Lee S, Plummer V. The effectiveness of orthopedic patient education in improving patient outcomes: a systematic review protocol. JBI Database System Rev Implement Rep. 2015;13(1):122–33.

60. Institute tJB: New JBI Levels of Evidence. 2013:1–6.

61. Goldsmith LJ, Suryaprakash N, Randall E, Shum J, MacDonald V, Sawatzky R, Hejazi S, Davis JC, McAllister P, Bryan S. The importance of informational, clinical and personal support in patient experience with total knee replacement: a qualitative investigation. BMC Musculoskelet Disord. 2017; 18(1):127.

20

Effect of bisphosphonates on periprosthetic bone loss after total knee arthroplasty

Mingmin Shi[1], Lei Chen[2], Haobo Wu[1], Yangxin Wang[1], Wei Wang[1], Yujie Zhang[1] and Shigui Yan[1*]

Abstract

Background: Aseptic loosening and osteolysis are the most common indications after TKA for revision surgery. This meta-analysis which included high-quality randomized controlled trials (RCTs) aimed to analyze the effect of bisphosphonates (BPs) on maintaining periprosthetic bone mineral density (BMD) after total knee arthroplasty.

Methods: PubMed, AMED, EMBASE, the Cochrane library, ISI Web of Science, and China National Knowledge Infrastructure were systematically searched, five RCTs were included and the total number of participants was 188. The weighted mean differences with 95% confidence interval were calculated to evaluate the efficacy of BPs on total BMD of knee and the BMD of different periprosthetic regions. A descriptive review was performed for BP-related adverse effects.

Results: The BPs group presented significantly higher total BMD in proximal part of the tibia than the control group at 3 and 6 months ($P < 0.05$), but no significant difference at 12 months ($P = 0.09$). The BPs group presented significantly higher BMD in the distal aspect of the femur than that in the control group at 3, 6, 12 months. The BPs group presented significantly higher periprosthetic BMD than that in the control group at 3, 6 and 12 months in tibial medial and lateral metaphyseal region, and femoral anterior, central and posterior metaphyseal region ($p < 0.05$), but no significant difference for tibial diaphyseal region at 3, 6, and 12 months. None of the included studies described severe or fatal adverse effects related to BPs.

Conclusion: BPs have a short-term effect on reducing periprosthetic bone loss after total knee arthroplasty. Compared with diaphyseal region, BPs are more effective on the preservation of BMD in medial lateral metaphyseal regions of proximal tibia and in anterior, central, and posterior metaphyseal region of distal femur.

Keywords: Bisphosphonates, Total knee arthroplasty, Bone mineral density, Meta-analysis randomized controlled trial

Background

Total knee arthroplasty (TKA) is a successful therapeutic option for the patients with knee osteoarthritis and rheumatoid arthritis. However, TKA changes the mechanical loads on the knee joint and causes bone mineral density and structure be adjusted to meet new mechanical demands surrounding the prosthesis and the new alignment of the lower legs [1–3]. Aseptic loosening and osteolysis are the most common indications after TKA for revision surgery [4–6]. Bone loss is mainly related to stress shielding, immobilization, and tissue damage due to surgical procedure [7, 8].

Previous studies reported a significant decrease in periprosthetic BMD after TKA [8–10].

Therefore, how to preserve the periprosthetic bone mass to improve the outcome of TKA has been an important subject [11].

Bisphosphonates (BPs) are widely used in the therapy of osteoporosis and other metabolic bone diseases. BPs

* Correspondence: zrjwsj@zju.edu.cn
[1]Department of Orthopaedic Surgery, Second Affiliated Hospital, School of Medicine, Zhejiang University, No.88 Jiefang Road, Hangzhou 310009, People's Republic of China
Full list of author information is available at the end of the article

are inhibitors of bone resorption which promote bone mineralization and inhibit farnesyl pyrophosphate synthase [12, 13]. Some studies revealed that bisphosphonates can decrease fracture risk and prolong survival time of implant [14, 15], and some randomized controlled trials have investigated the effect of reduce periprosthetic bone loss after total knee arthroplasty [16–20]. To confirm the effect of BPs on periprosthetic bone loss after total joint arthroplasty, we have made a previous meta-analysis [21], of which included 14 RCTs in 2012, and the result revealed that BPs could prevent bone loss after arthroplasty in medium-term follow-up. However, there were only 2 RCTs about TKA. Due to increased trend in recent investigations on effect of BPs on periprosthetic bone loss after TKA with large-scale and high quality, it is essential to update the analysis.

This meta-analysis of five high-quality RCTs aimed to analyze the effect of bisphosphonates on periprosthetic bone loss after TKA.

Methods

Literature search

Two independent investigators searched Electronic databases including PubMed, AMED, EMBASE, the Cochrane library, ISI Web of Science, and China National Knowledge Infrastructure from the inception dates to October 31, 2017. The search used the following keywords: (alendronate OR pamidronate OR etidronate OR zoledronate OR clodronate OR bisphosphonate) AND (arthroplasty OR knee arthroplasty OR joint prosthesis OR joint replacement OR knee replacement). To include additional eligible studies, citation lists of all the selected publications were searched by hand.

Selection criteria

The inclusion criteria were as follows: (1) the participants underwent total knee arthroplasty, (2) the intervention was administration of bisphosphonates after total knee arthroplasty, (3) the measurements must include periprosthetic BMD, and (4) the trial design was randomized and controlled. The exclusion criteria were as follows: (1) the participants had any history of bone metabolic diseases, (2) BMD data were not available, (3) the same participants reported in a short follow-up study duplicately.

Data extraction and outcome measures

For each initially screened trial, two independent investigators collected the information including name of first author, publication year, sample size, intervention, study duration, co-factors, measurements and loss-to-followup rate. If information was not described as text in the publications, we extracted it from the figures, tables, or other supplementary material. The characteristics of five finally included RCTs [16–20] were showed in Table 1. The primary outcome measurement was total periprosthetic BMD of knee. And the secondary measurement was the BMD of different periprosthetic regions of interest (ROIs), including the tibial regions and the femoral regions (Fig. 1). The tibial regions including medial metaphyseal region (R1), lateral metaphyseal region (R2), and diaphyseal region (R3). The femoral regions including anterior metaphyseal region (R4), central metaphyseal region (R5), and posterior region (R6). Because BMD levels are affected by gender, weight and general bone loss, the results were presented as a percentage of the BMD changing from the baseline. The percentage of BMD changing was used rather than the absolute numerical value to decrease the bias of different baseline. The percentage of BMD changing was calculated as follows: $100*(BMD_n-BMD_0)/BMD_0$. Here BMD_0 refers to the baseline BMD value, and BMD_n stands for the postoperative BMD at certain follow-up time point. Sensitivity analysis was performed for the effect size by omitting the studies for which data were imputed.

Table 1 Characteristics of the included studies

Study	Age (years), I/C	Sample Size, I/C	Intervention	Follow-up (month)	Outcome Measures
Soininvaara 2002	$83.5 \pm 19.9/ 79.7 \pm 8.7$	19 (8/11)	10 mg/day oral alendronate+ 500 mg/day calcium carbonate for 12 months vs. 500 mg/day calcium carbonate	12 months	Periprosthetic BMD: proximal femur
Han 2003	$63.6 \pm 4.1/ 65.2 \pm 5.6$	72 (36/36)	10 mg/day oral alendronate for 6 months vs. no placebo	12 months	Periprosthetic BMD: distal part of femur and proximal aspect of tibia
Wang 2006	$69.8 \pm 5.9/ 69.7 \pm 6.7$	60 (30/30)	10 mg/day oral alendronate for 6 months vs. no placebo	3 years	Periprosthetic BMD:distal part of femur and proximal aspect of tibia
Abu-Rajab 2009	$68 \pm 2.2/ 72 \pm 8.1$	11 (5/6)	70 mg/week oral alendronate for 6 months vs. a placebo	2 years	Periprosthetic BMD: distal part of femur and proximal aspect of tibia
Jaroma 2015	$66 \pm 7.0/ 68 \pm 8.2$	26 (14/12)	10 mg/day oral alendronate+ 500 mg/day calcium carbonate for 12 months vs. 500 mg/day calcium carbonate	7 years	Periprosthetic BMD: distal part of femur and proximal aspect of tibia

I/C intervention/control groups, BMD bone mineral density

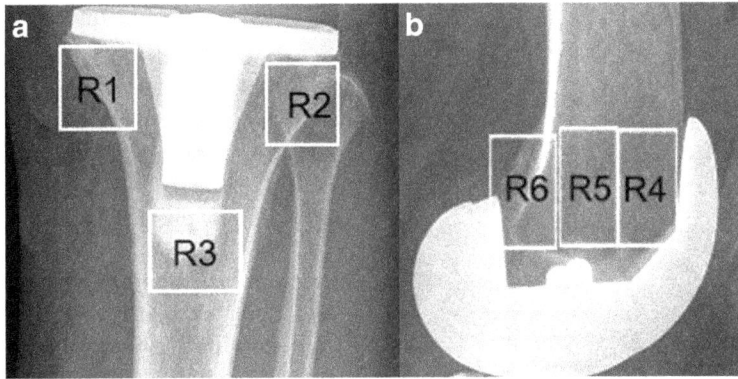

Fig. 1 Periprosthetic ROIs of knee. **a** periprosthetic ROIs of tibia: medial metaphyseal region (R1), diaphyseal region (R2), lateral metaphyseal region (R3), (**b**) periprosthetic ROIs of femur: anterior metaphyseal region (R4), central metaphyseal region (R5), posterior metaphyseal region (R6)

Methodological quality assessment

The methodologic quality of included trials were assessed the by two investigators independently with the Cochrane Collaboration tool for risk of bias, in which assessing factors included randomization, allocation concealment, and blinding etc. The weighted kappa for the agreement on the assessment of quality between all reviewers was 0.89 [95% confidence interval (CI), 0.80–0.99]. The criteria of the Grading of Recommendations Assessment, Development and Evaluation (GRADE) were used to assess the quality of evidence [22].

Statistical analysis

For data reported as continuous variables, means and standard deviations were extracted. All extracted data were input and analyzed in Review Manager 5.3.5 version (Cochrane Collaboration, London, England). Chi-square test and I^2 was used to assess heterogeneity the [23]. When there was no statistical heterogeneity ($P < 0.10$, or $I^2 < 50\%$), the fixed-effect (FE) model was used; otherwise ($P > 0.10$, or $I^2 > 50\%$), a random-effect (RE) model was chosen [24].

Sensitivity were evaluated by omitting some trials to assess whether specified factors (small sample size, randomization, intention-to-treat (ITT) analysis *etc*) could affect the overall result of analysis. The P value of heterogeneity less than 0.05 was considered as significant differences. The analyses of sensitive could not be performed when the number of trials was less than three in comparison.

Results

Trials selection

A flow diagram illustrating the study identification is shown in Fig. 2. There were 353 relevant trials selected by initially search, of which 269 trials were excluded because they were duplicated or non-clinical trial. Of the 84 remaining articles,

only 10 studies were on the main topic. Among the 10 studies, one trial [25] was excluded because there were longer follow-up and re-analyzed studies reported the same participants. But the data from these shorter-term follow-up trials were considered to be used when they were analyzed in other later trials. Two excluded trials had no available BMD data [26, 27]. Two trials were excluded because they were non-RCTs [14, 28]. Finally, 5 RCTs involving 188 participants were included in our meta-analysis (Fig. 1). The weighted kappa for agreement on eligibility between reviewers was 0.88 (95% CI, 0.80–0.96).

The characteristics of the included trials were summarized in Table 1. The BPs used in all the five trials were alendronate.

Methodological quality

A 6-item scale for assessing methodological quality was used (Fig. 3). All the 5 trials were RCTs. Three studies described adequate randomization, only one study

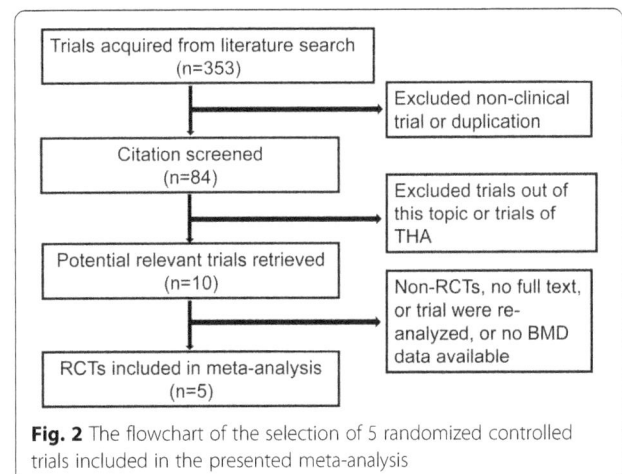

Fig. 2 The flowchart of the selection of 5 randomized controlled trials included in the presented meta-analysis

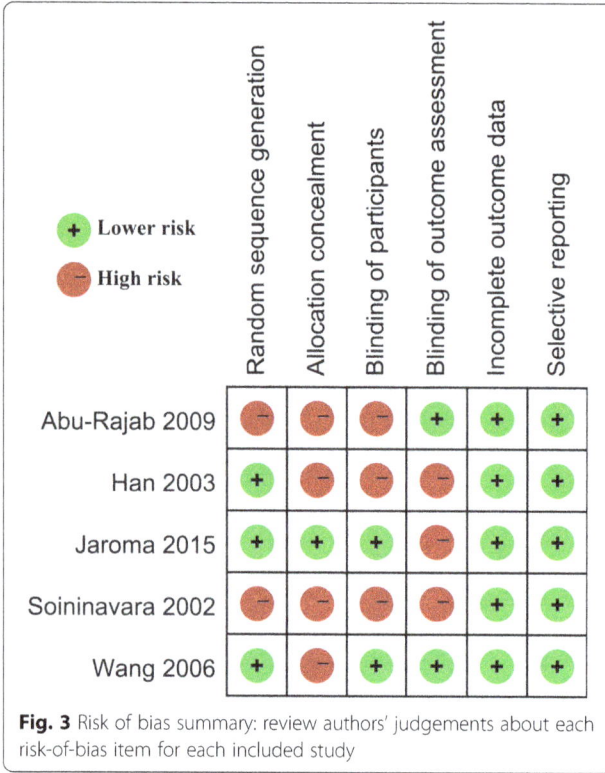

Fig. 3 Risk of bias summary: review authors' judgements about each risk-of-bias item for each included study

demonstrated sufficient allocation concealment, two studies described the blinding of outcome assessment and two studies described the blinding of participants. All the five studies retained complete outcome data, avoided selective reporting, and seemed to be free of other potential sources of bias. The investigators achieved good agreement in evaluating the methodological quality (0.86, 95% CI: 0.82–0.90).

Preservation of total periprosthetic BMD

It was illustrated that the BPs group presented significantly higher total BMD in proximal part of the tibia than the control group at 3 and 6 months respectively [(2 trials, WMD: 3.40, 95% CI: 2.06–4.73, $p < 0.05$); (3 trials, WMD: 2.66, 95% CI:1.63–3.69, $p < 0.05$)] (Fig. 4a and b). There was no significant difference of total BMD in proximal part of the tibia between the BPs group and the control group at 12 months (3 trials, WMD: -1.01, 95% CI: -2.19-0.17, $p = 0.09$) (Fig. 4c). The BPs group presented significantly higher BMD in the distal aspect of the femur than that in the control group at 3, 6, 12 months [(3 trials, WMD: 5.64, 95% CI: 4.42–6.85, $p < 0.05$); (5 trials, WMD: 7.22, 95% CI: 5.88–8.57, $p < 0.05$); (4 trials, WMD: 18.46, 95% CI:17.09–19.83, $p < 0.05$)] (Fig. 5).

Preservation of BMD in different knee regions

It was illustrated that the BPs group presented significantly higher periprosthetic BMD than that in the control

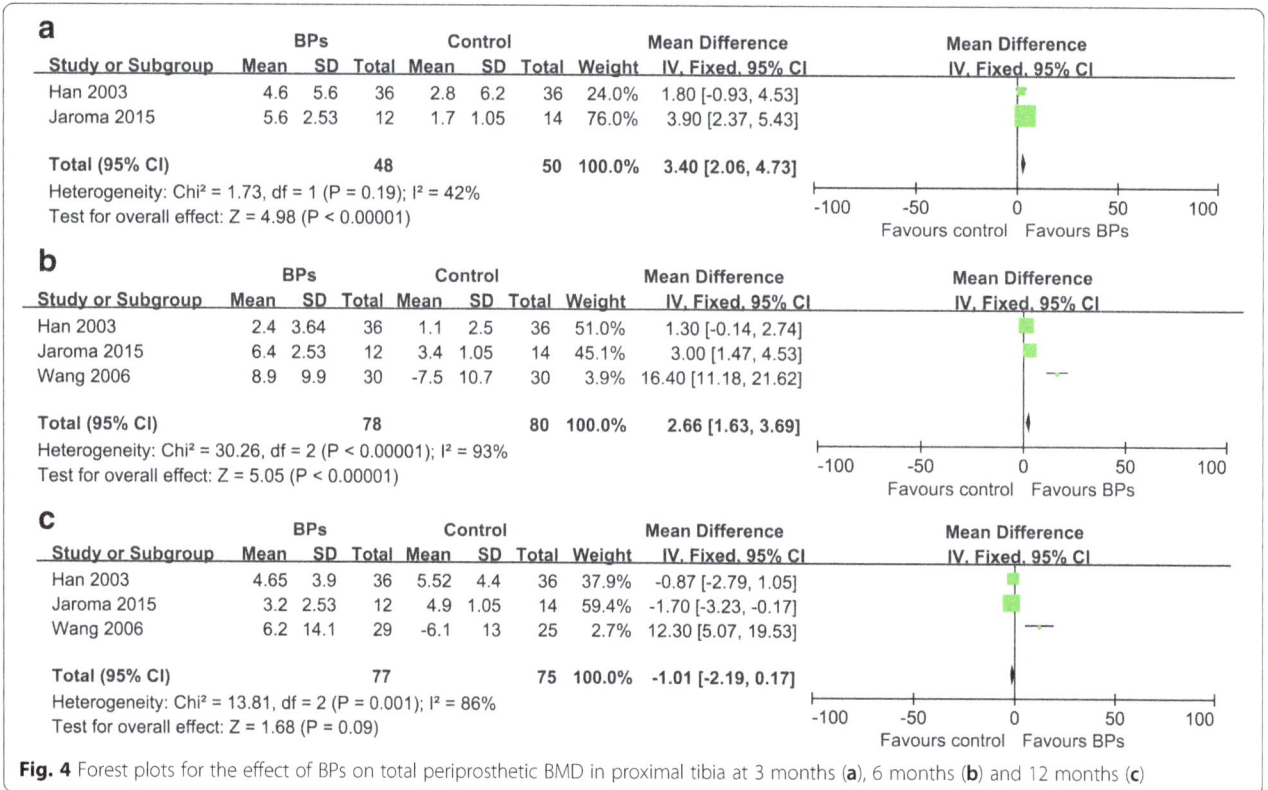

Fig. 4 Forest plots for the effect of BPs on total periprosthetic BMD in proximal tibia at 3 months (**a**), 6 months (**b**) and 12 months (**c**)

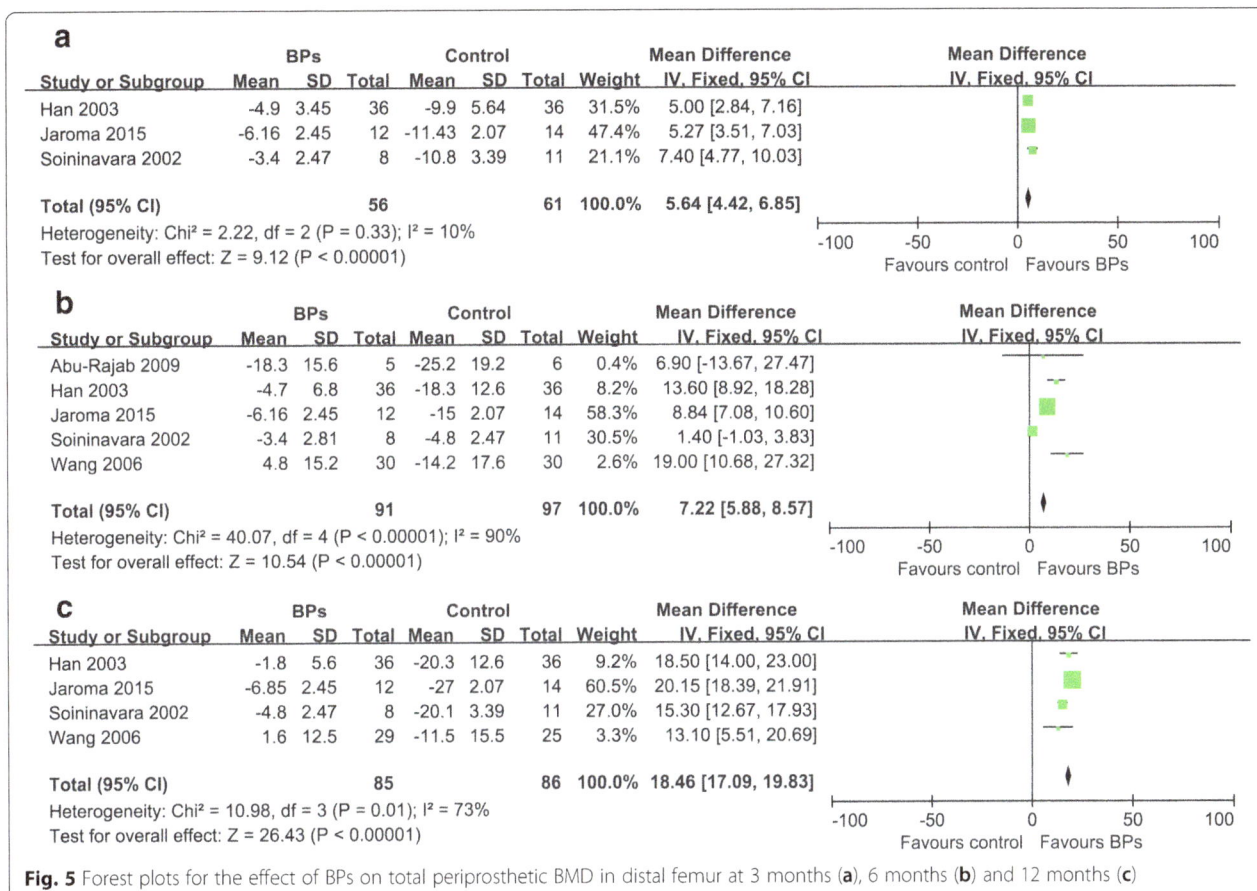

Fig. 5 Forest plots for the effect of BPs on total periprosthetic BMD in distal femur at 3 months (**a**), 6 months (**b**) and 12 months (**c**)

group at 3, 6 and 12 months in R1, R2, R4, R5 and R6 ($p < 0.05$) (Table 2). For R3, there was no significant difference of periprosthetic BMD between the BPs group and the control group at 3, 6, and 12 months ($p < 0.05$).

Heterogeneity and sensitivity analysis

The BMD in proximal part of the tibia and the distal aspect of the femur at different follow-up were statistically heterogeneous at 6 (tibia: $\chi^2 = 30.26$, $p < 0.00001$, $I^2 = 93\%$; femur: $\chi^2 = 40.07$, $p < 0.00001$, $I^2 = 90\%$) and 12 months respectively (tibia: $\chi^2 = 13.81$, $p < 0.00001$, $I^2 = 86\%$; femur: $\chi^2 = 10.98$, $p < 0.00001$, $I^2 = 73\%$) but not at 3 months (Fig. 4 and Fig. 5). The heterogeneity could not be minimized by omitting any trial. The overall effect was not significantly altered by omitting trials without the ITT analysis, those with small sample size (less than 20), or those funded by companies.

Strength of evidence.

Adverse reaction

No serious adverse effect was reported related to BPs in the 5 trials. The mostly reported adverse effect was digestive discomfort in 3 trials: 1 of 8 by Soininvaara [16]; 5 patients

Table 2 Meta-analyses of BMD of the different regions of knee at different time points

ROI		3 months WMD (95%CI)	6 months WMD (95%CI)	12 months WMD (95%CI)
Tibia	1	4.90 (3.53, 6.26)	6.63 (5.34, 7.93)	4.22 (2.92, 5.51)
		$P < 0.05$	$P < 0.05$	$P < 0.05$
	2	2.61 (1.32, 3.91)	5.86 (4.57, 7.16)	8.57 (7.28, 9.87)
		$P < 0.05$	$P < 0.05$	$P < 0.05$
	3	1.10 (−0.19, 2.40)	0.45 (−0.84, 1.75)	0.36 (0.94, 1.65)
		$P = 0.18$	$P = 0.39$	$P = 0.44$
Femur	4	4.10 (2.74, 5.46)	4.50 (3.13, 5.86)	5.70 (4.34, 7.06)
		$P < 0.05$	$P < 0.05$	$P < 0.05$
	5	6.90 (5.54, 8.27)	6.50 (5.14, 7.87)	7.02 (5.66, 8.39)
		$P < 0.05$	$P < 0.05$	$P < 0.05$
	6	4.34 (2.97, 5.70)	4.32 (2.96, 5.68)	5.25 (3.89, 6.62)
		$P < 0.05$	$P < 0.05$	$P < 0.05$

ROI: region of interest, WMD: weighted mean differences
A positive value of WMD means it favors experimental, and negative value means favoring control

by Wang [18]; 2 patients by Jaroma [20]. There was no severe side effect on renal, hepatic, or heart function.

Discussion

High BMD supports bone-implant fixation, and there have been several attempts to improve the quality of the primary arthroplasty and to reduce the incidence of failures caused by loss of BMD [29, 30]. A large population-based parallel-cohorts study [31] found that bisphosphonates could decrease the risk of periprosthetic fractures after THA. A larger retrospective cohort study on participants with primary total hip/knee arthroplasty showed that oral bisphosphonates reduced risk of revision surgery by 59% [32]. The present meta-analysis strengthened the evidence of BPs reducing periprosthetic bone loss.

Our previous meta-analyses based on 14 RCTs [21] found that BPs significantly preserved total periprosthetic BMD up to 10 years after joint arthroplasty. However, most included trials in that meta-analyses were in regards to THA, and there was only 2 RCTs about the TKA. More significant efficacy in proximal tibia was found at 3 and 6 months after arthroplasty in the BPs group compared with the control group. However, this difference was not significant at 12 months after arthroplasty. The reason that later stages after surgery have respectively lower efficacy may be the active bone resorption caused by the early iatrogenic damage and the late stress shielding induced osteolysis [33]. Meanwhile, more significant efficacy in distal femur was found at 3, 6 and 12 months after arthroplasty in the BPs group compared with the control group. Moreover, the secondary finding is that different femoral region has different response to bisphosphonates. In the proximal tibial region R1 and R2, BPs group presented significantly higher peripros-thetic BMD than that control group up to 12 months after arthroplasty, and in the proximal tibial region R3, the difference between BPs group and control group was not significantly at 3, 6 and 12 months after arthroplasty. The possible interpretation is that the medial and lateral

metaphyseal region have more stress shielding than diaph-yseal region [34]. In the distal femoral region R1, R2 and R3, BPs group presented significantly higher periprosthetic BMD than that control group at 3, 6 and 12 months after surgery. The possible interpretation is that these three regions have similar mechanical environment which provides similar stress shielding [35]. The present study showed there was no serious adverse effect related to BPs. It was reported a higher risk of periprosthetic fractures was found in TKA patients who used BPs, but the numbers were very small [36]. As there was no atypical femur fracture observed in this meta-analysis, there are likely to be a variety of factors involved in peri-prosthetic fracture, such as femoral geometry, prolonged duration of BP use, smoking, and activity level.

The strengths of our meta-analysis include the most included trials and largest sample size investigating the effect of BPs treatment following TKA. According to the GRADE system for evidence quality, all the included trials in the present meta-analysis began as high-quality or moderate-quality evidence, which was downgraded by five categories of limitations (Table 3). Inadequate blinding and substantial loss follow-up in some trials may raise risk of bias. Inconsistent reporting of outcomes and significant heterogeneity might reduce the quality. The number of included patients less than 150 is considered to be small and may cause imprecision and effect size more than 0.05 is considered to be large and strengthen the evidence.

The present meta-analysis has several limitations. Firstly, the limited number of trials and small sample size in some trials might reduce the precision of the pooled estimates. Secondly, the inclusion criteria and baseline characteristics of the included trials were heterogeneous, including the primary diseases, gender, ages of patients and the type of prosthesis, which would lead to bias. Thirdly, trials included in this meta-analysis only used alendronate. Finally, the presented study analyzed the short-term effect of BPs on periprosthetic bone loss after TKA, and

Table 3 GRADE evidence profile of RCTs for effect of BPs on periprosthetic bone loss after TKA

| | | Summary of findings | | Quality assessment | | | | | |
	Time points	n (treated/control)	WMD (95%CI, g/cm^2)	Limitations	Inconsistency	Indirectness	Imprecision	Others	Quality
Tibia	3 months	2 (48/50)	0.07 (0.04–0.10)	No serious[a]	No serious[b]	No serious	Serious[c]	Strong association[d]	Moderate
	6 months	3 (78/80)	0.12 (0.10–0.15)	No serious	No serious	No serious	No serious	Strong association[d]	High
	12 months	3 (77/75)	0.12 (0.10–0.15)	No serious	Serious	No serious	No serious	None	Moderate
Femur	3 months	3 (56/61)	0.07 (0.04–0.10)	No serious	No serious	No serious	Serious	Strong association	Moderate
	6 months	5 (91/97)	0.12 (0.10–0.15)	No serious	Serious	No serious	No serious	Strong association	Moderate
	12 months	4 (85/86)	0.12 (0.10–0.15)	No serious	Serious	No serious	No serious	Strong association	Moderate

[a]The inadequate blinding and substantial loss follow-up in some trials may raise risk of bias
[b]Inconsistent report of outcomes and significant heterogeneity existed across the trials
[c]The number of included patients less than 150 is considered to be small and may cause imprecision
[d]Effect size more than 0.05 is considered to be large and strengthen the evidence

the long-term effect remained unknown and required more clinical studies.

Conclusion

In the present meta-analysis of randomized clinical trials, BPs have a short-term effect on the preservation of periprosthetic BMD after total knee arthroplasty. Compared with diaphyseal region, BPs are more effective on the preservation of BMD in medial lateral metaphyseal regions of proximal tibia and in anterior, central, and posterior metaphyseal region of distal femur.

Abbreviations
BMD: Bone mineral density; BPs: Bisphosphonates; CI: Confidence interval; FE: Fixed-effect; GRADE: Grading of Recommendations Assessment, Development and Evaluation; ITT: Intention-to-treat; RCTs: Randomized controlled trials; RE: Random-effect; ROIs: Regions of interest; TKA: Total knee arthroplasty; WMD: Weighted mean difference

Acknowledgements
The corresponding author wishes to thank all the co-authors for their contributions.

Funding
This research was supported by National Natural Science Foundation of China under Grant No. 81772360, Zhejiang Province Natural Science Foundation of China under Grant No. LQ16H060002, Zhejiang Province Natural Science Foundation of China under Grant No. Y17H060027, Medical and Health Science and Technology Project of Zhejiang Province under Grant No. 2016KYB120, Health Foundation of Zhejiang Province under Grant No.2018263059 and China Postdoctoral Science Foundation under Grant No. 2017 M612012.

Authors' contributions
MS and LC searched the databases and performed data extraction and quality assessment; MS, WW and SY designed the study; MS, YW, WW, YZ and SY analyzed the data and wrote the manuscript. All authors read and approved the final content of the manuscript. HW and SY revised the manuscript.

Competing interests
The authors declare that they have no competing interests.

Author details
[1]Department of Orthopaedic Surgery, Second Affiliated Hospital, School of Medicine, Zhejiang University, No.88 Jiefang Road, Hangzhou 310009, People's Republic of China. [2]Department of Endocrinology and Metabolism, Sir Run Run Shaw Hospital Affiliated with School of Medicine, Zhejiang University, No. 3 Qingchun Road, Hangzhou 310009, People's Republic of China.

References
1. Huang CC, Jiang CC, Hsieh CH, Tsai CJ, Chiang H. Local bone quality affects the outcome of prosthetic total knee arthroplasty. J Orthop Res. 2016;34(2):240–8.
2. Winther N, Jensen C, Petersen M, Lind T, Schrøder H, Petersen M. Changes in bone mineral density of the proximal tibia after uncemented total knee arthroplasty. A prospective randomized study. Int Orthop. 2016;40(2):285–94.
3. van Loon CJ, Oyen WJ, de Waal Malefijt MC, Verdonschot N. Distal femoral bone mineral density after total knee arthroplasty: a comparison with general bone mineral density. Arch Orthop Trauma Surg. 2001;121(5):282–5.
4. Sundfeldt M, Carlsson LV, Johansson CB, Thomsen P, Gretzer C. Aseptic loosening, not only a question of wear: a review of different theories. Acta Orthop. 2006;77(2):177–97.
5. Munro JT, Pandit S, Walker CG, Clatworthy M, Pitto RP. Loss of tibial bone density in patients with rotating- or fixed-platform TKA. Clin Orthop Relat Res. 2010;468(3):775–81.
6. Järvenpää J, Soininvaara T, Kettunen J, Miettinen H, Kröger H. Changes in bone mineral density of the distal femur after total knee arthroplasty: a 7-year DEXA follow-up comparing results between obese and nonobese patients. Knee. 2014;21(1):232–5.
7. Spinarelli A, Petrera M, Vicenti G, Pesce V, Patella V. Total knee arthroplasty in elderly osteoporotic patients. Aging Clin Exp Res. 2011;23(2 Suppl):78–80.
8. Petersen MM, Lauritzen JB, Pedersen JG, Lund B. Decreased bone density of the distal femur after uncemented knee arthroplasty. A 1-year follow-up of 29 knees. Acta Orthop Scand. 1996;67(4):339–44.
9. Seki T, Omori G, Koga Y, Suzuki Y, Ishii Y, Takahashi HE. Is bone density in the distal femur affected by use of cement and by femoral component design in total knee arthroplasty? J Orthop Sci. 1999;4(3):180–6.
10. Soininvaara TA, Miettinen HJ, Jurvelin JS, Suomalainen OT, Alhava EM, Kröger HP. Periprosthetic femoral bone loss after total knee arthroplasty: 1-year follow-up study of 69 patients. Knee. 2004;11(4):297–302.
11. Cherian JJ, Jauregui JJ, Banerjee S, Pierce T, Mont MA. What host factors affect aseptic loosening after THA and TKA? Clin Orthop Relat Res. 2015;473(8):2700–9.
12. Cranney A, Wells G, Willan A, Griffith L, Zytaruk N, Robinson V, et al. Meta-analyses of therapies for postmenopausal osteoporosis. II. Meta-analysis of alendronate for the treatment of postmenopausal women. Endocr Rev. 2002;23(4):508–16.
13. Catterall JB, Cawston TE. Drugs in development: bisphosphonates and metalloproteinase inhibitors. Arthritis Res Ther. 2003;5(1):12–24.
14. Fu SH, Wang CY, Yang RS, Wu FL, Hsiao FY. Bisphosphonate use and the risk of undergoing Total knee arthroplasty in osteoporotic patients with osteoarthritis: a Nationwide cohort study in Taiwan. J Bone Joint Surg Am. 2017;99(11):938–46.
15. Khatod M, Inacio MC, Dell RM, Bini SA, Paxton EW, Namba RS. Association of Bisphosphonate use and Risk of revision after THA: outcomes from a US Total joint replacement registry. Clin Orthop Relat Res. 2015;473(11):3412–20.
16. Soininvaara TA, Jurvelin JS, Miettinen HJ, Suomalainen OT, Alhava EM, Kröger PJ. Effect of alendronate on periprosthetic bone loss after total knee arthroplasty: a one-year, randomized, controlled trial of 19 patients. Calcif Tissue Int. 2002;71(6):472–7.
17. Han H, Li X, Wang Y, Zeng X, Preventing XC. Prosthesis loose after joint replacement. Chinese journal of surgery of integrated traditional and western. Medicine. 2003;9(3):179–82.
18. Wang CJ, Wang JW, Ko JY, Weng LH, Huang CC. Three-year changes in bone mineral density around the knee after a six-month course of oral alendronate following total knee arthroplasty. A prospective, randomized study J Bone Joint Surg Am. 2006;88(2):267–72.
19. Abu-Rajab RB, Watson W, Gallacher P, Walker B, Meek RMD. The effect of 6 months oral alendronate treatment on periprosthetic bone loss after total knee arthroplasty. Eur J Orthop Surg Traumatol. 2009;19:231–5.
20. Jaroma AV, Soininvaara TA, Kröger H. Effect of one-year post-operative alendronate treatment on periprosthetic bone after total knee arthroplasty. A seven-year randomised controlled trial of 26 patients. Bone Joint J. 2015;97-B(3):337–45.
21. Lin T, Yan SG, Cai XZ, Ying ZM. Bisphosphonates for periprosthetic bone loss after joint arthroplasty: a meta-analysis of 14 randomized controlled trials. Osteoporos Int. 2012;23(6):1823–34.
22. Atkins D, Best D, Briss PA, Eccles M, Falck-Ytter Y, Flottorp S, et al. Grading quality of evidence and strength of recommendations. BMJ. 2004;328(7454):1490.
23. JPT H, Green S. Cochrane handbook for systematic reviews of interventions. Chichester, England: Wiley-Blackwell; 2008.
24. Higgins JP, Thompson SG, Deeks JJ, Altman DG. Measuring inconsistency in meta-analyses. BMJ. 2003;327(7414):557–60.0.
25. Wang CJ, Wang JW, Weng LH, Hsu CC, Huang CC, Chen HS. The effect of alendronate on bone mineral density in the distal part of the femur and proximal part of the tibia after total knee arthroplasty. J Bone Joint Surg Am. 2003;85-A(11):2121–6.

26. Lee JK, Lee CH, Choi CH. QCT bone mineral density responses to 1 year of oral bisphosphonate ate after total knee replacement for knee osteoarthritis. Osteoporos Int. 2013;24(1):287–92.
27. Hansson U, Toksvig-Larsen S, Ryd L, Aspenberg P. Once-weekly oral medication with alendronate does not prevent migration of knee prostheses: a double-blind randomized RSA study. Acta Orthop. 2009;80(1):41–5.
28. Prieto-Alhambra D, Javaid MK, Judge A, Murray D, Carr A, Cooper C, et al. Association between bisphosphonate use and implant survival after primary total arthroplasty of the knee or hip: population based retrospective cohort study. BMJ. 2011;343:d7222.
29. Jansen JP, Bergman GJ, Huels J, Olson M. The efficacy of bisphosphonates in the prevention of vertebral, hip, and nonvertebral-nonhip fractures in osteoporosis: a network meta-analysis. Semin Arthritis Rheum. 2011;40(4): 275–84. e1–2
30. Ji WP, Wang XL, Ma MQ, Lan J, Li H. Prevention of early bone loss around the prosthesis by administration of anti-osteoporotic agents and influences of collared and non-collared femoral stem prostheses on early periprosthetic bone loss. Eur J Orthop Surg Traumatol. 2013;23(5):565–71.
31. Prieto-Alhambra D, Javaid MK, Judge A, Maskell J, Kiran A, de Vries F, et al. Fracture risk before and after total hip replacement in patients with osteoarthritis: potential benefits of bisphosphonate use. Arthritis Rheum. 2011;63(4):992–1001.
32. Prieto-Alhambra D, Lalmohamed A, Abrahamsen B, Arden NK, de Boer A, Vestergaard P, et al. Oral bisphosphonate use and total knee/hip implant survival: validation of results in an external population-based cohort. Arthritis Rheumatol. 2014;66(11):3233–40.
33. Lee JK, Choi CH, Kang CN. Quantitative computed tomography assessment of bone mineral density after 2 years' oral bisphosphonate treatment in postmenopausal osteoarthritis patients who underwent total knee arthroplasty. J Int Med Res. 2013;41(3):878–88.
34. Jaroma A, Soininvaara T, Kröger H. Periprosthetic tibial bone mineral density changes after total knee arthroplasty. Acta Orthop. 2016;87(3):268–73.
35. Srinivasan P, Miller MA, Verdonschot N, Mann KA, Janssen D. Experimental and computational micromechanics at the tibial cement-trabeculae interface. J Biomech. 2016;49(9):1641–8.
36. Namba RS, Inacio MC, Cheetham TC, Dell RM, Paxton EW, Khatod MX. Lower Total knee arthroplasty revision risk associated with bisphosphonate use, even in patients with normal bone density. J Arthroplast. 2016;31(2):537–41.

21

Rationale, design and protocol of a longitudinal study assessing the effect of total knee arthroplasty on habitual physical activity and sedentary behavior in adults with osteoarthritis

Rebecca M. Meiring[1*], Emmanuel Frimpong[1], Lipalo Mokete[2], Jurek Pietrzak[2], Dick Van Der Jagt[2], Mohammed Tikly[3] and Joanne A. McVeigh[1,4]

Abstract

Background: Physical activity levels are decreased and sedentary behaviour levels are increased in patients with knee osteoarthritis (OA). However, previous studies have shown that following total knee arthroplasty (TKA), objectively measured physical activity levels do not change compared to before the surgery. Very few studies have objectively assessed sedentary behaviour following TKA. This study aims to assess patterns of objective habitual physical activity and sedentary behaviour in patients with knee OA and to determine whether these change following TKA.

Methods: Patients diagnosed with knee osteoarthritis and scheduled for unilateral primary total knee arthroplasty will be recruited from the Orthopaedic Division at the Charlotte Maxeke Johannesburg Academic Hospital. Eligible participants will have assessments completed one week before the scheduled arthroplasty, six weeks, and six months post-operatively. The primary outcomes are habitual physical activity and sedentary behaviour which will be measured using accelerometry (Actigraph GTX3+ and activPal monitors) at the specific time points. The secondary outcomes will be improvements in osteoarthritis-specific quality of life measures using the following questionnaires: Western Ontario and McMaster Universities Osteoarthritis Index (WOMAC), Knee injury and Osteoarthritis Outcome Score (KOOS), Oxford Knee Score (OKS), Knee Society Clinical Rating System (KSS), UCLA activity index; subjective pain scores, and self reported sleep quality.

Discussion: The present study will contribute to the field of musculoskeletal health by providing a rich detailed description of the patterns of accumulation of physical activity and sedentary behaviour in patients with knee OA. These data will contribute to existing knowledge using an objective measurement for the assessment of functional ability after total knee arthroplasty. Although studies have used accelerometry to measure physical activity in knee OA patients, the data provided thus far have not delved into the detailed patterns of how and when physical activity is accumulated before and after TKA. Accurate assessment of physical activity is important for physical activity interventions that target special populations.

Keywords: Accelerometery, Osteoarthritis, Sedentary behaviour, Physical activity, Knee arthroplasty

* Correspondence: Rebecca.Meiring@wits.ac.za
[1]Exercise Physiology Laboratory, School of Physiology, Faculty of Health Sciences, University of the Witwatersrand, 7 York Rd, Parktown, Johannesburg, South Africa
Full list of author information is available at the end of the article

Background

Osteoarthritis (OA), the most common joint disorder, causing disability and loss of function, affects over 40 % of adults (aged 70 years and older) worldwide [1]. Concomitant with disrupted sleep, depression, increased sedentary behaviour, less physical activity, obesity, and polypharmacy, OA is associated with a decreased quality of life. Most occurrences of OA (41 %) are in the knee [2]. Although data are lacking from low to middle income countries, the few studies that have been done have shown that similar to populations from the US, knee OA is more common than is hip OA in African populations [3–5].

Pain is often a major contributing factor that impedes physical activity and reduces functionality in patients with knee OA [6, 7]. Approximately 80 % of individuals with OA experience limitations in movement and 25 % of individuals with OA experience limitations in major activities in their daily lives [7, 8] and the more severe the pain, the greater the degree of physical disability [9]. Conversely higher physical activity is associated with a lower risk of OA related joint pain and stiffness [10].

People with knee OA are physically inactive and highly sedentary

Studies that have used objective measures to evaluate physical activity and sedentariness in patients with knee OA have found that 41.1 % of males and 56.5 % of females with knee OA are inactive [11], that is they do not meet the recommended physical activity guidelines [11–15]. In addition to the total amount of time spent in physical activity (PA) being important for health outcomes in adults [16, 17], there is an emerging body of evidence to show that the patterns of how physical activity and sedentary time are accumulated may also have implications for health. There remains a paucity of literature describing the detailed patterns of how physical activity is accumulated in patients with knee OA.

Sedentary behaviours (SBs) are those with an energy expenditure of less than 1.5 metabolic equivalents (METS) [18, 19]. In older men, interruptions to sedentary time is associated with better muscle quality in older men [20]. Adults with OA who are more sedentary experience a greater loss in functional capacity compared to adults who are less sedentary [12, 21–23], and this relationship appears to be independent of time spent in moderate to vigorous physical activity [21]. The number of daily hours patients with OA spend being sedentary (9.8 h) [12, 24] is similar to that reported in healthy adults (9.2 h) taking part in the European RISC study [25]. Additionally sedentary time in patients with knee OA is often elevated prior to knee replacement surgery [12, 26]. However detailed data describing how and when sedentary behaviour is accumulated are lacking in this population.

Physical activity and total knee arthroplasty

Compared to the other rheumatic diseases, pharmacological treatment for OA is relatively unsatisfactory [27]. Although non-surgical treatment is the primary choice of treatment in OA patients [28], the main indication for total knee arthroplasty (TKA) is failure of conservative treatment; essentially pain that is not responsive to both pharmacological and non-pharmacological measures together with an increasing difficulty with activities of daily life in the context of advanced degenerative changes of the knee. There are no accurate figures for the number of knee replacements done in South Africa as there are no established registries. The main aim of the surgery is to alleviate pain and restore quality of life. Generally, patients are being operated on earlier in the progressions of the disease as it is recognized that quality of life is more likely to be restored in those patients, as opposed to patients with advanced disease where quality of life can be improved but not necessarily restored. As such regaining of functional ability allowing for restoration of habitual activity levels as near to normal as possible and a reduction in sedentary time are important goals for post-operative knee OA patients. Hence a desirable outcome that could be considered useful in assessing the regaining of functional ability would be to determine the number of patients who meet current physical activity guidelines [29] (including a reduction in sedentary behaviour) following TKA.

Physical activity and functional ability outcomes have historically been measured using self-report, but a more objective and quantified understanding of the impacts of knee arthroplasty on physical and functional ability are needed. Studies using interview based questionnaires have shown improved mobility benefits of TKA in developed countries [30], although data in low to middle income countries are scarce.

Assessment of functional ability in knee OA patients following TKA

Studies using self-report have shown positive improvements in functional ability (ability to perform activities of daily living), pain and quality of life after TKA [31–33] while others have reported no significant improvements on health outcome measures following TKA [31, 34–36]. Self-report may also be open to bias and inaccuracy [37]. Thus there is a need for studies which use objective measures of physical activity as an important indicator of functional ability. Currently, habitual physical activity levels in large scale studies of healthy adult populations are most commonly objectively measured through the use of accelerometers [38].

Only nine studies since 2002 have used accelerometry as a measure of physical function in patients before and after TKA [39], some reporting little or no change in physical activity after surgery [24, 26, 33, 40] and others showing improvements in self-report measured functional ability [41, 42]. The variability in devices used to assess habitual physical activity before and after TKA makes the comparison of results across studies difficult. However, the ActiGraph GT1M accelerometer (an earlier version of the ActiGraph) has been used to assess the intensity and amount of physical activity occurring following TKA [26] but very small changes in activity were found. In addition, the timing and length of activity assessment is an important factor in determining changes in physical function in studies of TKA with some objectively measured studies showing improvements in physical activity six months after TKA [24, 43], and others showing very little or no improvement in daily activity at three or six months post-surgery [26, 41].

Recently, opportunities for measuring patterns of sitting and lying time have been made possible through the use of inclinometers e.g. the activPAL (PAL technologies Ltd, Glasgow, UK). The activPAL produces highly accurate and precise estimates of total sedentary time in free-living individuals [44] and has been validated to estimate time in different postures, step count, static and dynamic behaviours and sit-to-stand transitions in laboratory studies [44–46]. Only one study has used the activPAL in a cross-sectional assessment of energy expenditure in knee OA patients prior to arthroplasty [47]. The use of the activPAL to measure sedentary behaviour following TKA has not been done before.

The objective assessment of habitual physical activity may provide an alternative method of assessing whether functional ability is improved in OA patients following TKA, as a change in activities of daily living (assessed using sedentary behaviour and light activity measurements) without a change in moderate to vigorous physical activity may correspond to a patient's improved ability to function. Thus the aims of this study are to 1) describe habitual physical activity and sedentary behaviour patterns in knee OA patients scheduled for TKA, 2) to investigate the effects of unilateral primary TKA on objectively and subjectively measured habitual physical activity, sedentary behaviour and health outcomes of patients with knee OA and 3) to determine whether subjective measures of functional ability and sedentary behaviour (questionnaires) are correlated with objective measures of habitual physical activity and sedentary behaviour (accelerometry) before and after TKA. These data will help inform targeted interventions for the improvement and maintenance of physical activity.

Methods

Study participants

The study population will include all knee osteoarthritis patients receiving care at the Charlotte Maxeke Johannesburg Academic Hospital. Patients will be recruited from the Orthopaedic Division of the hospital. The participants for this study will be knee OA patients scheduled (on surgical waiting list) for a single primary total knee arthroplasty or replacement surgery. Knee OA will be diagnosed based on clinical criteria as defined by the American Rheumatism Association (ACR) [48]. Prospective participants will be given an information sheet describing the study and will have the study verbally explained to them prior to participation in the study. Participants will be required to sign a consent form should they wish to participate in the study. Participants will then complete a general health questionnaire in order to confirm eligibility in the study. Patients will be recruited to participate in the study if they have been diagnosed with knee OA and attended to by surgeons in the Orthopaedic Surgery Unit at the Hospital. Potential participants will be eligible to participate in the study by the attending orthopaedic surgeon. They will also be included if they have been refractory to analgesics for at least six months, are male or female between 55 and 80 years of age, are undergoing primary unilateral TKA surgery and are ambulant with or without assistive devices.

Patients will be excluded from participating in the study if they use assistive ambulatory devices for mobility problems other than knee OA, are scheduled for bilateral knee arthroplasty, a second knee arthroplasty or revision, or are scheduled for total hip replacement, or if they have co-morbidities or medical conditions that affect physical activity such as congestive heart failure, stroke and other neurological problems, chronic obstructive pulmonary disease (COPD), gout and/or sepsis, have been diagnosed with arthritis other than osteoarthritis (according to the 1987 American College of Rheumatology (ACR) criteria [48]), if further joint surgery is anticipated within six months of the index knee replacement or are non-ambulant or wheel chair-bound.

Study site

The study will be conducted at the Charlotte Maxeke Academic Hospital in Johannesburg, South Africa. It is an accredited central hospital with about 1088 beds serving patients from across Gauteng and neighbouring provinces. The hospital is situated in Parktown and also, serves as the main teaching hospital for the Faculty of Health Sciences, University of the Witwatersrand. Study participants will be recruited from the Division of Orthopaedics in the hospital. This hospital is chosen because: (1) it is a tertiary hospital that runs several specialist clinics including the Orthopaedic Division where TKA among several other surgeries are performed and (2) there is a collaboration between the Academic staff of the Faculty of Health Sciences of University of the Witwatersrand and the hospital Staff for teaching and research which will facilitate accessibility to patients.

Study design

This a longitudinal follow-up study of a cohort of participants who have been diagnosed with knee osteoarthritis and who are scheduled for TKA. After enrolment into the study, baseline assessments will be done prior to TKA. After TKA, participants will be followed-up and the same assessments done at baseline will also be done at six weeks, and six months post-operatively (Fig. 1). Habitual physical activity and sedentary behaviour will be measured using accelerometry (Actigraph GTX3+ and ActivPal monitors) at the specific time points. In addition, general health, functional ability, generic quality of life and pain questionnaires will be conducted at each time point on each participant.

Trial registration

This trial has been registered with the ClinicalTrials.gov registry (trial registration number: NCT02675062).

Outcomes

All outcomes will be measured at baseline, six weeks after surgery and again six months after the surgical

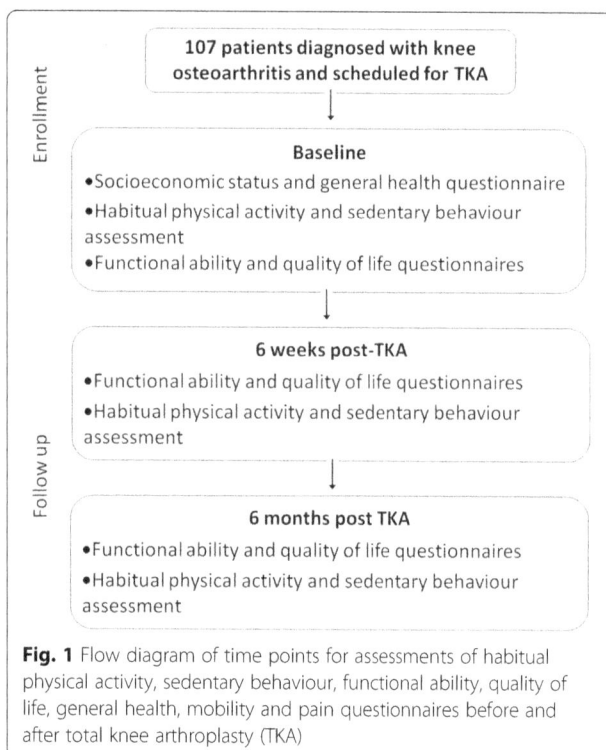

Fig. 1 Flow diagram of time points for assessments of habitual physical activity, sedentary behaviour, functional ability, quality of life, general health, mobility and pain questionnaires before and after total knee arthroplasty (TKA)

intervention (Table 1). The primary outcomes of this study will be an improvement habitual physical activity and a reduction in sedentary time after TKA. The secondary outcomes will be improvements in osteoarthritis-specific quality of life measures: Western Ontario and McMaster Universities Osteoarthritis Index (WOMAC), knee related quality of life from Knee injury and Osteoarthritis Outcome Score (KOOS), Knee Society Clinical Rating System (KSS), the Oxford Knee Score (OKS), self reported activity using the UCLA activity index; subjective pain scores, and self reported sleep quality.

Sample size determination

Time spent in bouts of sedentary activity longer than 20 min is associated with poorer health outcomes [49]. In order to achieve a 2 % (which, for an average 16 h day, equates to a 20 min) reduction in the time spent in sedentary behaviour per day [26], a total sample of 107 participants will be required in this study to detect a significant effect of knee arthroplasty on sedentary behaviour (power of 80 %).

Questionnaires
Socioeconomic Status (SES) and General Health Questionnaire (GHQ)

Socioeconomic status (SES) will be determined using a household amenity questionnaire [50]. Eligibility into the study will be determined using a GHQ in order to determine whether participants have any comorbidities that might exclude them from participation. Furthermore the GHQ will be used to record the health demographics of the participants, such as history of knee OA and medication use. The SES and general health questionnaires will be completed at the first visit only.

Functional ability questionnaires

Western Ontario and McMaster Universities Osteoarthritis Index (WOMAC) WOMAC assesses pain, stiffness, and physical function in patients with hip and knee OA (Bellamy, 2002). WOMAC consists of 24 items divided into 3 subscales: (1) 5 Pain items for assessing pain (2) 2 Stiffness items and (3) 17 Physical Function items. Each of the items requires the respondent to answer questions on 5-point Likert scale. These items request the respondent to indicate the degree of pain, stiffness, and physical functioning while engaging in specific activities, including walking, going upstairs, in bed at night, sitting, and standing upright. The scores for the items are summed and transformed to a 0-100 scale. Higher scores indicate improved pain, stiffness and physical function. Thus, a score of 0 represent the worst

Table 1 Summary of outcome measures and respective collection method

Outcome	Variables	Measurement method	Time points (months)
Primary	Habitual physical activity	Accelerometry (ActiGraph worn on the hip)	0, 1.5, 6
	Sedentary behaviour	Accelerometry (activPAL worn on thigh)	0, 1.5, 6
Secondary	Knee OA-specific functional ability and quality of life	WOMAC	0, 1.5, 6
		KOOS	
		KSS	
		OKS	
	Activity	UCLA activity index	0, 1.5, 6
	Pain	VAS	0, 1.5, 6
	Sleep quality	Sleep questionnaire	0, 1.5, 6

possible state while a score of 100 represents the best possible state.

Knee Injury and Osteoarthritis Outcome Score (KOOS)
The KOOS consists of 5 subscales: Pain, other symptoms, function in daily living, function in sport and recreation and knee-related quality of life. The previous week is the time period considered when answering the questions. Standardized answer options are given on five (5) Likert scales and each question is assigned a score from 0 to 4. The score is a percentage score from 0 to 100, with 0 representing extreme symptoms/problems and 100 representing no problems. The KOOS has been used in previous studies for evaluating outcome after TKA [51, 52].

Knee Society Clinical Rating System Score (KSS) The Knee Society Clinical Rating System is a rating system which consists of two scores: knee and patient functional scores. Both scores range from 0 (worst health or functioning) to 100 (best health or functioning). This instrument has been used for tracking and reporting outcomes after total and partial knee arthroplasty worldwide [53]. Fifty of 100 points in the knee score are allocated to pain assessment with 50 representing no pain whereas the other 50 points are allocated for a clinical assessment with 50 representing at least 0°-125°of knee flexion with no active lag, no instability and normal alignment. The function score reflects patient-reported walking distance and stairclimbing and makes deductions for use of a walking aid, with 100 representing unlimited walking distance and normal stair-climbing without use of an aid [54].

Oxford knee score (OKS) The OKS consists of 12 questions assessing pain and physical disability using a 5-point Likert scale and it generates a single score ranging from 0 (worst functional outcome) to 100 (best functional outcome) [55].

Physical activity questionnaire
The UCLA activity index is a scale from 1 to 10 with phrases ("no physical activity" to "regular participation in impact sports") which the patient chooses to best describe their most appropriate activity level. The UCLA has been shown to be the most appropriate subjective physical activity assessment for patients undergoing joint arthroplasty [56].

Pain and sleep questionnaires
Joint pain, sleep quality and morning vigilance at each time point of the study will be assessed on a 100-mm visual analogue scale (VAS). The pain and sleep questionnaires will be administered at each visit to the hospital. All questionnaires have been previously validated.

Anthropometric measurements
Height will be measured to the nearest millimetre with the participants bare foot using a stadiometer (Seca, model 202, Germany). Weight will be measured to the nearest gram using a scale (Mettler, Model TE120 ME36400, Switzerland) with the participants bare foot and wearing light clothing. Body mass index (BMI) will be calculated from the height and the weight (weight/square of height) for each participant.

Physical activity and sedentary behaviour measurements
ActiGraph GT3X+ Accelerometer
The ActiGraph GT3X+ is a small (4.6 cm × 3.3 cm × 1.5 cm) lightweight (19 g) tri-axial activity monitor that provides data on physical activity including activity counts, energy expenditure (kcal), steps and activity intensity (METs). The GT3X+ has an inclinometer to determine body position in sitting, lying and standing. The ActiGraph GT3X+ will be worn by participants for 24 h/day for seven days at each of the assessment time points. It will be attached to an elastic nylon strap which the participants can wear as a belt around the waist on the side of the affected knee. Participants will be asked

to remove the ActiGraph when showering, bathing or swimming. After seven days of accelerometer wear, the accelerometers will be collected at the next possible visit to the hospital or arrangement will be made for collection from participants at a location most convenient to them.

The data will be downloaded and processed using a custom built SAS program (v 9.3, SAS Institute, Cary, NC, USA) that implements a series of decision rules with user-modifiable thresholds to automatically identify waking wear data for continuously worn ActiGraph GT3X+ of 60 s epoch vertical axis data. Non-wear time will be classified as one minute intervals with consecutive zero counts for a minimum of 90 min (with an allowance of up to 3 min of counts between 0 and 50). For the day to be classified as valid, a minimum wear time of 10 h (600 min) is required. Each 60 s epoch of accelerometry data is classified according to calibration equations as sedentary if <100 counts per minute (cpm) [57], light intensity activity if between 100 and 1951 cpm, moderate-vigorous intensity activity if between 1952 and 5724 cpm and vigorous if >5724 cpm [58]. Adjacent epochs within the same intensity will be grouped into bouts. Only participants with four or more valid days of wear (including at least one weekend day) will be included in the analyses. Total daily time spent in the different PA intensities will be obtained by totalling the duration of all the bouts at each level for each day. The values will then be normalised to total wear time and averaged over the number of valid days to derive an estimate of the mean time spent within each intensity. A break in sedentary time will be counted as one minute or more where the counts per minute is greater than 100.

activPAL accelerometer

The activPAL is a small (2.0x1.4x0.3 in.) and light (20.1 g) single-unit accelerometer device worn on the mid-thigh fastened and secured by a non- allergenic adhesive tape and uses accelerometer-derived information about thigh position to estimate time spent in different body positions in lying, sitting and standing in 15 s epochs [44]. An activPAL will be taped to the thigh of the patient with waterproof taping and the patient will be asked to keep the activPAL on for the same amount of time as the ActiGraph. The activPAL can be covered with waterproof taping therefore, there will be no need to remove the activPAL when showering, bathing or swimming and therefore unless the device is reported to have fallen off by the patient, there will be no need for non-wear time classification for the activPAL data. The activPAL will be collected at the same time as the ActiGraph and data will be downloaded and analysed. The data are recorded in 15 s epochs and the manufacturer's software will be used to determine the variables of

interest from the downloaded activPAL data which will include the start time and duration of each sitting, lying, standing and stepping bout. Total sedentary time will be determined by summing the duration of all sitting/lying bouts. The interruption or break from sedentary time will be indicated at points where a sitting/lying bout is followed by a standing or stepping bout. Because the activPAL is worn for the same period as the ActiGraph, the same periods of sleep that are removed from the ActiGraph data, will also be removed from the activPAL data to be analysed. Further time-intensive methods of analysis will be employed according to current best practice guidelines [59].

Data analyses

Socioeconomic data will be summarised by descriptive statistics. Also, means and standard deviations will be used to summarise data for age, anthropometric (height, weight, BMI and %body fat), ActiGraph GT3X+ and ActivPAL.Scores for WOMAC, KOOS, OKS and KSS will be calculated by their respective scoring systems. Data will be analysed using SPSS v20 (SPSS Inc., Chicago, IL, USA).

Linear mixed models will be used to determine relationships between objectively measured habitual physical activity and sedentary behaviour, functional capacity and quality of life between pre-operative and 6 weeks and 6 months post-operatively. The model will be used to compare subjective measures of functional mobility (questionnaires) with objective measure of habitual physical activity. A multiple regression analysis will be used to describe the association between physical activity and/ or sedentary behaviour, functional capacity and quality of life of OA patients before and after TKA. Also, a multiple regression will be used to determine the relationship between habitual physical activity and sedentary behaviour on anthropometric parameters of OA patients before and after TKA. A p-value of less than 0.05 will be considered significant.

Discussion

The present study will contribute to the field of musculoskeletal health by providing a rich detailed description of the patterns of accumulation of physical activity and sedentary behaviour in patients with knee OA. These data will contribute to existing knowledge using an objective measurement for the assessment of functional ability after total knee replacement surgery. Although studies have used accelerometry to measure physical activity in knee OA patients, the data provided thus far have not delved into the detailed patterns of how and when the entire spectrum of physical activity is accumulated before and after TKA. Accurate assessment of physical activity is important for physical activity interventions that target special populations.

A key advantage of this study over previous studies includes the use of more than one monitor to objectively assess physical activity and sedentary behaviour. The activPAL may be used to capture the energy expenditure of habitual physical activity, however the real value of the tool is its ability to assess sedentary behaviour in terms of postural changes (lying/sitting). Furthermore, the way we wish to obtain a richer set of metrics to describe patterns and accumulation of physical activity is rather more than the activPAL is able to provide, hence the reason why both monitors will be used in this study. Detailed postural classifications of how patients with knee OA spend their time prior to and after surgery will be of interest to health care providers. An increase in sedentary behaviour leads to an increased risk of sarcopenia in healthy elderly populations [60]. The muscle degeneration that is associated with sedentary behaviour in an ageing population has implications for patients with knee OA, as the immobility and reduced functionality may be exacerbated by the knee OA. Furthermore greater levels of sedentary behaviour may occur at an earlier age in patients with knee OA predisposing these patients to an increased risk of sarcopenia as they age. No studies that we are aware of have investigated sedentary behaviour patterns (using the activPAL) in patients with knee OA therefore comprehensive measurement on patterns of sedentary behaviour in this population is needed to implement effective interventions aimed at decreasing sedentary behaviour levels.

Additionally, there are no data on objectively measured habitual physical activity or sedentary behaviour before and after total knee replacement on South African patients. Surgical intervention may be considered at an earlier stage of the disease in developed countries, compared to low to middle income countries such as South Africa where surgical intervention may often be delayed due to long waiting lists and budgetary constraints. Knowing more detailed information about how patterns of physical activity and sedentary time may change following surgical intervention will help inform best practices by providing clear information about whether patients can expect to improve their physical activity levels and decrease their time spent in sedentary behaviours by enough time so as to reduce their risk of cardiometabolic disease (which is a risk associated with a lack of activity). Describing changes in daily patterns of activity and sedentary behaviour may allow for further studies to target the timing and duration of physical activity interventions on a daily basis in order to attempt to increase the amount of physical activity patients with knee OA take part in.

As global populations age and in order to decrease the burden of the disease, there will be an increasing need for total knee replacements in adults affected by knee OA. This study will investigate the patterns by which habitual physical activity and sedentary behaviour are accumulated in patients with knee OA before and after surgery, and will therefore assist in informing targeting interventions to improve patterns of physical activity. Furthermore, a change in exercise guidelines from increasing the volume of exercise to offsetting the time spent in deleterious behaviours such as excessive time spent sitting, may contribute to developing more relevant criteria for physical activity prescription in patients with osteoarthritis.

Abbreviations
KOOS, Knee Injury and Osteoarthritis Outcome Score; KSS, Knee Society Clinical Rating System; METS, metabolic equivalents; OA, osteoarthritis; OKS, Oxford Knee Score; PA, physical activity; SB, sedentary behaviour; SES, socioeconomic status; TKA, total knee arthroplasty; WOMAC, Western Ontario and McMaster Universities Osteoarthritis Index

Acknowledgements
Not applicable.

Funding
There are no sources of funding to declare.

Authors' contributions
RM Conceptualization of study, development of study design, writing of drafts, editing of drafts. EF Development of study design, writing of drafts, editing of drafts. LM Development of study design, editing of drafts. JP Development of study design, editing of drafts. DVDJ Conceptualization of study, development of study design, editing of drafts. MT Conceptualization of study, development of study design, editing of drafts. JMcV Conceptualization of study, development of study design, writing of drafts, editing of drafts. All authors have read and approved the final version of the manuscript.

Authors' information
Not applicable.

Competing interests
The authors declare that they have no competing interests.

Consent for publication
Not applicable.

Author details
[1]Exercise Physiology Laboratory, School of Physiology, Faculty of Health Sciences, University of the Witwatersrand, 7 York Rd, Parktown, Johannesburg, South Africa. [2]Division of Orthopaedics, Faculty of Health Sciences, University of the Witwatersrand, 7 York Rd, Parktown, Johannesburg, South Africa. [3]Division of Rheumatology, Department of Medicine, Chris Hani Baragwanath Academic Hospital, Faculty of Health Sciences, University of the Witwatersrand, 7 York Rd, Parktown,

Johannesburg, South Africa. [4]School of Physiotherapy and Exercise Science, Curtin University, Kent St, Bentley, Western Australia.

References

1. Rousseau JC, Garnero P. Biological markers in osteoarthritis. Bone. 2012;51:265–77.
2. Felson DT, Lawrence RC, Dieppe PA, Hirsch R, Helmick CG, Jordan JM, Kington RS, Lane NE, Nevitt MC, Zhang Y, Sowers M, McAlindon T, Spector TD, Poole AR, Yanovski SZ, Ateshian G, Sharma L, Buckwalter JA, Brandt KD, Fries JF. Osteoarthritis: new insights. Part 1: the disease and its risk factors. Ann Intern Med. 2000;133:635–46.
3. Jenyo MS, Bamidele JO, Adebimpe WO. Pattern of arthralgia in an urban community in Southwestern Nigeria. Ann Afr Med. 2014;13:65–70.
4. Ouédraogo D-D, Ntsiba H, Tiendrébéogo Zabsonré J, Tiéno H, Bokossa LIF, Kaboré F, Drabo J. Clinical spectrum of rheumatologic diseases in a department of rheumatology in Ouagadougou (Burkina Faso). Clin Rheumatol. 2014;33:385–9.
5. Oniankitan O, Houzou P, Koffi-Tessio VES, Kakpovi K, Fianyo E, Tagbor KC, Mijiyawa M. Patterns of osteoarthritis in patients attending a teaching hospital clinic. Tunis Médicale. 2009;87:863–6.
6. Harding PA, Holland AE, Hinman RS, Delany C. Physical activity perceptions and beliefs following total hip and knee arthroplasty: a qualitative study. Physiother Theory Pract. 2015;31:107–13.
7. Sandell C-L. A multidisciplinary assessment and intervention for patients awaiting total hip replacement to improve their quality of life. J Orthop Nurs. 2008;12:26–34.
8. Ma VY, Chan L, Carruthers KJ. Incidence, prevalence, costs, and impact on disability of common conditions requiring rehabilitation in the United States: stroke, spinal cord injury, traumatic brain injury, multiple sclerosis, osteoarthritis, rheumatoid arthritis, limb loss, and back pain. Arch Phys Med Rehabil. 2014;95:986–95. e1.
9. Cubukcu D, Sarsan A, Alkan H. Relationships between pain, function and radiographic findings in osteoarthritis of the knee: a cross-sectional study. Arthritis. 2012;2012:984060.
10. Peeters GMEE, Pisters MF, Mishra GD, Brown WJ. The influence of long-term exposure and timing of physical activity on new joint pain and stiffness in mid-age women. Osteoarthritis Cartilage. 2015;23:34–40.
11. Dunlop DD, Song J, Semanik PA, Chang RW, Sharma L, Bathon JM, Eaton CB, Hochberg MC, Jackson RD, Kwoh CK, Mysiw WJ, Nevitt MC, Hootman JM. Objective physical activity measurement in the osteoarthritis initiative: Are guidelines being met? Arthritis Rheum. 2011;63:3372–82.
12. Lee J, Chang RW, Ehrlich-Jones L, Kwoh CK, Nevitt M, Semanik PA, Sharma L, Sohn M-W, Song J, Dunlop DD. Sedentary behavior and physical function: objective evidence from the Osteoarthritis Initiative. Arthritis Care Res. 2015; 67:366–73.
13. Semanik P, Lee J, Manheim L, Dipietro L, Dunlop D, Chang RW. Relationship between accelerometer-based measures of physical activity and the Yale Physical Activity Survey in adults with arthritis. Arthritis Care Res. 2011;63:1766–72.
14. Holsgaard-Larsen A, Roos EM. Objectively measured physical activity in patients with end stage knee or hip osteoarthritis. Eur J Phys Rehabil Med. 2012;48:577–85.
15. Farr JN, Going SB, Lohman TG, Rankin L, Kasle S, Cornett M, Cussler E. Physical activity levels in patients with early knee osteoarthritis measured by accelerometry. Arthritis Rheum. 2008;59:1229–36.
16. Buman MP, Winkler EAH, Kurka JM, Hekler EB, Baldwin CM, Owen N, Ainsworth BE, Healy GN, Gardiner PA. Reallocating time to sleep, sedentary behaviors, or active behaviors: associations with cardiovascular disease risk biomarkers, NHANES 2005-2006. Am J Epidemiol. 2014;179:323–34.
17. Carson V, Ridgers ND, Howard BJ, Winkler EAH, Healy GN, Owen N, Dunstan DW, Salmon J. Light-intensity physical activity and cardiometabolic biomarkers in US adolescents. PLoS One. 2013;8:e71417.
18. Owen N, Healy GN, Matthews CE, Dunstan DW. Too much sitting: the population health science of sedentary behavior. Exerc Sport Sci Rev. 2010;38:105–13.
19. Pate RR, McIver K, Dowda M, Brown WH, Addy C. Directly observed physical activity levels in preschool children. J Sch Health. 2008;78:438–44.
20. Chastin SFM, Ferriolli E, Stephens NA, Fearon KCH, Greig C. Relationship between sedentary behaviour, physical activity, muscle quality and body composition in healthy older adults. Age Ageing. 2012;41:111–4.
21. Semanik PA, Lee J, Song J, Chang RW, Sohn M-W, Ehrlich-Jones LS, Ainsworth BE, Nevitt MM, Kwoh CK, Dunlop DD. Accelerometer-monitored sedentary behavior and observed physical function loss. Am J Public Health. 2015;105:560–6.

22. Neto F, De EM, Queluz TT, Freire BFA. Physical activity and its association with quality of life in patients with osteoarthritis. Rev Bras Reumatol. 2011; 51:544–9.
23. Joubert J, Norman R, Lambert EV, Groenewald P, Schneider M, Bull F, Bradshaw D, South African Comparative Risk Assessment Collaborating Group. Estimating the burden of disease attributable to physical inactivity in South Africa in 2000. South Afr Med J. 2007;97(8 Pt 2):725–31.
24. Brandes M, Ringling M, Winter C, Hillmann A, Rosenbaum D. Changes in physical activity and health-related quality of life during the first year after total knee arthroplasty. Arthritis Care Res. 2011;63:328–34.
25. Balkau B, Mhamdi L, Oppert J-M, Nolan J, Golay A, Porcellati F, Laakso M, Ferrannini E, EGIR-RISC Study Group. Physical activity and insulin sensitivity: the RISC study. Diabetes. 2008;57:2613–8.
26. Harding P, Holland AE, Delany C, Hinman RS. Do activity levels increase after total hip and knee arthroplasty? Clin Orthop. 2014;472:1502–11.
27. Berenbaum F. Targeted therapies in osteoarthritis: a systematic review of the trials on www.clinicaltrials.gov. Best Pract Res Clin Rheumatol. 2010;24:107–19.
28. Van Manen MD, Nace J, Mont MA. Management of primary knee osteoarthritis and indications for total knee arthroplasty for general practitioners. J Am Osteopath Assoc. 2012;112:709–15.
29. World Health Organization. Global recommendations on physical activity for health. Geneva: World Health Organization; 2010.
30. Stenquist DS, Elman SA, Davis AM, Bogart LM, Brownlee SA, Sanchez ES, Santiago A, Ghazinouri R, Katz JN. Physical activity and experience of total knee replacement in patients one to four years postsurgery in the dominican republic: a qualitative study. Arthritis Care Res. 2015;67:65–73.
31. Ethgen O, Bruyère O, Richy F, Dardennes C, Reginster J-Y. Health-related quality of life in total hip and total knee arthroplasty. A qualitative and systematic review of the literature. J Bone Joint Surg Am. 2004;86–A:963–74.
32. Salaffi F, Carotti M, Grassi W. Health-related quality of life in patients with hip or knee osteoarthritis: comparison of generic and disease-specific instruments. Clin Rheumatol. 2005;24:29–37.
33. Vissers MM, Bussmann JB, de Groot IB, Verhaar JAN, Reijman M. Physical functioning four years after total hip and knee arthroplasty. Gait Posture. 2013;38:310–5.
34. Hoogeboom TJ, den Broeder AA, de Bie RA, van den Ende CHM. Longitudinal impact of joint pain comorbidity on quality of life and activity levels in knee osteoarthritis: data from the Osteoarthritis Initiative. Rheumatol Oxf Engl. 2013;52:543–6.
35. Muraki S, Akune T, Oka H, En-yo Y, Yoshida M, Saika A, Suzuki T, Yoshida H, Ishibashi H, Tokimura F, Yamamoto S, Nakamura K, Kawaguchi H, Yoshimura N. Association of radiographic and symptomatic knee osteoarthritis with health-related quality of life in a population-based cohort study in Japan: the ROAD study. Osteoarthr Cartil. 2010;18:1227–34.
36. Noble PC, Gordon MJ, Weiss JM, Reddix RN, Conditt MA, Mathis KB. Does total knee replacement restore normal knee function? Clin Orthop. 2005; 431:157–65.
37. Harris TJ, Owen CG, Victor CR, Adams R, Ekelund U, Cook DG. A comparison of questionnaire, accelerometer, and pedometer: measures in older people. Med Sci Sports Exerc. 2009;41:1392–402.
38. Bassett DR. Device-based monitoring in physical activity and public health research. Physiol Meas. 2012;33:1769–83.
39. Paxton RJ, Melanson EL, Stevens-Lapsley JE, Christiansen CL. Physical activity after total knee arthroplasty: A critical review. World J Orthop. 2015;6:614–22.
40. Kahn TL, Schwarzkopf R. Does Total Knee Arthroplasty Affect Physical Activity Levels? Data from the Osteoarthritis Initiative. J Arthroplasty. 2015;30:1521–5.
41. de Groot IB, Bussmann HJ, Stam HJ, Verhaar JA. Small increase of actual physical activity 6 months after total hip or knee arthroplasty. Clin Orthop. 2008;466:2201–8.
42. Tsonga T, Kapetanakis S, Papadopoulos C, Papathanasiou J, Mourgias N, Georgiou I, Fiska A, Kazakos K. Evaluation of improvement in quality of life and physical activity after total knee arthroplasty in Greek elderly women. Open Orthop J. 2011;5:343–7.
43. Walker DJ, Heslop PS, Chandler C, Pinder IM. Measured ambulation and self-reported health status following total joint replacement for the osteoarthritic knee. Rheumatology. 2002;41:755–8.
44. Kozey-Keadle S, Libertine A, Lyden K, Staudenmayer J, Freedson PS. Validation of wearable monitors for assessing sedentary behavior. Med Sci Sports Exerc. 2011;43:1561–7.
45. Ryde GC, Gilson ND, Suppini A, Brown WJ. Validation of a novel, objective measure of occupational sitting. J Occup Health. 2012;54:383–6.

46. Godfrey A, Culhane KM, Lyons GM. Comparison of the performance of the activPAL Professional physical activity logger to a discrete accelerometer-based activity monitor. Med Eng Phys. 2007;29:930–4.

47. Tonelli SM, Rakel BA, Cooper NA, Angstom WL, Sluka KA. Women with knee osteoarthritis have more pain and poorer function than men, but similar physical activity prior to total knee replacement. Biol Sex Differ. 2011;2:12.

48. Altman R, Asch E, Bloch D, Bole G, Borenstein D, Brandt K, Christy W, Cooke TD, Greenwald R, Hochberg M. Development of criteria for the classification and reporting of osteoarthritis. Classification of osteoarthritis of the knee. Diagnostic and Therapeutic Criteria Committee of the American Rheumatism Association. Arthritis Rheum. 1986;29:1039–49.

49. Dunstan DW, Kingwell BA, Larsen R, Healy GN, Cerin E, Hamilton MT, Shaw JE, Bertovic DA, Zimmet PZ, Salmon J, Owen N. Breaking up prolonged sitting reduces postprandial glucose and insulin responses. Diabetes Care. 2012;35:976–83.

50. Bradshaw D, Steyn K. Poverty and chronic disease in South Africa: Medical Research Council. 2001.

51. Stevens-Lapsley JE, Schenkman ML, Dayton MR. Comparison of self-reported knee injury and osteoarthritis outcome score to performance measures in patients after total knee arthroplasty. PM R. 2011;3:541–9.

52. Lygre SHL, Espehaug B, Havelin LI, Vollset SE, Furnes O. Does patella resurfacing really matter? Pain and function in 972 patients after primary total knee arthroplasty. Acta Orthop. 2010;81:99–107.

53. Insall JN, Dorr LD, Scott RD, Scott W. Rationale of the Knee Society clinical rating system. Clin Orthop. 1989;248:13–4.

54. Xie F, Lo N-N, Pullenayegum EM, Tarride J-E, O'Reilly DJ, Goeree R, Lee H-P. Evaluation of health outcomes in osteoarthritis patients after total knee replacement: a two-year follow-up. Health Qual Life Outcomes. 2010;8:87.

55. Dawson J, Carr A. Outcomes evaluation in orthopaedics. J Bone Joint Surg (Br). 2001;83:313–5.

56. Naal FD, Impellizzeri FM, Leunig M. Which is the best activity rating scale for patients undergoing total joint arthroplasty? Clin Orthop. 2009;467:958–65.

57. Matthews CE, Chen KY, Freedson PS, Buchowski MS, Beech BM, Pate RR, Troiano RP. Amount of time spent in sedentary behaviors in the United States, 2003-2004. Am J Epidemiol. 2008;167:875–81.

58. Freedson PS, Melanson E, Sirard J. Calibration of the Computer Science and Applications, Inc. accelerometer. Med Sci Sports Exerc. 1998;30:777–81.

59. Edwardson CL, Winkler EAH, Bodicoat DH, Yates T, Davies MJ, Dunstan DW, Healy GN. Considerations when using the activPAL monitor in field based research with adult populations. J Sport Health Sci. 2016. In Press.

60. Gianoudis J, Bailey CA, Daly RM. Associations between sedentary behaviour and body composition, muscle function and sarcopenia in community-dwelling older adults. Osteoporos Int. 2015;26:571–9.

22

Correlations between inflammatory cytokines, muscle damage markers and acute postoperative pain following primary total knee arthroplasty

Hai-bo Si[1,2], Ti-min Yang[1], Yi Zeng[1], Zong-ke Zhou[1], Fu-xing Pei[1], Yan-rong Lu[2], Jing-qiu Cheng[2*] and Bin Shen[1*]

Abstract

Background: Despite the success of total knee arthroplasty (TKA) in reducing knee pain and improving functional disability, the management of acute postoperative pain is still unsatisfactory. This study was aimed to quantitatively analyze the possible correlations between inflammatory cytokines, muscle damage markers and acute postoperative pain following primary TKA.

Methods: Patients scheduled for unilateral primary TKA were consecutively included, the serial changes of the numerical rating scale (NRS) at rest (NRSR) and at walking (NRSW), serum inflammatory cytokines and muscle damage markers were assessed before surgery (T0) and at postoperative day 1, 2, 3 and 5 (T1-T4, respectively); while pain disability questionnaire (PDQ) and synovial fluid inflammatory cytokines were evaluated at T0. The correlations between inflammatory cytokines, muscle damage markers and pain scores were examined, and Bonferroni correction was applied for multiple comparisons.

Results: Ninety six patients were included for serum markers and pain evaluations at T0-T4, while 54 (56.25%) for synovial fluid cytokines at T0. The NRSR at T1 and T2 were positively correlated with preoperative NRSW, while the NRSW at T1 to T4 were positively correlated with preoperative NRSR, NRSW and PDQ (all $p < 0.05$). The NRSR was positively correlated with serum PGE2, IL-6, and CK at T1; the NRSW was positively correlated with serum CRP at T1, with PGE2 and IL-6 at T1 to T3, with CK at T2 and T4, and with Mb and LDH at T1 to T4 (all $p < 0.003$). Meanwhile, positive correlations were observed between preoperative NRSW and synovial fluid PGE2, IL-6, IL-8, or TNF-α, as well as between PDQ and PGE2 (all $p < 0.003$), but no associations between postoperative pain scores and preoperative synovial fluid cytokines was found (all $p \geq 0.003$). Additionally, the NRSR at T1 and T2, and NRSW at T1 to T4 were positively correlated with body mass index (all $p < 0.05$).

Conclusions: Serum inflammatory cytokines and muscle damage markers are positively correlated with acute postoperative pain following primary TKA, and the key cytokines (CRP, PGE2, and IL-6) and markers (Mb, CK and LDH) may serve as the targets for developing novel analgesic strategies.

Keywords: Total knee arthroplasty, Acute postoperative pain, Inflammatory cytokines, Muscle damage markers, Body mass index

* Correspondence: jqcheng@scu.edu.cn; shenbin_1971@163.com
[2]Key Laboratory of Transplant Engineering and Immunology, West China Hospital, Sichuan University, No.1 Keyuan 4th Road, Chengdu, Sichuan 610041, China
[1]Department of Orthopedic Surgery, West China Hospital, Sichuan University, 37th Guoxue Road, Chengdu, Sichuan 610041, China

Background

A growing prevalence of knee osteoarthritis (OA), one of the most common age-related knee diseases characterized by cartilage degradation leading to progressive joint pain and disability [1, 2], is expected with the aging of population, and various interventions, aiming at alleviating pain and improving joint function and quality of life, have been developing for OA treatment [3–5]. Total knee arthroplasty (TKA) is one of the most frequently performed surgical procedures, and the incidence of postoperative pain to vary degrees is also expected [6, 7]. Indeed, acute postoperative pain, being defined as an expected physiological response to surgery, is the most common and predicted problem following TKA [8, 9]. High level of acute postoperative pain have deleterious effects on individuals, it impedes short- and long-term functional rehabilitation, extends length of hospital stay and increases the risk of chronic postoperative pain [10–12]. Despite lots of original studies and guidelines regarding pain management have been reported, postoperative pain management following primary TKA is far from optimal and TKA is considered among the most painful surgeries [12–14]. Therefore, exploring the possible contributing factors and how relevant the factors are to the acute postoperative pain will be helpful for treatment modalities and development of new analgesic strategies.

It is commonly known that the body mass index (BMI), gender and surgical approach are associated with acute postoperative pain after TKA [15–19], and many studies reported that the serum inflammatory cytokines, including erythrocyte sedimentation rate (ESR), C-reactive protein (CRP), prostaglandin E2 (PGE2), interleukins (ILs), and tumor necrosis factor alpha (TNF-α), might also be related to postoperative pain [20–24], but few studies have detected the levels of the inflammatory cytokines in synovial fluid. Meanwhile, some researchers have used serum muscle damage markers, including myoglobin (Mb), creatinine (Cre), creatine kinase (CK), lactate dehydrogenase (LDH) and aspartate transaminase (AST), to compare different approaches in orthopedic surgeries [25, 26], but whether these markers were associated with acute postoperative pain following primary TKA is less known. Moreover, few studies have quantitatively analyzed the possible correlations between inflammatory cytokines, muscle damage markers and acute postoperative pain after primary TKA.

To address these questions, we first examined the serial changes of acute postoperative pain scores, serum and synovial fluid inflammatory cytokines, and serum muscle damage markers in patients with severe knee OA before surgery and in subsequent periods after primary TKA in this study. Then, we quantitatively investigated whether the inflammatory cytokines and muscle damage markers were significantly correlate with acute postoperative pain.

Methods

Study participants

From October 2014 to December 2015, consecutive patients were evaluated for primary knee OA and scheduled for a TKA at the Department of Orthopedic Surgery, West China Hospital, Sichuan University. Patients eligible for this study should be: (1) more than 18 years old, and able to understand the nature of this study (informed consent); (2) without any infectious, psychiatric or neurologic pathologies (e.g., psychosis and dementia); (3) with a diagnosis of OA with a severity grade ≥ 3 according to the Kellgren-Lawrence (KL) classification [27], and with a varus or valgus angle ≤30°; (4) undergoing elective, unilateral and primary TKA. Patients who met the following conditions were excluded: (1) allergy to nonsteroidal anti-inflammatory drugs (NSAIDs) because parecoxib and celecoxib would be sequentially administered after surgery (described below); (2) history of gastrointestinal ulcer or bleeding; (3) alcohol and medical abuse within the 3 months preceding the inclusion; (4) being treated with corticosteroids, or hyaluronic acid within 6 months preceding the study, or systemic NSAIDs within 15 days before the study; (5) with progressive serious comorbidities (such as AIDS, malignant tumor, or end-stage renal or liver diseases), or with other painful conditions, or on medication that could possibly confound the evaluation of pain. Those who do not follow the study scheme, take other analgesics, withdraw the informed content, and are diagnosed with postoperative infection or other complications that will confound the results would be dropped out.

All procedures performed in this study were approved by the Ethical Committee of West China Hospital, Sichuan University, and with the 1964 Helsinki declaration and its later amendments or comparable ethical standards. Informed consent was obtained from all participants included in this study.

Total knee arthroplasty and postoperative pain management

All patients were classified according to the ASA (physical status classification of the American Society of Anesthesiologists) scoring system and underwent general anesthesia with same anesthesia protocols by a same senior anesthetist. All surgeries were performed by the same senior joint surgeon (Bin Shen), who had performed more than 1000 TKAs, through the standard medial parapatellar approach in the same laminar air flow operating room, and posterior stabilized total knee prosthesis system (DePuy, New Jersey, USA) was used in all included patients. A pneumatic tourniquet was used in all patients, inflating before skin incision and releasing after prosthesis placement, and a suction drainage was indwelled before suture and removed on the first morning after surgery. All patients began ambulation on the postoperative day (POD) 1. As an alternative multimodal analgesic protocols, all patients were sequentially treated with intravenous parecoxib (40 mg/q12h), the first injectable cyclooxygenase-2 (COX-2) selective inhibitor with approved indication of postoperative pain [28], for the first three postoperative days and followed by oral celecoxib (200 mg/q12h) which could relieve pain superior to low doses of morphine (4 mg iv) for further analgesia [29]. Tramadol (100 mg/tablet, per os) or dolantin (10 mg, intramuscular injection) was used as rescue analgesic when the NRS at rest ≥4 [30].

Pain assessment

Joint pain at rest (supine) and at walking (5 min after walk) were assessed 24 h before (T0), 24 h after (POD1, T1), 48 h after (POD2, T2), 72 h after (POD3, T3) and 5 days (POD5, T4) after surgery by 2 investigators using the numerical rating scale (NRS, with 0 represents no pain, and 10 represents the worst possible pain) [31]. Pain disability status was also assessed using the Pain Disability Questionnaire (PDQ), which is well validated in patients with musculoskeletal disorders compared with normal asymptomatic participants [32, 33]. The PDQ include 9 functional status items and 6 psychosocial items, and each was answered on a scale from 0 to 10, with 0 representing no disability and 10 representing maximal disability.

Quantification of inflammatory cytokines and muscle damage markers

Venous blood samples were collected at T0 - T4, and synovial fluid specimens were collected before exposure of the capsule intraoperatively (considered as preoperative sampling). The levels of inflammatory cytokines, including ESR, CRP, PGE2, IL-6, IL-8 and TNF-α, and muscle damage markers, including Mb, Cre, CK, LDH and AST, in serum were measured by the Department of Laboratory Medicine of our hospital certified by the College of American Pathologists. Additionally, PGE2, IL-6, IL-8 and TNF-α in synovial fluid were detected as well.

Statistical analysis

The demographics, operative information, NRS scores, values of inflammatory cytokines and muscle damage markers were collected. All statistical analyses were performed using the Statistical Package for Social Sciences (SPSS) software for Windows, version 22.0 (IBM, New York, USA). All continuous data were checked for normality first using Kolmogorov-Smirnov and Shapiro-Wilk tests. Comparisons between two groups (male and female) were conducted using the Student t-test for normally distributed data and Mann-Whitney U-test for non-normally distributed data, while comparisons among three groups (obese, overweight, and normal weight) were conducted using the one-way analysis of variance (ANOVA) with $post$-hoc analysis for normally distributed data, while Kruskal-Wallis H and Mann-Whitney U tests for non-normally distributed data. Spearman's rank-based correlation coefficient was used to quantify the correlations between inflammatory cytokines, muscle damage markers and pain scores, as well as between BMI and pain scores. A p-value <0.05 was considered to indicate statistical significance. Since 15 markers (PGE2, IL-6, IL-8 and TNF-α were evaluated in both the serum and synovial fluid) were assessed, the statistical significance for multiple correlations between inflammatory cytokines, muscle damage markers and pain scores were further evaluated using the conservative Bonferroni p value (0.05/15 = 0.003) to control the family-wise error rate.

Results

Fig. 1 provides the full details of the study flow, 96 patients completed the study and included in the final analyses, and the raw data were shown in the Additional file 1. The overall mean age of the population was 65.96 ± 5.44 years with a mean body mass index (BMI) of 25.68 ± 2.80 kg/m^2. The mean ASA was 1.75 ± 0.68, incision length was 15.21 ± 0.62 cm, operative time (from skin incision to the end of skin suture) was 58.20 ± 4.40 min, and the length of postoperative hospital stay (LPHS) was 7.11 ± 1.84 days. There was no significant differences in these characteristics between male (n = 18) and female (n = 78) patients. Additionally, synovial fluid inflammatory cytokines were detected in 54 patients (56.25%, Fig. 1).

Correlations between pre- and postoperative pain

The serial changes of NRS pain scores following primary TKA are shown in Fig. 2a, and there was no significant differences in NRS, both at rest (NRSR) and at walking (NRSW), between male and female patients. However, obese patients (BMI ≥ 30 kg/m^2 [34], n = 5) tended to report higher NRS than overweight (25 ≤ BMI < 30 kg/m^2, n = 48) and normal weight (BMI < 25 kg/m^2, n = 43) patients, although not all of the differences were statistically significant (Fig. 2b and c). Associations between pre- and postoperative pain scores are shown in Table 1. Postoperative NRSW at T1 to T4 were positively correlated with preoperative NRSR, NRSW and PDQ (all p < 0.05), while postoperative NRSR at T1 and T2 were positively correlated with preoperative NRSW (all p < 0.001). These results remained significant even if after adjusting for multiple comparisons (Bonferroni p

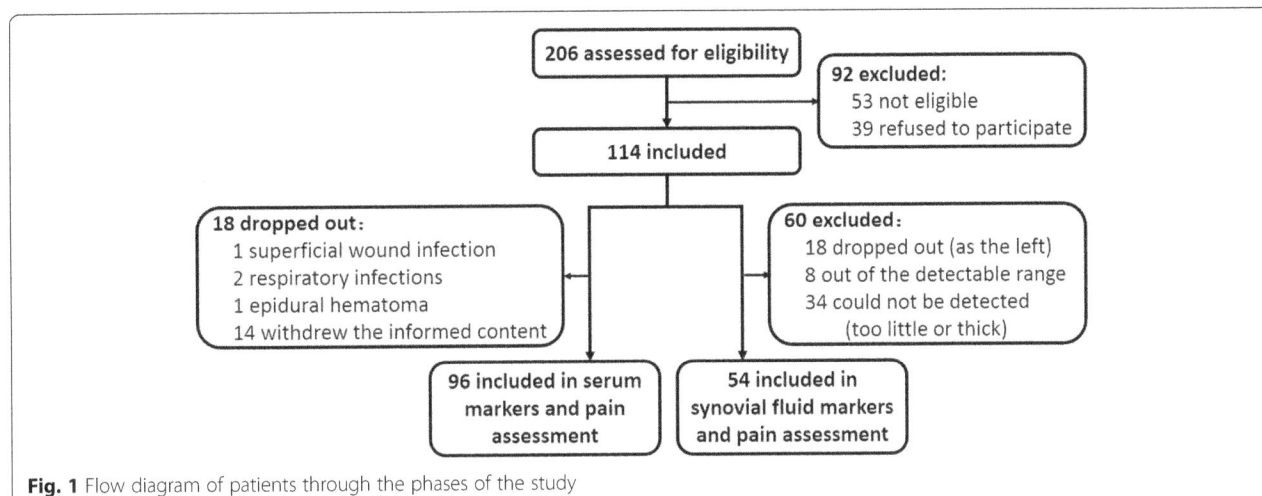

Fig. 1 Flow diagram of patients through the phases of the study

value, $0.05/3 = 0.017$). Furthermore, the preoperative NRSW was positively correlated with NRSR and PDQ ($r = 0.30$, $p = 0.003$; $r = 0.40$, $p < 0.001$, respectively), while no significant correlation between preoperative NRSR and PDQ was found.

Correlations between inflammatory cytokines and acute postoperative pain

The serial changes of serum inflammatory cytokines are shown in Fig. 3a and b, and the associations between serum inflammatory cytokines and pain scores are shown in Table 2. Before surgery (at T0), the NRSR was positively correlated with ESR and IL-6; the NRSW was positively correlated with ESR, CRP, PGE2 and IL-6; and the PDQ was positively correlated with ESR, CRP and PGE2 (all $p < 0.003$, with Bonferroni correction). Postoperatively, the NRSR was positively correlated with PGE2 and IL-6 at T1; and the NRSW was positively correlated with CRP at

T1, and with PGE2 and IL-6 at T1 to T3 (all $p < 0.003$).

The overall mean values of preoperative PGE2, IL-6, IL-8 and TNF-α in synovial fluid ($n = 54$) were 43.73 ± 17.85 ng/ml, 128.29 ± 104.2 pg/ml, 41.74 ± 21.58 pg/ml and 22.44 ± 11.34 pg/ml, respectively. Associations between synovial fluid inflammatory cytokines and pain scores are shown in Table 3. Preoperatively, the NRSW was positively correlated with PGE2, IL-6, IL-8 and TNF-α; the PDQ was positively correlated with PGE2 (all $p < 0.003$); while no significant correlations between preoperative NRSR and cytokines was found (all $p \geq 0.003$). Furthermore, there was also no significant correlations between postoperative NRS, both NRSR and NRSW at T1 to T4, and preoperative synovial fluid cytokines (all $p \geq 0.003$). Additionally, the preoperative PGE2, as well as IL-6, in serum and synovial fluid were also positively correlated ($r = 0.54$, $p < 0.001$; and $r = 0.33$, $p = 0.014$, respectively).

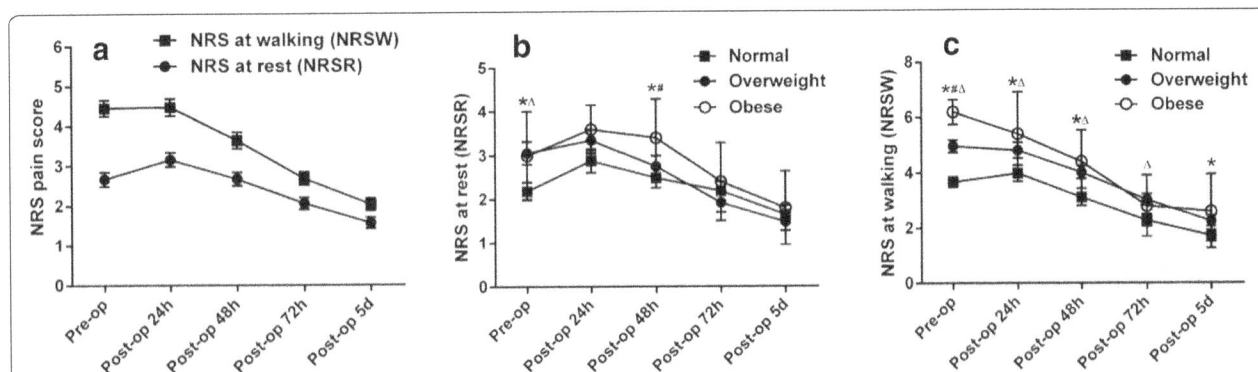

Fig. 2 The serial changes of NRS pain scores after primary total knee arthroplasty (Mean ± 95% confidence intervals). **a** The serial changes of total NRS at rest and at walking following primary TKA. **b, c** Comparisons of NRS at rest (**b**) and at walking (**c**) among obese, overweight, and normal weight patients. *, the difference between obese and overweight patients was significant, $p < 0.05$; #, the difference between obese and normal weight patients was significant, $p < 0.05$; ▵, the difference between overweight and normal weight patients was significant, $p < 0.05$

Table 1 Correlations between pre- and postoperative pain, $n = 96$ (*Spearman's correlation coefficients, p*)

Pre-op scores	Post-op NRSR				Post-op NRSW			
	T1	T2	T3	T4	T1	T2	T3	T4
Pre-op NRSR	0.01, 0.911	0.04, 0.706	−0.14, 0.182	−0.07, 0.482	0.34, 0.001*	0.37, <0.001*	0.25, 0.013*	0.26, 0.010*
Pre-op NRSW	0.40, <0.001*	0.37, <0.001*	−0.001, 0.995	−0.06, 0.595	0.30, 0.003*	0.38, <0.001*	0.39, <0.001*	0.34, 0.001*
Pre-op PDQ	0.08, 0.432	0.06, 0.587	−0.12, 0.240	0.04, 0.697	0.75, <0.001*	0.52, <0.001*	0.47, <0.001*	0.36, <0.001*

Abbreviations: NRSR numerical rating scale at rest, *NRSW* numerical rating scale at walking, *PDQ* pain disability questionnaire, *T1-T4* 1, 2, 3 and 5 days after surgery, respectively. The significant correlations according $p < 0.05$ (*) remained significant after Bonferroni correction ($p = 0.05/3$).

Correlations between muscle damage markers and acute postoperative pain

The serial changes of serum muscle damage markers are shown in Fig. 3c, and the correlations between serum muscle damage markers and pain scores are shown in Table 4. Preoperative PDQ was positively correlated with Cre ($p = 0.001$), while no correlations between NRS and muscle damage markers was observed (all $p \geq 0.003$). Postoperatively, the NRSR was positively correlated with CK at T1 ($p < 0.001$); the NRSW was positively correlated with Mb and LDH at T1 to T4, and with CK at T2 and T4 (all $p < 0.003$).

Correlations between BMI and acute postoperative pain

Because the obese patients tended to report higher NRS than overweight and normal weight patients (see above), the correlations between BMI and pain scores were further evaluated. As a result, preoperative NRSR, NRSW and PDQ were positively correlated with BMI ($r = 0.56$, 0.80, and 0.37, respectively; and all $p < 0.001$). Meanwhile, the NRSW at T1 to T4 ($r = 0.80$, 0.44, 0.53, and 0.44, respectively; and all $p < 0.001$), as well as the NRSR at T1 and T2 ($r = 0.56$, $p = 0.001$; and $r = 0.26$, $p = 0.010$, respectively), were also positively correlated with BMI.

Discussion

TKA is a successful procedure aiming to ultimately alleviate pain and restore joint function in patients suffering from end-stage knee diseases [1, 32, 35]. The management of acute postoperative pain, however, is still far from optimal, and TKA is among the most painful surgeries [19, 36]. In this study, we quantitatively assessed the possible correlations between inflammatory cytokines, muscle damage markers and acute postoperative pain, which few studies have reported, in 96 consecutive primary TKA patients. As a result, we found that the rest pain of the operated knee was positively correlated with serum PGE2, IL-6, and CK at POD 1; while the walking pain was positively correlated with serum CRP at POD 1, with PGE2 and IL-6 at POD 1 to POD 3, with CK at POD 2 and POD 5, and with Mb and LDH at POD 1 to POD 5, indicating that some inflammatory cytokines (CRP, PGE2, IL-6) and muscle damage markers (Mb, CK, and LDH) are indeed interacted with acute postoperative pain after primary TKA.

Inflammatory cytokines, including PGE2, ILs (mainly IL-6) and TNF-α, presented in serum and synovial fluid in OA pathogenesis [37, 38], and it raises the question that whether these cytokines associated with acute postoperative pain after TKA. It has been proved that surgery and trauma are often accompanied by changes in serum levels of certain cytokines and markers, including

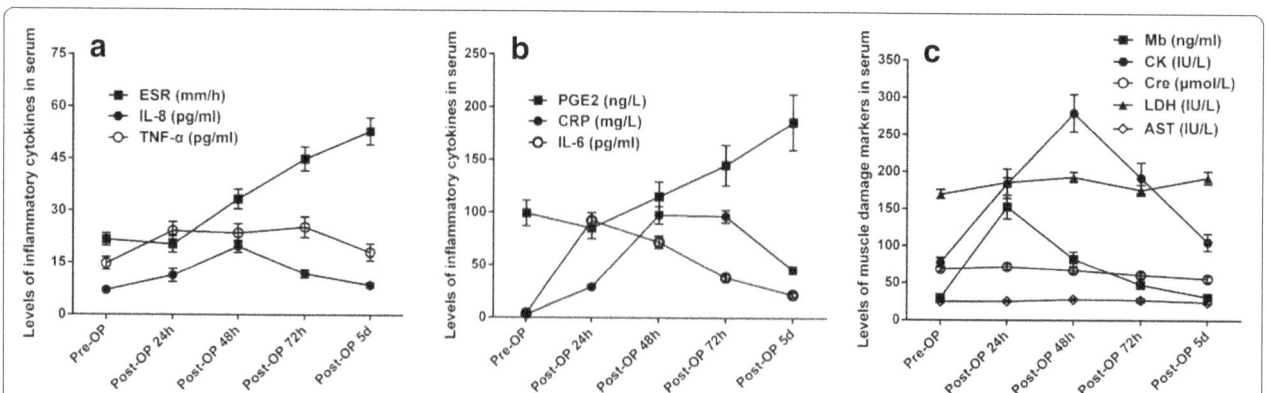

Fig. 3 The serial changes of serum inflammatory cytokines and muscle damage markers after primary total knee arthroplasty. **a, b** The serial changes of serum inflammatory cytokines, including erythrocyte sedimentation rate (ESR); C-reactive protein (CRP), prostaglandin E2 (PGE2), interleukin-6 and -8 (IL-6 and IL-8), tumor necrosis factor alpha (TNF-α). **c** The serial changes of serum muscle damage markers, including myoglobin (Mb), creatinine (Cre), creatine kinase (CK), lactate dehydrogenase (LDH), and aspartate transaminase (AST)

Table 2 Correlations between serum inflammatory cytokines and pain scores, n = 96 (*Spearman's correlation coefficients, p*)

	PDQ	NRSR					NRSW				
		T0	T1	T2	T3	T4	T0	T1	T2	T3	T4
ESR	0.31, 0.002*	0.44, <0.001*	0.04, 0.691	−0.13, 0.203	−0.04, 0.718	−0.10, 0.339	0.53, <0.001*	0.13, 0.192	0.15, 0.142	0.04, 0.670	0.04, 0.672
CRP	0.37, <0.001*	0.24, 0.017	0.04, 0.689	−0.08, 0.446	0.00, 0.982	−0.02, 0.814	0.34, 0.001*	0.38, <0.001*	0.29, 0.004	0.15, 0.134	−0.03, 0.743
PGE2	0.44, <0.001*	0.24, 0.017	0.37, <0.001*	0.29†, 0.005	0.06, 0.584	−0.02, 0.824	0.67, <0.001*	0.35, 0.001*	0.42, <0.001*	0.39, <0.001*	0.29, 0.004
IL-6	0.26, 0.009	0.34, 0.001*	0.31, 0.002*	0.28, 0.007	−0.07, 0.474	−0.20, 0.047	0.33, 0.001*	0.41, <0.001*	0.40, <0.001*	0.37, <0.001*	0.22, 0.034
IL-8	−0.05, 0.641	−0.10, 0.314	−0.13, 0.224	−0.07, 0.520	−0.20, 0.055	−0.04, 0.709	−0.03, 0.782	−0.17, 0.107	−0.24, 0.020	0.21, 0.041	−0.07, 0.937
TNF-α	0.09, 0.404	0.16, 0.110	−0.01, 0.907	−0.14, 0.186	−0.11, 0.302	−0.06, 0.583	0.18, 0.080	0.05, 0.619	0.06, 0.576	−0.01, 0.944	−0.04, 0.737

Abbreviations: NRSR numerical rating scale at rest, NRSW numerical rating scale at walking, PDQ pain disability questionnaire, ESR erythrocyte sedimentation rate; CRP C-reactive protein, PGE2 prostaglandin E2, IL interleukin, TNF-α tumor necrosis factor alpha, T0 24 h before surgery, T1-T4 1, 2, 3 and 5 days after surgery, respectively. The p-values are presented in their raw, uncorrected form, but the statistical significance for multiple comparisons were further corrected using the conservative Bonferroni p value (0.05/15 = 0.003) to control the family-wise error rate, and p < 0.003 are deemed significant (*).

inflammatory cytokines and muscle damage markers [39, 40]. However, to our knowledge there is no studies investigated the associations between these markers and acute postoperative pain following primary TKA. Large amounts of IL-6 are produced at the surgical site and enter the systemic circulation, where its concentrations correlate with the severity of surgery and the magnitude of the tissue injury [41]. After surgery or injury, IL-6 levels were detectable in the systemic circulation at 60 min, it reached to a peak value between 4 to 6 h, and could persist for as long as 10 days [20]. We were not able to specify the exact time of peak value of IL-6 in this study, but we found that the IL-6 value was significant elevated within the first postoperative day and then began to decline. We also observed that the serum IL-6 levels were positively correlated with the acute postoperative pain, with rest pain at POD 1 and with walk pain at POD 1 to POD 3, following primary TKA. Similar correlations was also found between acute postoperative pain and PGE2, which could (indirectly) increase the sensitization of nociceptors and acute postoperative pain [38]. TNF-α has been shown to influence and coordinate the inflammatory response in almost all tissues, it can influence the excitability of nociceptors either directly or through the expression of downstream cytokines, or both, and play a crucial role in the pathophysiology of injury-related pain. However, no significant correlations between acute postoperative pain and TNF-α, both in serum and in synovial fluid, was found in our study. Additionally, it would be specially mentioned that we initially detected the IL-1β, which was reported as a strong pro-inflammatory cytokine [42, 43], but its level was very low and difficult to be detected in the systemic circulation, as well as in synovial fluid, even in subsequent periods following surgery, and this was also been reported by other researchers [24, 44].

ESR is a non-specific hematological marker routinely used as an indirect parameter of increased acute phase reactants, and CRP is a major acute phase reactant and produced by the liver in response to inflammation, infection, malignancy or tissue damage [23]. Honsawek et al. reported that ESR was increased with a peak value reached 2 weeks after TKA and reduced to its preoperative level at 26 weeks postoperatively, while the CRP was elevated on the POD 1 and decreased to its preoperative value at 2 weeks postoperatively [24]. However, this

Table 3 Correlations between synovial fluid inflammatory cytokines and pain scores, n = 54 (*Spearman's correlation coefficients, p*)

	PDQ	NRSR					NRSW				
		T0	T1	T2	T3	T4	T0	T1	T2	T3	T4
PGE2	0.43, 0.001*	0.08, 0.588	0.38, 0.004	0.36, 0.007	0.03, 0.806	0.15, 0.286	0.52, <0.001*	0.33, 0.017	0.29, 0.032	0.26, 0.055	0.14, 0.317
IL-6	0.34, 0.011	0.08, 0.577	0.17, 0.225	0.09, 0.542	−0.22, 0.115	−0.12, 0.409	0.47, <0.001*	0.31, 0.021	0.27, 0.051	0.25, 0.065	0.07, 0.625
IL-8	0.15, 0.264	0.32, 0.019	0.10, 0.464	0.04, 0.763	−0.16, 0.254	−0.21, 0.122	0.74, <0.001*	0.16, 0.235	0.22, 0.109	0.20, 0.157	0.13, 0.350
TNF-α	0.28, 0.043	0.30, 0.029	0.19, 0.159	0.30, 0.028	−0.05, 0.740	−0.15, 0.295	0.76, <0.001*	0.25, 0.069	0.22, 0.116	0.22, 0.111	0.26, 0.062

Abbreviations: NRSR numerical rating scale at rest, NRSW numerical rating scale at walking, PDQ pain disability questionnaire, PGE2 prostaglandin E2, IL interleukin, TNF-α tumor necrosis factor alpha, T0 24 h before surgery, T1-T4 24, 48, 72 h and 5 days after surgery, respectively. The p-values are presented in their raw, uncorrected form, but the statistical significance for multiple comparisons were further corrected using the conservative Bonferroni p value (0.05/15 = 0.003) to control the family-wise error rate, and p < 0.003 are deemed significant (*)

Table 4 Correlations between serum muscle damage markers and pain scores, n = 96 (*Spearman's correlation coefficients, r*)

	PDQ	NRSR					NRSW				
		T0	T1	T2	T3	T4	T0	T1	T2	T3	T4
Mb	0.19, 0.059	0.28, 0.006	0.11, 0.278	0.06, 0.535	0.04, 0.688	0.16, 0.121	0.20, 0.051	0.46, <0.001*	0.32, 0.001*	0.36, <0.001*	0.35, <0.001*
Cre	0.33, 0.001*	0.09, 0.398	−0.12, 0.981	0.16, 0.111	0.22, 0.028	−0.05, 0.653	0.07, 0.531	−0.16, 0.110	−0.11, 0.297	−0.09, 0.409	0.07, 0.475
CK	0.06, 0.554	0.27, 0.007	0.39, <0.001*	0.14, 0.189	−0.02, 0.850	0.01, 0.910	0.25, 0.014	0.24, 0.019	0.34, 0.001*	0.29, 0.004	0.34, 0.001*
LDH	0.23, 0.022	0.26, 0.011	0.25, 0.016	0.10, 0.330	0.04, 0.683	−0.07, 0.513	0.30, 0.003	0.32, 0.001*	0.41, <0.001*	0.47, <0.001*	0.36, <0.001*
AST	0.12, 0.240	0.21, 0.039	0.07, 0.504	0.001, 0.991	−0.002, 0.986	−0.13, 0.198	0.25, 0.013	0.09, 0.399	0.10, 0.314	0.28, 0.005	0.18, 0.075

Abbreviations: NRSR numerical rating scale at rest, *NRSW* numerical rating scale at walking, *PDQ* pain disability questionnaire, *Mb* myoglobin, *Cre* creatinine, *CK* creatine kinase, *LDH* lactate dehydrogenase, *AST* aspartate transaminase, *T0* 24 h before surgery, *T1-T4* 1, 2, 3 and 5 days after surgery, respectively. The *p*-values are presented in their raw, uncorrected form, but the statistical significance for multiple comparisons were further corrected using the conservative Bonferroni *p* value (0.05/15 = 0.003) to control the family-wise error rate, and *p* < 0.003 are deemed significant (*)

study showed that the values of ESR were slightly declined on POD 1, and then evaluated with a continuously slow rise, while the CRP values were increased to peak on POD 2, and then began to decline. We further found that the postoperative walking pain at POD 1 were positively correlated with the CRP, but no correlation between postoperative pain and ESR was found. Overall, these results demonstrate that acute postoperative pain after TKA was indeed associated with inflammatory cytokines, in which CRP, PEG2, and IL-6 are the key ones.

We further quantitatively analyzed the correlations between muscle damage markers and acute postoperative pain following primary TKA, and identified that Mb, CK and LDH were the key markers in systemic circulation which positively correlated with acute postoperative pain. Muscle damage could occurred not only intraoperatively, but also postoperatively. The medial parapatellar retinacular incision and release of medial collateral ligament (MCL) were inevitable in TKA, and contribute to the intraoperative muscle damage. Niki et al. reported that the levels of muscle-related enzymes were affected by the degree of medial release for appropriate soft-tissue balancing [26]. Despite the medial collateral ligament (MCL) and semimembranosus muscle were intraoperatively released from the tibia by subperiosteal dissection, which could avoid damage to the actual muscle fibers theoretically, Niki et al. reported that such release appear to elevate muscle damage marker levels [26]. Meanwhile, postoperative functional exercise, including walking and flexing, in the early stage after surgery might also cause potential muscle fiber injury and subsequent elevations in relative markers in serum. Additionally, it is still debated whether tourniquet-induced ischemia represents a substantial contributor to inflammatory response and muscle damage, as well as subsequent release of relative markers. Clementsen et al.

investigated the release of inflammatory cytokines, including IL-1β, IL-6, IL-8, and TNF-α, after tourniquet use in TKA, but levels of these cytokines did not change regardless of tourniquet use [44]. Laurence et al. evaluated tourniquet-induced ischemia during TKA and reported that no significant difference in Mb between patients with and without tourniquet (less than 150 min), and the elevation of serum Mb associated with tourniquet was negligible [45].

In this study, obese patients tended to report higher pain scores than overweight and normal weight patients, and the rest pain at POD1 and POD2, as well as the walking pain at POD1 to POD 5, were positively correlated with BMI. Although these results further supported our previous finding that a BMI ≥ 30 kg/m^2 have a negative influence on the outcomes of primary TKA [34], but whether obese patients should be encouraged to lose weight before TKA is still controversial, and many other factors, such as age, physical condition and the feasibility of losing weight, should be taken into account [46]. Moreover, more than half of the patients included in this study with a BMI ≥ 25 kg/m^2 (*n* = 53), in which only 5 were obese, the unbalanced sample size might introduce a bias, and further studies with more subjects and appropriate BMI constitution were needed to further illustrate the effects of BMI on acute postoperative pain after primary TKA.

Additionally, although the overall walking pain was more severe than rest pain, some patients reported a more severe rest pain than walking pain in the same day. There is only one relative study, by Lunn et al., reported that acute postoperative pain at rest and during hip and knee flexion after TKA was significantly reduced 5 min and 20 min after walk compared with that before walk, and pain was further reduced during the second walk compared with the first walk [47]. We assessed NRSW 5 min after walk and similar results were obtained in partial patients, indicating that mobilization might be able to promote analgesic effects. Future studies with a randomized, controlled design on exercise dose-response effects after primary TKA were necessary to illustrate this phenomenon.

However, several limitations must be taken into account in this study. Firstly, the subjects included in this study were confined to OA patients, and therefore it could not be generalized to other types of knee arthrosis, such as rheumatoid arthritis. Secondly, only 54 out of 96 (56.25%) patients had the synovial fluid data collected for preoperative analyses because the synovial fluid in some patients was too little or viscous and could not be detected, and the postoperative synovial fluid cytokines were also not assessed because the drainage tube was removed on the first morning after surgery. Thirdly, no control group, such as unicompartmental knee arthroplasty or minimally invasive approach, was established, and the joint function was not reported in this study. Finally, other confounding factors, such as fear or anxiety, articular nerves, implant type, and anticoagulant used for prophylaxis of postoperative venous thromboembolism [48–50], might also affected the acute postoperative pain following TKA.

Conclusions

We demonstrate in this study that serum inflammatory cytokines and muscle damage markers are positively correlated with acute postoperative pain following primary TKA, and the key serum cytokines (CRP, PGE2, and IL-6) and markers (Mb, CK and LDH) may serve as the targets for developing novel analgesic strategies.

Abbreviations

AST: Aspartate transaminase; BMI: Body mass index; Cre: Creatinine; CK: Creatine kinase; CRP: C-reactive protein; ESR: Erythrocyte sedimentation rate; IL: Interleukin; LDH: Lactate dehydrogenase; Mb: Myoglobin; NRS: Numerical rating scale; NRSR: NRS at rest; NRSW: NRS at walking; PDQ: Pain disability questionnaire; PGE2: Prostaglandin E2; POD: Postoperative day; TKA: Total knee arthroplasty; TNF-α: Tumor necrosis factor alpha

Acknowledgements
Many thanks to the Department of Laboratory Medicine of West China Hospital, Sichuan University for their technical help in the detection of serum and synovial fluid samples; and Dr. Hu Qin-sheng for help in the analyses of the data. Also, the authors would like to thank all participants who took part in the study and people who helped us with the study.

Funding
This research was supported by the China Health Ministry Program (201302007).

Authors' contributions
SB and SHb conceived, designed and coordinated the experiments. SHb, ZZk and PFx contributed to acquisition of data. SHb, YTm and ZY analyzed and interpreted the data. SHb, YTm, CJq and LYr drafted and revised the manuscript. All authors read and approved the final manuscript.

Authors' information
Not applicable.

Competing interests
The authors declare that they have no competing interests.

Consent for publication
Not applicable.

References
1. Glyn-Jones S, Palmer AJ, Agricola R, Price AJ, Vincent TL, Weinans H, et al. Osteoarthritis Lancet. 2015;386(9991):376–87.
2. Jakob R. The management of early osteoarthritis. Knee. 2014;21(4):799–800.
3. Kurtz S, Ong K, Lau E, Mowat F, Halpern M. Projections of primary and revision hip and knee arthroplasty in the United States from 2005 to 2030. J Bone Joint Surg Am. 2007;89(4):780–5.
4. Pinto PR, McIntyre T, Ferrero R, Almeida A, Araujo-Soares V. Predictors of acute postsurgical pain and anxiety following primary total hip and knee arthroplasty. J Pain. 2013;14(5):502–15.
5. Lizaur-Utrilla A, Gonzalez-Parreno S, Miralles-Munoz FA, Lopez-Prats FA. Ten-year mortality risk predictors after primary total knee arthroplasty for osteoarthritis. Knee Surg Sports Traumatol Arthrosc. 2015;23(6):1848–55.
6. Schache MB, McClelland JA, Webster KE. Lower limb strength following total knee arthroplasty: a systematic review. Knee. 2014;21(1):12–20.
7. Huang YM, Wang CM, Wang CT, Lin WP, Horng LC, Jiang CC. Perioperative celecoxib administration for pain management after total knee arthroplasty - a randomized, controlled study. BMC Musculoskelet Disord. 2008;9:77.
8. Carr DB, Goudas LC. Acute pain. Lancet. 1999;353(9169):2051–8.
9. Chan EY, Blyth FM, Nairn L, Fransen M. Acute postoperative pain following hospital discharge after total knee arthroplasty. Osteoarthr Cartil. 2013;21(9): 1257–63.
10. Morrison RS, Magaziner J, McLaughlin MA, Orosz G, Silberzweig SB, Koval KJ, et al. The impact of post-operative pain on outcomes following hip fracture. Pain. 2003;103(3):303–11.
11. Brander VA, Stulberg SD, Adams AD, Harden RN, Bruehl S, Stanos SP, et al. Predicting total knee replacement pain: a prospective, observational study. Clin Orthop Relat Res. 2003;416:27–36.
12. Wu CL, Raja SN. Treatment of acute postoperative pain. Lancet. 2011; 377(9784):2215–25.
13. Gerbershagen HJ, Pogatzki-Zahn E, Aduckathil S, Peelen LM, Kappen TH, van Wijck AJ, et al. Procedure-specific risk factor analysis for the development of severe postoperative pain. Anesthesiology. 2014;120(5):1237–45.
14. Piscitelli P, Iolascon G, Innocenti M, Civinini R, Rubinacci A, Muratore M, et al. Painful prosthesis: approaching the patient with persistent pain following total hip and knee arthroplasty. Clin Cases Miner Bone Metab. 2013;10(2):97–110.
15. Beswick AD, Wylde V, Gooberman-Hill R, Blom A, Dieppe P. What proportion of patients report long-term pain after total hip or knee replacement for osteoarthritis? A systematic review of prospective studies in unselected patients. BMJ Open. 2012;2(1):1–12.
16. Parvizi J, Bloomfield MR. Multimodal pain management in orthopedics: implications for joint arthroplasty surgery. Orthopedics. 2013;36(2 Suppl):7–14.
17. Thomas T, Robinson C, Champion D, McKell M, Pell M. Prediction and assessment of the severity of post-operative pain and of satisfaction with management. Pain. 1998;75(2–3):177–85.

18. Wylde V, Rooker J, Halliday L, Blom A. Acute postoperative pain at rest after hip and knee arthroplasty: severity, sensory qualities and impact on sleep. Orthop Traumatol Surg Res. 2011;97(2):139–44.

19. Gerbershagen HJ, Aduckathil S, van Wijck AJ, Peelen LM, Kalkman CJ, Meissner W. Pain intensity on the first day after surgery: a prospective cohort study comparing 179 surgical procedures. Anesthesiology. 2013;118(4):934–44.

20. Watkins LR, Maier SF, Goehler LE. Immune activation: the role of pro-inflammatory cytokines in inflammation, illness responses and pathological pain states. Pain. 1995;63(3):289–302.

21. Ohtori S, Takahashi K, Moriya H, Myers RR. TNF-alpha and TNF-alpha receptor type 1 upregulation in glia and neurons after peripheral nerve injury: studies in murine DRG and spinal cord. Spine. 2004;29(10):1082–8.

22. Takeshita M, Nakamura J, Ohtori S, Inoue G, Orita S, Miyagi M, et al. Sensory innervation and inflammatory cytokines in hypertrophic synovia associated with pain transmission in osteoarthritis of the hip: a case-control study. Rheumatology (Oxford). 2012;51(10):1790–5.

23. Chen X, Bai C, Xie L, Zhang Y, Wang K. Inflammatory response to orthopedic biomaterials after total hip replacement. J Orthop Sci. 2012;17(4):407–12.

24. Honsawek S, Deepaisarnsakul B, Tanavalee A, Sakdinakiattikoon M, Ngarmukos S, Preativatanyou K, Bumrungpanichthaworn P. Relationship of serum IL-6, C-reactive protein, erythrocyte sedimentation rate, and knee skin temperature after total knee arthroplasty: a prospective study. Int Orthop 2011;35(1):31-5.

25. Huang Z, Shen B, Ma J, Yang J, Zhou Z, Kang P, et al. Mini-midvastus versus medial parapatellar approach in TKA: muscle damage and inflammation markers. Orthopedics. 2012;35(7):e1038–45.

26. Niki Y, Mochizuki T, Momohara S, Saito S, Toyama Y, Matsumoto H. Is minimally invasive surgery in total knee arthroplasty really minimally invasive surgery? J Arthroplast. 2009;24(4):499–504.

27. Kellgren JH, Lawrence JS. Radiological assessment of osteo-arthrosis. Ann Rheum Dis. 1957;16(4):494–502.

28. Zhu Y, Wang S, Wu H, Wu Y. Effect of perioperative parecoxib on postoperative pain and local inflammation factors PGE2 and IL-6 for total knee arthroplasty: a randomized, double-blind, placebo-controlled study. Eur J Orthop Surg Traumatol. 2014;24(3):395–401.

29. Kiefer W, Dannhardt G. Novel insights and therapeutical applications in the field of inhibitors of COX-2. Curr Med Chem. 2004;11(24):3147–61.

30. Gerbershagen HJ, Rothaug J, Kalkman CJ, Meissner W. Determination of moderate-to-severe postoperative pain on the numeric rating scale: a cut-off point analysis applying four different methods. Br J Anaesth. 2011;107(4):619–26.

31. Hawker GA, Mian S, Kendzerska T, French M. Measures of adult pain: visual analog scale for pain (VAS pain), numeric rating scale for pain (NRS pain), McGill pain questionnaire (MPQ), short-form McGill pain questionnaire (SF-MPQ), chronic pain grade scale (CPGS), short form-36 bodily pain scale (SF-36 BPS), and measure of intermittent and constant osteoarthritis pain (ICOAP). Arthritis Care Res. 2011;63(Suppl 11):S240–52.

32. Azim S, Nicholson J, Rebecchi MJ, Galbavy W, Feng T, Reinsel R, et al. Endocannabinoids and acute pain after total knee arthroplasty. Pain. 2015; 156(2):341–7.

33. Anagnostis C, Gatchel RJ, Mayer TG. The pain disability questionnaire: a new psychometrically sound measure for chronic musculoskeletal disorders. Spine. 2004;29(20):2290–302. discussion 303

34. Si HB, Zeng Y, Shen B, Yang J, Zhou ZK, Kang PD, et al. The influence of body mass index on the outcomes of primary total knee arthroplasty. Knee Surg Sports Traumatol Arthrosc. 2014;23(6):1824–32.

35. Si HB, Yang TM, Zeng Y, Shen B. No clear benefit or drawback to the use of closed drainage after primary total knee arthroplasty: a systematic review and meta-analysis. BMC Musculoskelet Disord. 2016;17:183.

36. Lunn TH, Husted H, Laursen MB, Hansen LT, Kehlet H. Analgesic and sedative effects of perioperative gabapentin in total knee arthroplasty: a randomized, double-blind, placebo-controlled dose-finding study. Pain. 2015;156(12):2438–48.

37. Chen X, Tanner K, Levine JD. Mechanical sensitization of cutaneous C-fiber nociceptors by prostaglandin E2 in the rat. Neurosci Lett. 1999;267(2):105–8.

38. Miller RE, Miller RJ, Malfait AM. Osteoarthritis joint pain: the cytokine connection. Cytokine. 2014;70(2):185–93.

39. Lisowska B, Maslinski W, Maldyk P, Zabek J, Baranowska E. The role of cytokines in inflammatory response after total knee arthroplasty in patients with rheumatoid arthritis. Rheumatol Int. 2008;28(7):667–71.

40. Mjaaland KE, Kivle K, Svenningsen S, Pripp AH, Nordsletten L. Comparison of markers for muscle damage, inflammation, and pain using minimally invasive direct anterior versus direct lateral approach in total hip arthroplasty: a prospective, randomized, controlled trial. J Orthop Res. 2015; 33(9):1305–10.

41. Lin E, Calvano SE, Lowry SF. Inflammatory cytokines and cell response in surgery. Surgery. 2000;127(2):117–26.

42. Matute Wilander A, Karedal M, Axmon A, Nordander C. Inflammatory biomarkers in serum in subjects with and without work related neck/shoulder complaints. BMC Musculoskelet Disord. 2014;15:103.

43. Papathanasiou I, Michalitsis S, Hantes ME, Vlychou M, Anastasopoulou L, Malizos KN, et al. Molecular changes indicative of cartilage degeneration and osteoarthritis development in patients with anterior cruciate ligament injury. BMC Musculoskelet Disord. 2016;17:21.

44. Clementsen T, Reikeras O. Cytokine patterns after tourniquet-induced skeletal muscle ischaemia reperfusion in total knee replacement. Scand J Clin Lab Invest. 2008;68(2):154–9.

45. Laurence AS, Norris SH. Serum myoglobin following tourniquet release under anaesthesia. Eur J Anaesthesiol. 1988;5(2):143–50.

46. Bordini B, Stea S, Cremonini S, Viceconti M, De Palma R, Toni A. Relationship between obesity and early failure of total knee prostheses. BMC Musculoskelet Disord. 2009;10:29.

47. Lunn TH, Kristensen BB, Gaarn-Larsen L, Kehlet H. Possible effects of mobilisation on acute post-operative pain and nociceptive function after total knee arthroplasty. Acta Anaesthesiol Scand. 2012;56(10):1234–40.

48. Witt KL, Vilensky JA. The anatomy of osteoarthritic joint pain. Clin Anat. 2014;27(3):451–4.

49. Nashi N, Hong CC, Krishna L. Residual knee pain and functional outcome following total knee arthroplasty in osteoarthritic patients. Knee Surg Sports Traumatol Arthrosc. 2015;23(6):1841–7.

50. Hovik LH, Winther SB, Foss OA, Gjeilo KH. Preoperative pain catastrophizing and postoperative pain after total knee arthroplasty: a prospective cohort study with one year follow-up. BMC Musculoskelet Disord. 2016;17:214.

23

Differences between native and prosthetic knees in terms of cross-sectional morphology of the femoral trochlea: a study based on three-dimensional models and virtual total knee arthroplasty

Zhe Du[1†], Shichang Chen[2†], Mengning Yan[2], Bing Yue[1] and You Wang[1*] (ID)

Abstract

Background: The cross-sectional morphology of the prosthetic knee is crucial to understanding patellar motion and quadriceps strength after total knee arthroplasty. However, few comparative evaluations of the cross-sectional morphology of the femoral trochlea have been performed in the native knee and currently available femoral implants, and the relationship between the trochlear anatomy of prosthetic components and post-operative patellofemoral complications remains unclear. We aimed to investigate the differences in cross-sectional morphology of the femoral trochlea between native knees and prosthetic femoral components.

Methods: Virtual total knee arthroplasty was performed, whereby four different femoral components (medial-pivot, Triathlon, NRG and NexGen) were virtually superimposed onto three-dimensional models of 42 healthy femurs. The following morphological parameters were measured in three cross-sections (0, 45 and 90°) of the femoral trochlea: sulcus height, lateral tilt angle, medial tilt angle and sulcus angle. Only statistically significant differences are described further ($p < 0.05$).

Results: In the 0° cross-section, sulcus height was smaller in the native knee than in the Triathlon, NRG and NexGen components; all prosthetic components had smaller lateral tilt angles and larger medial tilt angles. In the 45° cross-section, sulcus height was larger in the native knee than in the medial-pivot, Triathlon and NexGen components; both lateral and medial tilt angles were smaller in the prosthetic components. In the 90° cross-section, sulcus height was smaller in the native knee than in the medial-pivot component; all prosthetic components had a larger lateral tilt angle and smaller medial tilt angle. In all cross-sections, the sulcus angle was smaller in the native knee.

Conclusions: The discrepancy between native and prosthetic trochlear geometries suggests altered knee mechanics after total knee arthroplasty, but further cadaveric, computational or fluoroscopic investigations are necessary to clarify the implications of this observation. Our findings can be used to optimize biomechanical guidelines for total knee arthroplasty (patellar resurfacing or non-resurfacing) in Chinese individuals so as to decrease the risk of patellar lateral dislocation, to maintain stability and to optimize extensor kinematics.

Keywords: Total knee arthroplasty, Femoral trochlea, Morphology, Prosthesis design

* Correspondence: drwangyou@163.com

†Equal contributors

[1]Department of Bone and Joint Surgery, Renji Hospital, School of Medicine, Shanghai Jiaotong University, 145 Middle Shandong Road, Shanghai 200001, China

Full list of author information is available at the end of the article

Background

The most common complications after total knee arthroplasty (TKA) are related to femoropatellar problems, with residual pain in the anterior knee manifested in 5–45% of patients [1–3]. It has been proposed that excessive quadriceps load and altered patellar kinematics contribute to the development of patellar complications after TKA [3, 4]. Previous findings suggest that limitations of the implant design may result in such complications [5–7], and numerous authors have emphasized the changes in knee kinematics following TKA. Merican et al. [8] noted that TKA led to significant changes in patellofemoral kinematics, with significant increases in lateral shift, tilt and rotation compared to those characteristic to the native knee. Similarly, Akbari et al. [9] reported that the postoperative patella was more inferiorly positioned and tilted laterally in mid-flexion. It was speculated that these kinematic changes were due to trochlear dysplasia, since appropriate design for the prosthetic trochlea was accepted as the main determinant of patellofemoral outcome in TKA [10]. Previous evidence of trochlear dysplasia in the design of the femoral component was obtained based on 14 digital TKA models, but these findings were not evaluated in the context of the clinical outcomes achieved with the evaluated implants [7]. Saffarini et al. [11] highlighted the influence of patellofemoral geometry on mid-flexion kinematics after comparing two different knee components (HLS Noetos® and KneeTec®). In their simulation study, Varadarajan et al. [6] also measured the trochlear geometry before and after TKA, but did not discuss the effect of TKA on patellar motion and soft-tissue changes. To our knowledge, few comparative evaluations of the cross-sectional morphology of the femoral trochlea have been performed in the native knee and currently available femoral implants, and the relationship between the trochlear anatomy of prosthetic components and post-operative patellofemoral complications remains unclear.

In the present study based on virtual TKAs, whereby femoral implants were superimposed onto three-dimensional (3D) models of healthy femurs, we provide a detailed comparison between native and prosthetic knees regarding the cross-sectional morphology of the femoral trochlea, evaluated in terms of the sulcus height (H), lateral tilt angle (α), medial tilt angle (β) and sulcus angle. We aimed to investigate potential differences between the native knee and currently available prosthetic knee designs, and subsequently analyze the effects of prosthetic trochlear design on quadriceps strength and retinacula tension following TKA. The findings of our study are relevant for optimization of implant design, patient diagnosis and surgical technique. Our original hypothesis was that patellar kinematic changes and quadriceps weakness after TKA were due to irrational prosthetic trochlear design.

Methods

The study included 42 healthy Chinese participants (10 male and 32 female), with an average age of 45.8 years (range, 34–57 years), an average height of 161.4 cm (range, 150–179 cm), an average body mass index of 23.7 kg/m^2 (range, 16.5–29.6 kg/m^2), and an average mechanical axis of the lower limb of 179.7° (range, 174.7–184.4°). Only participants with healthy knees were included. The exclusion criteria were previous knee trauma or knee pain; soft tissue injury; osteoarthritis; and other chronic diseases of the musculoskeletal system.

Obtaining the 3D models of the native and prosthetic knee

Computed tomography (CT) images (Light speed 16; GE Medical Systems, Milwaukee, WI) were used to create 3D knee models. Only models of the right knee were included in the analysis. To reduce radiographic exposure, CT slices were acquired at intervals of 0.6 mm for the knee joint, and at intervals of 2 mm for the hip and ankle joints (resolution, 512 × 512 pixels). Four types of prosthetic components were evaluated in the present study, namely the Advance Medial-Pivot (MP) Knee System, (MicroPort Orthopedics Co., Arlington, TN), the Triathlon® Knee System (Stryker Co., Kalamazoo, MI), the NRG® Knee System (Stryker Co., Mahwah, NJ) and the NexGen® Complete Knee Solution (Zimmer Inc., Warsaw, IN). A 3D laser scanner (KLS-171; Kreon Technologies, Limoges, France) was used to create 3D models of the metal femoral components for the right knee. CT and laser scanning data were imported into Geomagic Studio version 10.0 (Geomagic Inc., Research Triangle Park, NC) in order to reconstruct the 3D models of the native knee and prosthetic components, respectively.

Selecting a suitable size of the prosthetic component for virtual TKA

According to the general principles of TKA, the size of the femoral component was chosen based on the difference between the anteroposterior dimensions of the 3D models of the knee and prosthetic component in the sagittal plane [12]. In the model of the native knee, the anteroposterior dimension APk was defined as the distance between the anterior femoral cortex and the posterior condyle. In the model of the prosthetic component, the anteroposterior dimension APc was defined as the distance between the most proximal point of the backside of the anterior flange and the posterior condyle (Fig. 1). The criterion for selecting an appropriate size of the prosthetic component was set at |APk – APc| < 2 mm. For example, if APk was 54.5–58.5 mm, an MP component of size 3 (APc = 56.5 mm) was selected, whereas if APk was < 54.5 mm or > 58.5 mm, MP components of size 2 or 4, respectively, were selected.

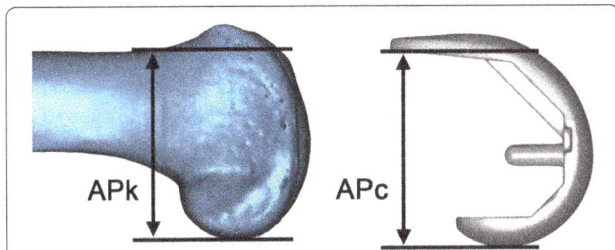

Fig. 1 Approach for selecting prosthetic components for performing virtual total knee arthroplasty. The size of the femoral component used in the simulation was chosen so that the three-dimensional models of the native knee and prosthetic components have similar anteroposterior dimensions in the sagittal plane (|APk − Apc| < 2 mm; APk, distance between the anterior femoral cortex and posterior condyle in the model of the native femur; APc, distance between the most proximal point of the backside of the anterior flange and the posterior condyle in the model of the prosthetic component)

Superimposing the prosthetic component model onto the knee model

We performed virtual surgery (virtual TKA) with the purpose of detecting the appropriate size of the implant (i.e., to size the implant). The following 3D planes were established for the virtual TKAs. The coronal plane was defined as the plane passing through the farthest posterior points of the medial and lateral condyles and those of the greater trochanter. The sagittal plane was defined as the plane passing through the center of the femoral head and the center of the intercondylar notch of the knee, perpendicularly to the coronal plane. The transverse plane was defined as the plane perpendicular to both the coronal and sagittal planes. The model of the selected prosthetic component was then positioned with its coronal plane parallel to the coronal plane of the native-knee model. Next, the model of the prosthetic component was oriented with its distal condyles parallel to the transverse plane, and its posterior condyles at 3° of external rotation from the coronal plane of the native-knee model. The model of the prosthetic component was translated in the 3D space until it overlapped with the native-knee model, such that: the medial-lateral center of the prosthetic component reached the sagittal plane of the native knee; the backside of the most proximal point of the anterior flange of the prosthetic component reached the anterior cortex of the native femur; and the distal medial condyle of the prosthetic component reached the surface of the medial condyle of the native knee [12].

Cutting planes and parameters of the cross-sectional morphology

In the sagittal plane, a cylinder was established with its axis parallel to both the coronal and transverse planes, and its radius was adjusted to allow the cylindrical surface to closely fit the trochlear groove of the bone

(Fig. 2); the axis of the cylinder was represented by the axis of the trochlear groove (Figs. 2 and 3). The fit of this cylindrical region of interest was first performed by the eye, based on experience, provided that we could clearly identify the groove of the prosthesis and the groove of the native knee (Fig. 2). Then, the radius of the cylinder and the position (coordinates) of its center were recorded; this measurement was performed twice to test the repeatability and sensitivity of the results. Once the cylinder was fitted, the geometrical parameters could be established. Starting from a plane parallel to the transverse plane (0° cutting plane), cutting planes were established in 45° increments towards the distal end of the trochlear groove, resulting in three cross-sections (0, 45 and 90°; Fig. 2). In each cross-section (Fig. 3), the deepest point in the trochlear groove (a) and the highest point on each condyle facet (b, c) were identified in both the native- and prosthetic-knee models. The following parameters characterizing the cross-sectional morphology of the femoral trochlea were defined: sulcus height (H), as the distance between point a and the groove axis; lateral tilt angle (α), as the angle between segment ab and the groove axis; medial tilt angle (β), as the angle between segment ac and the groove axis; sulcus angle, as the angle between segments ab and ac (Fig. 3). In order to obtain the values of the cross-sectional morphology parameters for angles, the following geometric parameters were defined: $h1$ and $h2$, representing the distances between a line parallel to the groove axis that passes through point a, and points b and c, respectively; $w1$ and $w2$, representing the distances between sulcus height (H) and $h1$ and $h2$, respectively (Fig. 3). Subsequently, the lateral and medial tilt angles were calculated as $\alpha = \arctan(h1/w1)$ and $\beta = \arctan(h2/w2)$. The morphological parameters were measured or calculated, as appropriate, for each of the 3D models used (i.e., 42 models of the native knee, and 42×4 models of prosthetic components).

To eliminate inter-observer bias, all measurements were performed by the same surgeon. To assess the repeatability of the measurements, each parameter was measured two times in one randomly selected model of the native knee. A test-retest analysis was performed to determine intra-observer reliability between the initial measurements and a repeat measurement performed over a month later. The low standard deviation of the two measurements indicated high repeatability of the measurements.

Statistical analysis

One-way analysis of variance (Fisher's Least Significant Difference and Student-Newman-Keuls) was used to compare the measurements for different cross-sections. The Student's t test was used to compare the native and

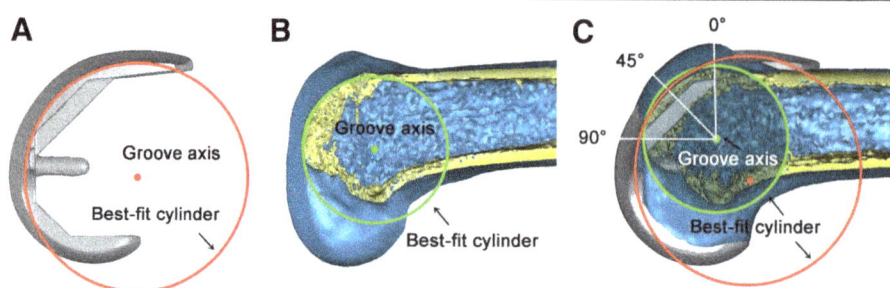

Fig. 2 Definition of the three cross-sections of the femoral trochlea in a three-dimensional model of the knee. **a, b** To help define the geometrical parameters of interest, a cylinder was established in the sagittal plane, with its axis represented by the axis of the trochlear groove, and its radius adjusted to allow the cylindrical surface to closely fit the trochlear groove of the prosthesis (**a**) or that of the bone (**b**). The fit was first performed by eye, provided that the trochlear groove was clearly visible in both the model of the prosthesis (**a**) and in that of the native knee (**b**). **c** Cutting planes were defined at 0, 45 and 90° starting form a plane parallel to the transverse plane, and rotating in 45° increments towards the distal end of the trochlear groove. The cutting planes were applied to the cylinder whose surface best fit the trochlear groove (**a, b**). The axis of the best-fit cylinder for the native knee (*green circle*) corresponds to the groove axis (**b**). The axis of the best-fit cylinder for the prosthetic knee (*red circle*) may not coincide with that of the best-fit cylinder for the native knee (*green*), as the radius was adjusted to allow the cylindrical surface to closely fit the trochlear groove of the prosthesis, leading to variations in sulcus height for the three cross-sections analyzed

prosthetic knees in terms of sulcus height (H), lateral tilt angle (α), medial tilt angle (β) and sulcus angle in each cross-section. A *p*-value less than 0.05 was considered to indicate statistical significance.

Results

The APk for all right knees included in the study was 55.4–58.4 mm. Based on the criterion |APk – Apc| < 2 mm, we selected the following components: MP of size 3 (APc = 56.5 mm), Triathlon of size 7+ (APc = 57 mm), NRG of size 7+ (APc = 55.8 mm), and NexGen of size E (APc = 56.9 mm).

There was no significant difference among the values measured for sulcus height (H) (average, 18 mm) in the in three cross-sections of the native-knee model (Table 1, Fig. 4). In the 0° cross-section, sulcus height (H) was

18.52 mm in the native knee, which was significantly smaller than that noted for the Triathlon, NRG and Nex-Gen components ($p < 0.05$; Table 1, Fig. 4). Concerning angles, only 28 knee models were included in the analysis, because the beginning of trochlear groove varied significantly with each individual; as such, the trochlear groove, lateral tilt angle (α) and medial tilt angle (β) could not be identified in this cross-section for all models. Compared to the native knees, prosthetic components showed significantly smaller lateral tilt angle (α), and significantly larger medial tilt angle (β) ($p < 0.05$; Table 2, Fig. 4). In the 45° cross-section, the sulcus height (H) was 18.24 mm in the native knee, which was significantly larger than that noted for the MP, Triathlon and NexGen components ($p < 0.05$). Both lateral tilt angle (α) and medial tilt angle (β) were significantly

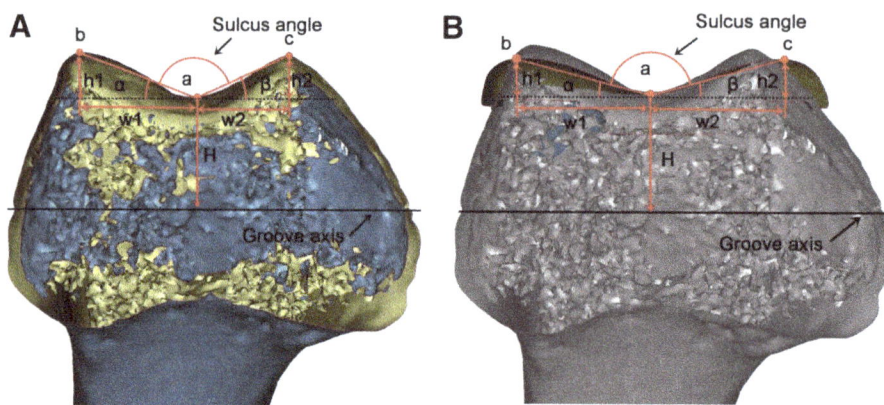

Fig. 3 Definition of parameters characterizing the cross-sectional morphology of the femoral trochlea (transverse plane) in three-dimensional models of the native (**a**) and prosthetic knee (**b**). The lateral tilt angle (α) could be calculated as arctan (h1/w1), while the medial tilt angle (β) could be calculated as arctan (h2/w2)

Table 1 Sulcus height (mm) in cross-sections of the femoral trochlea, as measured in threedimensional models of native and prosthetic knees ($n = 42$)

	0° cross-section	45° cross-section	90° cross-section
MP	18.5 (1.4)	16.8 (1.5)[*]	20.3 (1.8)[*]
Triathlon	19.2 (1.4)[*]	17.0 (1.5)[*]	-
NRG	20.1 (1.4)[*]	17.8 (1.5)	-
NexGen	19.3 (1.5)[*]	16.9 (1.5)[*]	-
Native knee	18.5 (1.4)[*a]	18.2 (1.3)[*a]	18.8 (1.2)[*a]

All parameters are reported as mean (standard deviation)
[*] Significant difference ($p < 0.05$) when comparing against the native knee
[a] Native knee taken as reference

lower in the prosthetic than in the native knees ($p < 0.05$; Table 3, Fig. 4). In the 90° cross-section, only data regarding the MP component were collected, as most prosthetic trochlear grooves of the other knee components (Triathlon, NRG and NexGen) were not long enough to be intersected with the 90° cutting plane (cross section), and point a could not be identified in this cross-section for prosthetic components other than MP. For the native knee, sulcus height (H) was 18.78 mm, which was significantly smaller than that noted for the MP component ($p < 0.05$); the native knee showed significantly smaller lateral tilt angle (α) and significantly larger medial tilt angle (β) ($p < 0.05$; Table 4, Fig. 4). In all cross-sections, the sulcus angle was significantly smaller in the native than the prosthetic knees ($p < 0.05$; Tables 2, 3 and 4, Fig. 4).

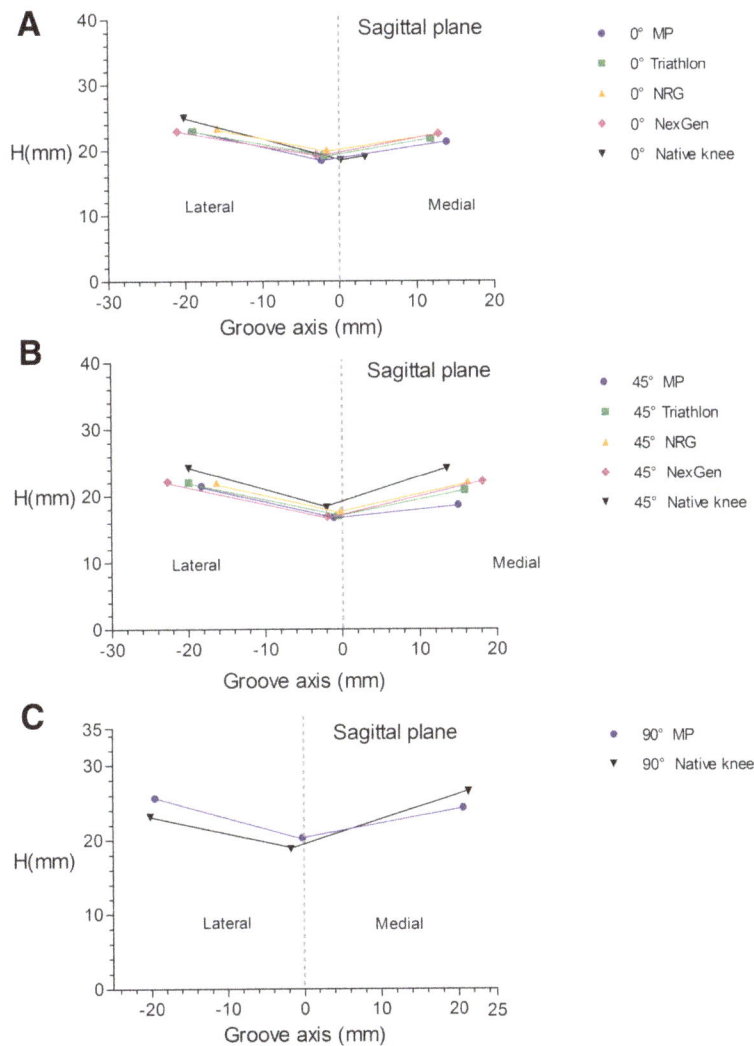

Fig. 4 Sulcus height (H) as a key geometric feature of the patellofemoral articular surface. In each case, the line describes the overall profile of the patellofemoral articular surface, characterized by the deepest point in trochlear groove (*a; midpoint of the line*) and the highest point on each condyle facet (*b, c; outer points of the line*). See Fig. 4a for an explanation of each parameter. **a** 0° cross-section; **b** 45° cross-section; **c** 90° cross-section

Table 2 The lateral tilt, medial tilt and sulcus angles of the femoral trochlea calculated based on 0° cross-sections of three-dimensional models of native and prosthetic knees ($n = 28$)

0° cross-section	Lateral tilt angle (°)	Medial tilt angle (°)	Sulcus angle (°)
MP	15.5	9.8	172.6
Triathlon	13.3	11.4	173.2
NRG	13.9	12.1	173.5
NexGen	12.5	13.2	172.3
Native knee	16.4 (2.9)	4.5 (5.3)	159.1 (6.7)

All parameters are reported as mean or mean (standard deviation)
Significant differences ($p < 0.05$) between the native and prosthetic knees were noted for all angles evaluated

Discussion

In the present study, we performed a detailed comparison of the cross-sectional morphology of the femoral trochlea in native and prosthetic knees. We based our choice of cutting planes on the previous report that 20° of patellofemoral flexion occurs for every 30° of knee flexion [13]. Thus, 0, 45 and 90° cross-sections of the trochlear groove are roughly representative of 0, 67.5 and 135° knee flexion [14]. Importantly, as there are differences in femur geometry parameters between Asian and Caucasian populations [15], and our findings were obtained based on measurements in Chinese subjects, it should be kept in mind that our findings are applicable to the Chinese population, and caution should be exerted when extrapolating our conclusions to non-Asian populations.

In our definition, sulcus height (H) represented the distance between the rotating axis and the trochlear groove. Since we found no significant variation among the three cross-sections in terms of sulcus height (H) values for the native knee models, we concluded that the surface of the cylinder defined in our assessment was indeed a close fit to the trochlear groove (Fig. 2). For the prosthetic knees, sulcus height (H) was comparatively higher in the 0° cross-section (by 0.76 mm), lower in the 45° cross-section (by 1.12 mm), then again higher in the

Table 3 The lateral tilt, medial tilt and sulcus angles of the femoral trochlea calculated based on 45° cross-sections of three-dimensional models of native and prosthetic knees ($n = 42$)

45° cross-section	Lateral tilt angle (°)	Medial tilt angle (°)	Sulcus angle (°)
MP	15.5	6.8	157.7
Triathlon	15.4	14.3	150.3
NRG	15.5	15.6	148.9
NexGen	14.8	15.4	149.8
Native knee	18.5 (2.6)	20.8 (2.8)	140.7 (4.4)

All parameters are reported as mean or mean (standard deviation)
Significant differences ($p < 0.05$) between the native and prosthetic knees were noted for all angles evaluated

Table 4 The lateral tilt, medial tilt and sulcus angles of the femoral trochlea calculated based on 90° cross-sections of three-dimensional models of native and prosthetic knees ($n = 42$)

90° cross-section	Lateral tilt angle (°)	Medial tilt angle (°)	Sulcus angle (°)
MP	15.2	11.7	153.1
Native knee	13.5 (2.8)	18.4 (3.2)	148.0 (4.8)

All parameters are reported as mean or mean (standard deviation)
Significant differences ($p < 0.05$) between the native and prosthetic knees were noted for all angles evaluated

90° cross-section (by 1.53 mm) (Table 1, Fig. 4). Therefore, the native and prosthetic knees differ in terms of the best cylinder radius that would allow the cylindrical surface to closely fit the trochlear groove (Fig. 2). The discrepancies between the native and prosthetic knees in terms of sulcus height (H) values, which are exemplified in Fig. 2, may be related to different positioning of the patella following TKA; as the position of the patella determines the lever arm of the extensor mechanism, such inappropriate design of the prosthetic components is likely to influence quadriceps efficiency as well as joint reaction forces and contact levels on the femoral trochlea or condyles [11]. Such differences might also cause the component to become anteriorly displaced, as evident in the higher sulcus height (H) values noted for the 0 and 90° cross-sections. Richard et al. [16] reported that, with increasing knee flexion, patellar tilt angle in the sagittal plane was substantially greater in prosthetic than in native knees, which might be related to anterior displacement of the implant. Indeed, Mihalko et al. [17] reported that a 2- and 4-mm build-up in the patellofemoral compartment resulted in flexion loss of 1.8 and 4.4°, respectively. Therefore, prosthetic trochlear design should be modified to avoid irritation of the soft tissue during initial and late knee flexion.

In the native knee, we noted that the sulcus angle first decreased and then increased when moving forward through the cross-sections (i.e., 159.11°, 140.66°, 148.04° in the 0°, 45° and 90° cross-sections, respectively), indicating that the bony structure may give more freedom for the patella to engage into the groove, but may hold the patella during knee flexion. This observation should be considered in the context of the patella-femoral reaction force (PRF), which represents the resultant vector of the quadriceps tendon strain force and the patellar tendon strain force, and is oriented inward in the coronal and axial views. The inward vector of PRF, occurring on the slope of the lateral femoral trochlea, neutralizes the lateral vector produced by the Q-angle of the knee [18, 19]. Therefore, the inward vector of PRF increases with the lateral tilt angle (α), stabilizing the patella. In the 0° cross-section, the PRF is relatively small, and thus the decrease in lateral tilt angle (α) has little effect on the PRF vector or the stability of the patella. However, recent studies revealed that quadriceps forces are highest between 70 and 110° [11, 20, 21]. In the 45° cross-section (67.5° of knee flexion), the PRF is relatively high, and thus the decrease in lateral tilt angle (α) might result in a decrease in the PRF vector and subsequent patellar instability. In the 90° cross-section (135° knee flexion), even though the lateral tilt angle (α) in the MP component is higher than that noted in the native knee, the patella transits over the intercondylar notch [11, 22, 23], and it is the retinacula, rather than the bony structure, that might serve as the main factor maintaining patellar stability. As the patella tilts laterally from 0 to 75° of knee flexion [24], the contact area is mainly on the lateral side; however, the medial tilt (β) might affect patellar tilting during knee flexion, together with the sulcus angle, and does not represent the main factor regulating patellar motion in the 0 and 45° cross sections. Additionally, the sulcus angle was larger in the prosthetic components in all cross-sections, which represents an adverse factor for patellar restraint. Therefore, after TKA, patellar stability might be more dependent on the static and dynamic stability of soft tissues rather than on the bony structure.

The present study showed that the prosthetic trochlear design does not correspond to the morphology of the native trochlea. In mid-flexion, the sulcus height (H), sulcus angle and lateral tilt angle (α) were all significantly lower in the prosthetic components, which might cause lever arm shortening, extensor weakness and decrease in the inward vector of PRF. These changes in anatomy might provide explanations for the clinical prevalence of relative quadriceps weakness [12, 25] and potential patellar dislocation after TKA. Hence, the current prosthetic trochlea might not facilitate patellar motion and quadriceps strength in mid-knee flexion.

In a well-aligned and balanced total knee prosthesis, the resurfaced patella will present a complex 3D movement pattern, broadly similar to that noted in the native knee, as discussed above. The behavior of a particular patellar component is dependent on the surface geometry variables of the mating femoral component, as well as the extrinsic stability provided by muscle and soft tissue support. Articular surface geometries of patellar components vary greatly, and each implant design bears particular advantages, with none being ultimately superior [19]. For example, the majority of currently available patellar components are of the all-polyethylene, dome-shaped type, which may compensate for limited degrees of patellar tilt and rotation by maintaining acceptable contact congruency. Regarding femoral components, on the one hand, the MP, Triathlon and NexGen prostheses evaluated provide deepened central femoral grooves in the 45° cross-section, and the MP component has a distal extension of the trochlear groove. For patella resurfacing or non-resurfacing, such designs would be patella-friendly and provide more stability. On the other hand, all four prostheses provide larger sulcus angles than those in the native knee in all three cross-sections examined; for this reason, we speculate that, other than the native patella, the resurfaced patella would maintain stability better than the non-surfaced patella because of improved contact congruency. By contrast, if undergoing arthroplasty, native knees with similar angles would provide more stability if the native patella were retained.

There were some limitations in this study. First, the data regarding three prosthetic systems were not complete for the 90° cross-sections, as the prosthetic groove of the posterior stabilized component was not long enough to be identified in this cross-section. Therefore, more appropriate components should be included in a future study. Second, the geometry of the cartilage surface differed from that of the bone in the trochlea, although the difference was small [14]. Third, this study only focused on the anatomical parameters of the femoral trochlea obtained from 3D-CT images, to provide some explanations with clinical implications. However, the dynamic performance of the implant and its effect on patellar motion and ligament tension should be studied in the future. Finally, only one implant size was included for each prosthetic component, even though most components are available in several sizes. Nevertheless, the implants were sized according to well-established protocols and criteria (e.g., |APk – APc| < 2 mm) and commonly used based on our experience. Moreover, the study participants were selected from an imaging database with data regarding the lower extremities of 100 healthy Chinese individuals (50 males, 50 females). Furthermore, since implants of different sizes are manufactured in the same shape, our findings regarding shape-specific parameters are relevant even if they were obtained based on one implant size.

Conclusions

Our study revealed that the discrepancy between the trochlear geometries of the native and prosthetic knee may alter knee mechanics. Nevertheless, these observations should be further investigated through cadaveric, computational or fluoroscopic studies. Our findings can be used to optimize biomechanical guidelines for total knee arthroplasty (patellar resurfacing or non-resurfacing) in Chinese individuals so as to decrease the risk of patellar lateral dislocation, maintain stability and optimize extensor kinematics.

Abbreviations
3D: Three-dimensional; CT: Computed tomography; PRF: Patella-femoral reaction force; TKA: Total knee arthroplasty

Acknowledgement
We thank Mr. Jason Du for support with expert language editing of our manuscript.

Funding
This study was supported by the National Natural Science Foundation of China (Grant No.81272037). The funders had no role in study design, data collection and analysis, decision to publish or preparation of the manuscript.

Authors' contributions
YW designed the study, analyzed the data and wrote and revised the manuscript. ZD designed the study, performed measurements and reviewed the manuscript. MNY and BY performed measurements. SCC designed the study and reviewed the manuscript. All authors read and approved the final manuscript.

Competing interest
The authors declare that they have no competing interests.

Consent for publication
Not applicable.

Author details
[1]Department of Bone and Joint Surgery, Renji Hospital, School of Medicine, Shanghai Jiaotong University, 145 Middle Shandong Road, Shanghai 200001, China. [2]Department of Orthopaedic Surgery, Ninth People's Hospital, Shanghai Jiaotong University School of Medicine, Shanghai, China.

References
1. Armstrong AD, Brien HJ, Dunning CE, King GJ, Johnson JA, Chess DG. Patellar position after total knee arthroplasty: influence of femoral component malposition. J Arthroplasty. 2003;18:458–65.
2. Skwara A, Tibesku CO, Ostermeier S, Stukenborg-Colsman C, Fuchs-Winkelmann S. Differences in patellofemoral contact stresses between mobile-bearing and fixed-bearing total knee arthroplasties: a dynamic in vitro measurement. Arch Orthop Trauma Surg. 2009;129:901–7.
3. Kainz H, Reng W, Augat P, Wurm S. Influence of total knee arthroplasty on patellar kinematics and contact characteristics. Int Orthop. 2012;36:73–8.
4. Boyd Jr AD, Ewald FC, Thomas WH, Poss R, Sledge CB. Long-term complications after total knee arthroplasty with or without resurfacing of the patella. J Bone Joint Surg Am. 1993;75:674–81.
5. Varadarajan KM, Freiberg AA, Gill TJ, Rubash HE, Li G. Relationship between three-dimensional geometry of the trochlear groove and in vivo patellar tracking during weight-bearing knee flexion. J Biomech Eng. 2010;132:061008.
6. Varadarajan KM, Rubash HE, Li G. Are current total knee arthroplasty implants designed to restore normal trochlear groove anatomy? J Arthroplasty. 2011;26:274–81.
7. Dejour D, Ntagiopoulos PG, Saffarini M. Evidence of trochlear dysplasia in femoral component designs. Knee Surg Sports Traumatol Arthrosc. 2014;22:2599–607.
8. Merican AM, Ghosh KM, Baena FR, Deehan DJ, Amis AA. Patellar thickness and lateral retinacular release affects patellofemoral kinematics in total knee arthroplasty. Knee Surg Sports Traumatol Arthrosc. 2014;22:526–33.
9. Akbari Shandiz M, Boulos P, Saevarsson SK, Yoo S, Miller S, Anglin C. Changes in knee kinematics following total knee arthroplasty. Proc Inst Mech Eng H. 2016;230:265–78.
10. Kulkarni SK, Freeman MA, Poal-Manresa JC, Asencio JI, Rodriguez JJ. The patellofemoral joint in total knee arthroplasty: is the design of the trochlea the critical factor? J Arthroplasty. 2000;15:424–9.
11. Saffarini M, Zaffagnini S, Bignozzi S, Colle F, Marcacci M, Dejour D. Does patellofemoral geometry in TKA affect patellar position in mid-flexion? Knee Surg Sports Traumatol Arthrosc. 2015;23:1799–807.
12. Chen S, Zeng Y, Yan M, Yue B, Zhang J, Wang Y. Morphological evaluation of the sagittal plane femoral load-bearing surface in computer-simulated virtual total knee arthroplasty implantation at different flexion angles. Knee Surg Sports Traumatol Arthrosc. 2016. doi:10.1007/s00167-016-3997-1.
13. Lee TQ, Gerken AP, Glaser FE, Kim WC, Anzel SH. Patellofemoral joint kinematics and contact pressures in total knee arthroplasty. Clin Orthop Relat Res. 1997;340:257–66.
14. Chen S, Du Z, Yan M, Yue B, Wang Y. Morphological classification of the femoral trochlear groove based on a quantitative measurement of computed tomographic models. Knee Surg Sports Traumatol Arthrosc. 2016. doi:10.1007/s00167-016-4236-5.
15. Yue B, Varadarajan KM, Ai S, Tang T, Rubash HE, Li G. Differences of knee anthropometry between Chinese and white men and women. J Arthroplasty. 2011;26:124–30.
16. Komistek RD, Dennis DA, Mabe JA, Walker SA. An in vivo determination of patellofemoral contact positions. Clin Biomech. 2000;15:29–36.
17. Mihalko W, Fishkin Z, Krackow K. Patellofemoral overstuff and its relationship to flexion after total knee arthroplasty. Clin Orthop Relat Res. 2006;449:283–7.
18. Schindler OS, Scott WN. Basic kinematics and biomechanics of the patello-femoral joint. Part 1: The native patella. Acta Orthop Belg. 2011;77:421–31.
19. Schindler OS. Basic kinematics and biomechanics of the patellofemoral joint part 2: the patella in total knee arthroplasty. Acta Orthop Belg. 2012;78:11–29.
20. Calliess T, Schado S, Richter BI, Becher C, Ezechieli M, Ostermeier S. Quadriceps force during knee extension in different replacement scenarios with a modular partial prosthesis. Clin Biomech. 2014;29:218–22.
21. Mason JJ, Leszko F, Johnson T, Komistek RD. Patellofemoral joint forces. J Biomech. 2008;41:2337–48.
22. Clarke HD, Fuchs R, Scuderi GR, Mills EL, Scott WN, Insall JN. The influence of femoral component design in the elimination of patellar clunk in posterior-stabilized total knee arthroplasty. J Arthroplasty. 2006;21:167–71.
23. Hozack WJ, Rothman RH, Booth Jr RE, Balderston RA. The patellar clunk syndrome. A complication of posterior stabilized total knee arthroplasty. Clin Orthop Relat Res. 1989;241:203–8.
24. Nha KW, Papannagari R, Gill TJ, Van de Velde SK, Freiberg AA, Rubash HE, Li G. In vivo patellar tracking: clinical motions and patellofemoral indices. J Orthop Res. 2008;26:1067–74.
25. Mizner RL, Stevens JE, Snyder-Mackler L. Voluntary activation and decreased force production of the quadriceps femoris muscle after total knee arthroplasty. Phys Ther. 2003;83:359–65.

24

Total knee arthroplasty: risk factors for allogeneic blood transfusions in the South Asian population

Syed Hamza Mufarrih[1*], Nada Qaisar Qureshi[1], Arif Ali[3], Azeem Tariq Malik[1], Huda Naim[2] and Shahryar Noordin[3]

Abstract

Background: Total knee arthroplasty (TKA) is the recommended treatment for end-stage knee osteoarthritis. Considering the various risks associated with intra and postoperative blood transfusions, better understanding is required with respect to the risk factors contributing to a greater possibility of blood transfusion during or after surgery. Although literature highlights several such factors, our study is among the first to identify these risk factors in the South Asian population which differs from other populations in several ways.

Methods: The study consists of a review of 658 patients undergoing TKA from 2005 to 2015. Data was obtained from patient medical records and was analysed using logistic regression analysis. The relationship between each predictor and the outcome variable was calculated as an Odds ratio (OR), the threshold of significance for which was $p = 0.25$ and $p = 0.05$ for univariate and multivariable analysis respectively.

Results: The mean age of the patient population was 63 years (78% female), 25% of whom received one or more blood transfusions. Multivariable analysis revealed 5 significant independent predictors for increased risk of blood transfusions including bilateral knee surgery (OR:5.51), preoperative anemia (OR:4.15), higher ASA (American Society of Anaesthesiologists) status (3–4) (OR:1.92), female sex (OR:3.44) and BMI (Body mass index) ≤30 (OR:1.79) while increasing co-morbidities and age (>60) were found to be insignificant.

Conclusions: The factors identified for the South Asian population are largely similar to those for other populations. Identification of high risk patients will permit the application of an international multipronged approach which not only targets the modifiable risk factors but also the decision making process and blood management protocols in order to minimize the transfusion associated risks for a patient undergoing a TKA.

Keywords: Blood transfusion, Total knee Arthroplasty, Risk factors

Background

Total Knee Arthroplasty (TKA) is the treatment of choice for several end stage knee diseases. The aim of the procedure is to relieve pain and restore the mobility of the patient and has been proven to have excellent results [1]. Intra and post-operative blood transfusions increase the cost of surgery, not only directly but also through the use of staff time and hospital resources and prolonging hospital stay [2]. In developing countries, the chance of acquiring blood borne infections is an added risk associated with blood transfusions [3]. Previous

literature identifies, estimated blood loss, preoperative anemia, bilateral procedures, advancing age, female sex, higher ASA (American Society of Anesthesiologists) status and low BMI (Body mass index) among others as significant predictors for blood transfusions following TKA [4–8]. To our knowledge, there has been no publication which assesses these risks in patients from South Asia. The genetic variation between different ethnicities has significant medical implications. The rationale for this is population-specific mutations, linkage disequilibrium and different selecting pressures [9]. This leads to the basis of unequal disease-associated and risk-associated allele distribution in different populations which results in discrete findings in different populations [9]. Similarly,

* Correspondence: hamzamufarrih@live.com
[1]Aga Khan University, Karachi, Pakistan
Full list of author information is available at the end of the article

literature highlights several other differences between populations worldwide for instance lower anti-coagulant requirements in Asian population suggests differences in the coagulation factors between different ethnicities [10–12] which would affect intra operative blood loss. South Asia also has one of the highest rates of anemia secondary to increased prevalence of carrier state of haemoglobinopathies and micronutrient deficiencies [13–17]. In addition to higher prevalence of anaemia, studies have also shown that Asians have a higher bleeding tendency [18]. While the rates of obesity in many Asian countries are similar to those in USA, the predisposition to developing obesity related non-communicable diseases such as osteoarthritis is higher is Asians [18, 19]. An important non-communicable disease prevalent in Asians is diabetes which alters haemostatic and thrombotic state of the body [20]. Along with this, ethnicity also plays a role when it comes to sociocultural beliefs regarding lifestyle modifications including dietary habits and physical activity along with poor accessibility to self-care facilities [21]. These factors, together with others such as a longer mean operative duration make it imperative to study blood transfusions intra and post-surgery in the Asian population. The aim of our study was to identify the factors which increase the risk of blood transfusions during and after total knee arthroplasty surgery in the South Asian population.

Methods

Study design and patient population

We conducted a retrospective review of the hospital course of 658 patients who underwent Total Knee Arthroplasty (TKA) between May 2005 and December 2015 at our University Hospital. All patients admitted for an elective TKA with a primary diagnosis of advanced osteoarthritis or rheumatoid arthritis refractory to conservative management were included in the study. Patients undergoing revision arthroplasty or having another orthopaedic procedure in addition to a TKA during one anaesthetic session, as well as patients with missing relevant clinical information were excluded from the study. Unilateral surgeries and staged bilateral procedures were included in the unilateral category while the simultaneous bilateral procedure patients were included in the bilateral category. Data was obtained from the medical record files of all patients included in the study. Data variables studied were patient demographics, body mass index (BMI), concomitant co-morbidities including Diabetes mellitus (DM), Hypertension (HTN), Asthma and chronic obstructive pulmonary disease (COPD), Thyroid Disease, Coronary artery disease (CAD), dyslipidaemia, Chronic kidney disease (CKD), preoperative and postoperative haemoglobin levels, length of hospital stay,

type of anaesthesia, American Society of Anaesthesiologists (ASA) score, Anaesthesia and Operative time, estimated intraoperative blood loss, and any intra and post-operative blood transfusions received by the patient.

Clinical course

Prior to the surgical procedure, every patient visited the orthopaedic clinic where a thorough evaluation and all preoperative investigations were done. The patients were also preoperatively evaluated by anaesthesia and relevant services depending on their co-morbidities in conjunction with anaesthesia. Patients received routine postoperative physiotherapy. Along with being vitally monitored, post-operative day one measurements of blood haemoglobin levels were requested to access the need for blood transfusions. There are 8 major societies who have published transfusion criteria. In general, the different guidelines have recommended that transfusion is not indicated for haemoglobin >10 g/dL, but the lower threshold varies from 6 g/dL to 8 g/dL [22, 23]. In our setup, patients were transfused blood after written consent, based on the criteria of either experiencing persistent symptoms such as dizziness, tachycardia, hypotension or shortness of breath with a haemoglobin level of less than 9 g/dl or asymptomatic anaemia with a blood haemoglobin level of less than 7 g/dl. Discharge was based on the attainment of a stable hemodynamic status and independent mobilization with support.

Statistical analysis

Data analysis was performed using SPSS Version 22. Descriptive analyses were conducted on all study measures, including patient characteristics and features of their hospital stay, using measures of central tendency for continuous measures and proportions for binary measures. Before stating central tendencies, normality test was run on the data. For normally distributed data, mean was used as the measure of central tendency while median was used as the measure of central tendency for skewed data. The relationship between blood transfusion as the outcome variable with various predictors such as age, sex, type of surgery, ASA, number of co-morbidities, obesity, preoperative haemoglobin levels and operative time was analysed by fitting a logistic regression model. The outcome variable was treated as binary, by use of the following categories: no transfusions versus 1 or more transfusions. The threshold for statistical significance was set at $p = 0.25$ for univariate analysis and $p = 0.05$ for multivariable analyses. The variables found to be insignificant in univariate analysis were excluded from the multivariable analysis.

Results

Patient characteristics and features of hospital stay

The mean age of the patient population was 62.5 years with 78% female. Most patients had at least 1 but not more than 2 comorbid conditions, with hypertension and diabetes being the more prominent ones. The mean BMI of the patients was 30.95, categorized as obese in our study, supporting the well-established relationship between obesity and development and progression of osteoarthritis [24], which was also the most common diagnosis of the patients selected for surgery. More patients underwent simultaneous bilateral TKA (58.7%) in comparison to unilateral (41.3%) procedures. The mean preoperative hemoglobin level was in the normal range for females according to the cutoff value of >11, but was low for males (cutoff > 13.6). The mean operative duration for unilateral and bilateral surgeries was 146 and 257 min respectively. The co-morbidities found prevalent were hypertension (58.2%), diabetes (28.1%) and CAD (8.5%) among others. Most patients were diagnosed with Osteoarthritis (95.6%) while a small proportion suffered from other diseases such Rheumatoid arthritis (3.6%). The most common type of anesthesia used was General (45.5%), followed by epidural combined with general (34.4%) and epidural alone (20.1%). Out of the 658 patients, 25% received blood transfusions. Descriptive analysis for the above mentioned and additional measures are given in Tables 1 and 2.

Effect of predictors on blood transfusions

The findings of our study have been tabulated in Table 3 as odds ratio (with 95% confidence interval) for univariate analysis and adjusted odds ratio (with 95% confidence interval) for multivariable analysis along with the significance of each finding as a p-value, the threshold

Table 1 Patient Characteristics (continuous variables)

Variable	Central Tendency
Age (y)	62.5 ± 9.7
BMI (kg/m2)	30.47 ± 5.36
Pre-op Haemoglobin (g/dL)	
Male	13.16 ± 1.43
Female	12.11 ± 1.27
Operative Duration (min)	
Unilateral	143 ± 37
Bilateral	254 ± 56
Estimated Blood Loss (ml)	153 ± 124
Post-op Haemoglobin (g/dL)	
Male	11.14 ± 1.39
Female	10.17 ± 1.34
Length of Stay (days)	9.00 ± 3

Table 2 Patient Characteristics (non-continuous variables)

Variable	Categories	Percentage (%)
Gender	Male	21.9
	Female	78.1
No. of co-morbidities	0	29.8
	1–2	63.4
	≥3	6.84
ASA	Low risk (1–2)	77.5
	High risk (3–4)	22.5
Type of Surgery	Unilateral	41.3
	Bilateral	58.7
Transfusions	Received	25.1

for which is 0.25 for univariate analysis and 0.05 for multivariable analysis. Univariate analysis shows 6 significant variables for increased risk of blood transfusions: bilateral surgery (OR: 4.34), preoperative anaemia (OR: 2.20), higher ASA status (OR: 1.73), female gender (OR: 1.59), BMI ≤30 (OR: 1.37) and increasing number of co-morbidities (OR-1: 0.88, OR-2: 1.32, OR-3: 1.54, OR-4: 5.44). The effect of advancing age on the outcome variable was insignificant and was excluded from the multivariable analysis. Multivariable analysis revealed 5 significant variables increasing blood transfusions: bilateral surgery (OR: 5.51), preoperative anaemia (OR: 4.15), higher ASA status (OR: 1.92), female gender (OR: 3.44) and BMI ≤30 (OR: 1.79) while increasing number of co-morbidities was deemed insignificant.

Discussion

Our study identified bilateral Total knee arthroplasty surgery, preoperative anemia, the female sex, higher ASA grade (3–4) and lower BMI (≤30) as independent predictors for increased intra and post-operative blood transfusions. However, advancing age (>60) did not affect the outcome variable significantly. Increasing number of co-morbidities, although not an independent risk factor, also contributed to an increased risk of blood transfusions. These findings are mainly similar to those of previous studies done for other populations as discussed below except for the effect of increasing age. This encourages the use of international practices regarding blood loss and transfusion for the South Asian population despite the differences in genetics and lifestyle in comparison to other ethnicities.

Total Knee arthroplasty is now considered the gold standard for the treatment of end stage osteoarthritis [25]. With primary osteoarthritis being the most prevalent joint disease worldwide [26], it is crucial to study the factors affecting the outcomes of this surgery. While many studies have been done to study the long term

Table 3 Risk factors for allogeneic blood transfusions

Variable	Odds Ratio (95% CI) Univariate analysis	p-value	Adjusted Odds Ratio (95% CI) Multivariate analysis	p-value
Type of Surgery		<0.001		<0.001
Unilateral	1		1	
Bilateral	4.34 (2.81, 6.69)		5.51 (3.34, 9.01)	
ASA		0.007		0.009
Low Risk (1–2)	1		1	
High Risk (3–4)	1.73 (1.16, 2.58)		1.92 (1.18, 3.14)	
Pre-op Haemoglobin		<0.001		<0.001
Normal	1		1	
Low	2.20 (1.52, 3.20)		4.15 (2.48, 6.96)	
Sex		0.049		<0.001
Male	1		1	
Female	1.59 (1.00, 2.52)		3.44 (1.84, 6.43)	
BMI		0.098		0.008
> 30 (Obese)	1		1	
≤ 30 (non-Obese)	1.37 (0.94, 2.00)		1.79 (1.17, 2.76)	
No. of co-morbidities		0.048		0.379
None	1		1	
1	0.88 (0.56, 1.38)		0.84 (0.49, 1.42)	
2	1.32 (0.82, 2.12)		1.06 (0.60, 1.87)	
3	1.54 (0.79, 2.99)		1.15 (0.51, 2.58)	
4	5.44 (1.25, 23.61)		4.10 (0.81, 20.77)	
Age		0.825		
< 60 years	1			
≥ 60 years	1.04 (0.72, 1.50)			

outcomes of total knee arthroplasty surgery in terms of pain relief, restoration of mobility and overall quality of life [27, 28], lesser data is available on the improvement of the intra and postoperative course of the patient. Our study targets one aspect of the latter by studying the factors contributing to an increased risk of blood transfusion in patients undergoing Total Knee arthroplasty surgery.

Allogeneic blood transfusion can be a life-saving modality in the setting of acute blood loss as it is the fastest way to increase blood hemoglobin levels. Even though the process has evolved to much safer levels [29], statistics show the occurrence of side effects in 10% of the blood transfusions with 1/5000 transfusions suffering from serious adverse reactions, including hemolytic reactions, acute lung injury and multi organ failure secondary to bacterial contamination [30]. Additionally, allogeneic blood transfusions have been associated with an increased risk of complications including infections, fluid overload and an increased length of stay at the hospital [31, 32].

Our findings of simultaneous bilateral TKA being an independent risk factor blood transfusions is consistent with several findings in the past [2, 7, 33]. The greater amounts of blood loss may be due to simultaneous bilateral bone cuts and surgical trauma [5]. Research also shows that the second knee in bilateral sequential TKAs bleeds significantly more than the first one due to the hypothesized decrease in clotting factors following release of the first tourniquet and perioperative hypothermia as suggested by animal models and in vitro studies [34]. However, even with the benefit of decreased risk of blood transfusions in staged bilateral total knee arthroplasty (BTKA) (categorized as unilateral TKA in our study), there is evidence to suggest that the combined cost and duration of hospital stay together with the doubled risk of exposure to hospital environment and anesthesia for those undergoing staged BTKA overcome the advantage of requiring less blood transfusions. [35–38].

Results also revealed pre-operative hemoglobin to be a significant risk factor for allogeneic blood transfusions. These findings were consistent with numerous studies done in the past which have identified pre-operative hemoglobin as an independent risk factor for postoperative blood transfusions. [7, 39–46]. Because patients with low preoperative hemoglobin have a low reserve of red blood cells that are further lowered after the surgical procedure, they are at a higher risk of developing life-threatening anemia and therefore require blood transfusion to increase the hemoglobin level to an optimum level. Given this, correction of preoperative anemia by stimulating erythropoiesis through administration of iron and recombinant erythropoietin among other techniques has also been suggested [47–49].

High-risk patients (ASA > 3) were also at a higher risk of transfusions than low-risk (ASA 1–2) patients. Previous studies have agreed with this finding [8, 31, 39, 41, 50, 51]. This may be due to the association of ASA levels 3 and 4 with greater number of co-morbidities and a greater amount of intra operative blood loss [52].

Findings that females are at a higher risk of receiving blood transfusions have been supported by previous studies [2, 8]. Apart from the higher prevalence of iron deficiency anemia in women [53], this could be due to having the same cutoff value of 9 g/dl as the criteria for blood transfusion for both sexes while having a normal range of hemoglobin lower than that of men.

Even though most studies show no correlation between BMI and risk of blood transfusions [43–46, 54], few studies have stated that a lower BMI (<30) serves as an independent factor for increased risk of blood transfusions in comparison to obese individuals who have larger volume and a lower percentage of estimated blood loss (EBL) volume [39–42, 55]. Our findings agree with this as the results show that a BMI ≤ 30 acts as an independent factor for increased risk of blood transfusions.

Our study also identifies increasing number of comorbid conditions to increase the risk of blood transfusions, although not independently. We did not find any studies which have made the same comparison. Our findings may be due the association of comorbid conditions with higher ASA status which has been shown to be an independent predictor for blood transfusions.

Previous studies have shown advancing age (>60) to be a significant predictor of increased risk of blood transfusions following TKA surgery [2, 7, 8, 45, 51]. Diminished postoperative hematopoietic regenerative capacity secondary to advancing age could account for these findings [56]. Our findings do not demonstrate this relationship. This may be due to the fact that the mean age of the population being studied was 62.5 years, thus decreasing the sensitivity of our study to the effects of advancing age (≥60).

Having stated the risks associated with blood transfusions and the factors contributing to increased chances of receiving them, it is crucial to apply methods of minimizing their occurrence during the intra and postoperative course of the patient's experience. A multipronged approach can be adopted to target not only the various risk factors, but also the decision making process and

blood management protocols following identification of high risk patients [57].

Caveats
As a single centre study, the number of patients studied is not the true representation for the said population, which is the primary focus of our study. To our knowledge, this research is the first to study the South Asian population which differs from other populations in several ways, as discussed earlier. For greater accuracy and generalizability, multi-centred studies should be carried out including hospitals from several countries of South Asia.

Conclusions
Our study identifies simultaneous bilateral TKA surgery, preoperative anaemia, higher ASA grade (3 and above), female gender, and lower BMI (≤30) as independent predictors for an increased risk of blood transfusions during and following knee arthroplasty surgery in South Asian patients. These factors are similar to those for other populations thus encouraging the use of international guidelines for blood management protocols despite the differences in the genetic makeup and lifestyle between South Asians and other populations. This information will help us in identification of high risk patients and correction of modifiable risk factors to minimize the need for blood transfusions in South Asian patients undergoing TKA.

Abbreviations
ASA: American society of anaesthesiologists; BMI: Body Mass Index; BTKA: Bilateral total knee arthroplasty; CAD: Coronary artery disease; CI: Confidence interval; CKD: Chronic kidney disease; OR: Odds ratio; COPD: Chronic obstructive pulmonary disease; DM: Diabetes mellitus; EBL: Estimated blood loss; HTN: Hypertension; TKA: Total knee arthroplasty

Acknowledgements
Not applicable.

Funding
No funding required or received.

Authors' contributions
Analysed the data: SHM. Wrote the first draft of the manuscript: SHM. Contributed to the writing of the manuscript: NQQ. Agree with manuscript results and conclusions: SN. Jointly developed the structure and arguments for the paper: SHM, NQQ. Made critical revisions and approved final version: SN. Data collection: AA, AT, HN, SHM, NQQ. All authors reviewed and approved of the final manuscript.

Consent for publication
Not applicable.

Competing interests

The authors declare that they have no competing interests.

Author details

[1]Aga Khan University, Karachi, Pakistan. [2]Dow International Medical College, Karachi, Pakistan. [3]Aga Khan University Hospital, Karachi, Pakistan.

References

1. Moran CG, Horton TC. Total knee replacement: the joint of the decade. A successful operation, for which there's a large unmet need. 2000;320(7238): 820. http://www.bmj.com/content/320/7238/820?variant=full.
2. Nichols CI, Vose JG. Comparative risk of transfusion and incremental Total hospitalization cost for primary unilateral, bilateral, and revision Total knee Arthroplasty procedures. J Arthroplast. 2016;31(3):583–9. e1
3. Mahmood MA, Khawar S, Anjum AH, Ahmed SM, Rafiq S, Nazir I, et al. Prevalence of hepatitis B, C and HIV infection in blood donors of Multan region. Ann King Edward Med Univ. 2016;10(4). http://www.annalskemu. org/journal/index.php/annals/article/view/1264.
4. Romagnoli S, et al. Onsets of complications and revisions are not increased after simultaneous bilateral unicompartmental knee arthroplasty in comparison with unilateral procedures. Int Orthop. 2015;39(5):871–7.
5. Bohm ER, et al. Outcomes of unilateral and bilateral total knee arthroplasty in 238,373 patients. Acta Orthop. 2016;87(Suppl 1):24–30.
6. Brito SA, Rankin EA, McNear M. Acute blood loss anemia in the octogenarian Total knee Arthroplasty, estimated blood loss and transfusions rates. J Natl Med Assoc. 2016;108(1):86–9.
7. Hatzidakis AM, et al. Preoperative autologous donation for total joint arthroplasty. An analysis of risk factors for allogenic transfusion. J Bone Joint Surg. 2000;82(1):89–100.
8. Hart A, et al. Blood transfusion in primary total hip and knee arthroplasty. Incidence, risk factors, and thirty-day complication rates. J Bone Joint Surg Am. 2014;96(23):1945–51.
9. Ntzani EE, et al. Consistency of genome-wide associations across major ancestral groups. Hum Genet. 2012;131(7):1057–71.
10. Ma C. Current antithrombotic treatment in East Asia: some perspectives on anticoagulation and antiplatelet therapy. Thromb Haemost. 2012;107(6): 1014.
11. Ross AM, et al. A randomized trial confirming the efficacy of reduced dose recombinant tissue plasminogen activator in a Chinese myocardial infarction population and demonstrating superiority to usual dose urokinase: the TUCC trial. Am Heart J. 2001;142(2):244–7.
12. Addition of clopidogrel to aspirin in 45 852 patients with acute myocardial infarction. Randomised placebo-controlled trial. Lancet. 2005;366(9497): 1607–21.
13. Flint J, et al. 1 the population genetics of the haemoglobinopathies. Baillière's Clin Haematol. 1998;11(1):1–51.
14. DeMaeyer E, Adiels-Tegman M. *The prevalence of anaemia in the world. La prevalence de lanemie dans le monde*. World health statistics quarterly. Rapport Trimestriel de Stat Sanitaires Mondiales. 1985;38(3):302–16.
15. Weatherall DJ. The inherited diseases of hemoglobin are an emerging global health burden. Blood. 2010;115(22):4331–6.
16. Angastiniotis M, Modell B. Global epidemiology of hemoglobin disorders. Annals New York Acad Sci. 1998;850(1):251–69.
17. McLean E, et al. Worldwide prevalence of anaemia, WHO vitamin and mineral nutrition information system, 1993–2005. Public Health Nutr. 2009; 12(4):444.
18. Dodani S. Excess coronary artery disease risk in south Asian immigrants: can dysfunctional high-density lipoprotein explain increased risk? Vascular Health Risk Manag. 2008;4(5):953.
19. Misra A, Khurana L. Obesity-related non-communicable diseases: south Asians vs white Caucasians. Inter J Obes. 2011;35(2):167–87.
20. Grant P. Diabetes mellitus as a prothrombotic condition. J Int Med. 2007; 262(2):157–72.
21. Davidson EM, et al. Consideration of ethnicity in guidelines and systematic reviews promoting lifestyle interventions: a thematic analysis. European J Public Health. 2014;24(3):508–13.
22. Stehling L, et al. Practice guidelines for blood component therapy-a report by the American Society of Anesthesiologists Task Force on blood component therapy. Anesthesiol. 1996;84(3):732–47.
23. Retter A, et al. Guidelines on the management of anaemia and red cell transfusion in adult critically ill patients. British J Haematol. 2013;160(4):445–64.
24. Sekar S, et al. Dietary fats and osteoarthritis: insights, evidences, and new horizons. J Cell Biochem. 2017;118(3):453–63.
25. Carr AJ, et al. Knee replacement. Lancet. 2012;379(9823):1331–40.
26. Pereira D, et al. The effect of osteoarthritis definition on prevalence and incidence estimates: a systematic review. Osteoarthr Cartil. 2011;19(11):1270–85.
27. Anderson JG, et al. Functional outcome and patient satisfaction in total knee patients over the age of 75. J Arthropl. 11(7):831–40.
28. Wylde V, et al. Total knee replacement: is it really an effective procedure for all? Knee. 2007;14(6):417–23.
29. Ngo LT, Bruhn R, Custer B. Risk perception and its role in attitudes toward blood transfusion: a qualitative systematic review. Transfus Med Rev. 2013; 27(2):119–28.
30. Schoettker P, et al. Revisiting transfusion safety and alternatives to transfusion. Presse Med. 2016;45(7–8):e331–40. Pt 2
31. Bierbaum BE, et al. An analysis of blood management in patients having a total hip or knee arthroplasty. J Bone Joint Surg Am. 1999;81(1):2–10.
32. Husted H, Holm G, Jacobsen S. Predictors of length of stay and patient satisfaction after hip and knee replacement surgery: fast-track experience in 712 patients. Acta Orthop. 2008;79(2):168–73.
33. Rasouli MR, et al. Blood management after total joint arthroplasty in the United States: 19-year trend analysis. Transfusion. 2016;56(5):1112–20.
34. Bould M, et al. Blood loss in sequential bilateral total knee arthroplasty. The Journal Arthroplasty. 1998;13(1):77–9.
35. March LM, et al. Two knees or not two knees? Patient costs and outcomes following bilateral and unilateral total knee joint replacement surgery for OA. Osteoarthr Cartil. 2004;12(5):400–8.
36. Reuben JD, et al. Cost comparison between bilateral simultaneous, staged, and unilateral total joint arthroplasty. J Arthroplast. 1998;13(2):172–9.
37. Restrepo C, et al. Safety of simultaneous bilateral total knee arthroplasty. A meta-analysis. J Bone Joint Surg Am. 2007;89(6):1220–6.
38. Ritter MA, et al. Simultaneous bilateral, staged bilateral, and unilateral total knee arthroplasty. A survival analysis. J Bone Joint Surg Am. 2003;85-A(8): 1532–7.
39. Morais S, et al. Blood transfusion after primary total knee arthroplasty can be significantly minimised through a multimodal blood-loss prevention approach. Int Orthop. 2014;38(2):347–54.
40. Salido JA, et al. Preoperative hemoglobin levels and the need for transfusion after prosthetic hip and knee surgery: analysis of predictive factors. J Bone Joint Surg Am. 2002;84-A(2):216–20.
41. Rashiq S, et al. Predicting allogeneic blood transfusion use in total joint arthroplasty. Anesth Analg. 2004;99(4):1239–44. table of contents
42. Larocque BJ, Gilbert K, Brien WF. A point score system for predicting the likelihood of blood transfusion after hip or knee arthroplasty. Transfusion. 1997;37(5):463–7.
43. Ogbemudia AE, et al. Preoperative predictors for allogenic blood transfusion in hip and knee arthroplasty for rheumatoid arthritis. Arch Orthop Trauma Surg. 2013;133(9):1315–20.
44. Jiganti JJ, Goldstein WM, Williams CS. A comparison of the perioperative morbidity in total joint arthroplasty in the obese and nonobese patient. Clin Orthop Relat Res. 1993;289:175–9.
45. Noticewala MS, et al. Predicting need for allogeneic transfusion after total knee arthroplasty. J Arthroplast. 2012;27(6):961–7.
46. Park JH, et al. Predictors of perioperative blood loss in total joint arthroplasty. J Bone Joint Surg Am. 2013;95(19):1777–83.
47. Na HS, et al. Effects of intravenous iron combined with low-dose recombinant human erythropoietin on transfusion requirements in iron-deficient patients undergoing bilateral total knee replacement arthroplasty. Transfusion. 2011;51(1):118–24.
48. Cuenca J, et al. Preoperative haematinics and transfusion protocol reduce the need for transfusion after total knee replacement. Int J Surg. 2007;5(2):89–94.
49. Mercuriali F, et al. Use of recombinant human erythropoietin to assist autologous blood donation by anemic rheumatoid arthritis patients undergoing major orthopedic surgery. Transfusion. 1994;34(6):501–6.
50. Keating EM, et al. Predictors of transfusion risk in elective knee surgery. Clin Orthop Relat Res. 1998;357:50–9.
51. Bong MR, et al. Risks associated with blood transfusion after total knee arthroplasty. J Arthroplast. 2004;19(3):281–7.
52. Daabiss M. American Society of Anaesthesiologists physical status classification. Indian Journal Anaesthesia. 2011;55(2):111.

53. Agarwalla R, et al. Assessment of prevalence of anemia in and its correlates among community-dwelling elderly of Assam, India: a cross-sectional study. Int J Nutrition, Pharmacol, Neurological Diseases. 2016;6(1):23–7.
54. Sehat KR, Evans RL, Newman JH. Hidden blood loss following hip and knee arthroplasty. Correct management of blood loss should take hidden loss into account. J Bone Joint Surg Br. 2004;86(4):561–5.
55. Frisch N, et al. Effect of body mass index on blood transfusion in Total hip and knee Arthroplasty. Orthopedics. 2016;39(5):e844–9.
56. Tsuboi I, Harada T, Aizawa S. Age-related functional changes in hematopoietic microenvironment. J Physical Fitness Sports Med. 2016;5(2):167–75.
57. Goodnough LT, et al. Transfusion medicine. Second of two parts–blood conservation. N Engl J Med. 1999;340(7):525–33.

25

Surgically modifiable factors measured by computer-navigation together with patient-specific factors predict knee society score after total knee arthroplasty

Frank Lampe[1,3], Franziska Fiedler[2], Carlos J. Marques[1*], Anusch Sufi-Siavach[2] and Georg Matziolis[4]

Abstract

Background: The purpose was to investigate whether patient-specific factors (PSF) and surgically modifiable factors (SMF), measured by means of a computer-assisted navigation system, can predict the Knee Society Scores (KSS) after total knee arthroplasty (TKA).

Methods: Data from 99 patients collected during a randomized clinical trial were used for this secondary data analysis. The KSS scores of the patients were measured preoperatively and at 4-years follow-up. Multiple regression analyses were performed to investigate which combination of variables would be the best to predict the 4-years KSS scores.

Results: When considering SMF alone the combination of four of them significantly predicted the 4-years KSS-F score ($p = 0.009$), explaining 18 % of its variation. When considering only PSF the combination of age and body weight significantly predicted the 4-years KSS-F ($p = 0.008$), explaining 11 % of its variation. When considering both groups of predictors simultaneously the combination of three PSF and two SMF significantly predicted the 4-years KSS-F ($p = 0.007$), explaining 20 % of its variation.

Conclusions: Younger age, better preoperative KSS-F scores and lower BMI before surgery, a positive tibial component slope and small changes in femoral offset were predictors of better KSS-F scores at 4-years.

Keywords: Total knee replacement, Computer-assisted surgery, Prognosis, Outcome assessment

Background

Total knee arthroplasty (TKA) is an effective and cost-efficient [1–3] intervention for end-stage knee osteoarthritis (OA). The outcomes by which the success of TKA can be measured are different. Pain relief and the restoration of functional activities have been reported as the main outcomes after primary TKA [4]. Other authors have focused on aspects influencing health-related quality of life (HRQL) [5–9] or patient satisfaction [10–12].

In the field of outcome-research there is an increasing interest in understanding the factors that influence and may predict the results after TKA. In this context there are patient-specific factors (PSF) and surgically modifiable factors (SMF) that can be considered as potential predictors of outcomes. Examples of PSF are the preoperative range of movement (ROM) [13, 14], body mass index (BMI) [15] and the presence or absence of co-morbidities [16, 17]. Under SMF one could consider, among others, the type of prosthesis used [18, 19], changes in posterior tibial slope (PTS) [14] and changes in posterior condylar offset (PCO) [14]. In the past these factors could only be assessed by radiographs, with the well-known limitations of radiometric morphometry. Using computer-navigation systems a large variety of biomechanical parameters can be monitored and saved intra-operatively. Several meta-analyses have shown that navigated TKA can reduce the number of radiographic

* Correspondence: cmarques@schoen-kliniken.de
[1]Research Center of the Department of Orthopedics and Joint Replacement at the Schoen Klinik Hamburg Eilbek, Dehnhaide 120, D-22081 Hamburg, Germany
Full list of author information is available at the end of the article

outliers compared with traditional techniques, leading to significant improvements in prosthesis alignment and positioning [20–24].

From a clinician perspective, clinical scores are of great importance as endpoints because they are easy to apply. Their use is widespread, allowing comparisons between different populations. The knee society score (KSS) [25] is a validated rating system generally used to evaluate both the knee function and patient functional ability before and after TKA. With its KSS-Knee and KSS-Function sub-scores, it combines an objective physician-derived with a patient-subjective component. Pain relief, function and patient satisfaction can be evaluated.

The purpose of this study was to investigate the predictive value of PSF and SMF measured by means of a computer-assisted navigation system on the KSS ratings. It was hypothesized that a combination of PSF and SMF could explain a proportion of KSS variability at 4-years after surgery.

Methods
Subjects

This study is a secondary analysis of data obtained during a prospective randomized clinical trial designed to investigate the effects of mobile bearing (MB) vs. fixed-bearing (FB) TKA implants on clinical scores [26].

Ninety-nine patients (100 knees) scheduled for primary bicondylar, posterior cruciate retaining TKA at the Schoen Klinik Hamburg Eilbek were informed about the study and agreed to participate.

All patients met the following inclusion criteria: clinical and radiological signs of osteoarthritis of the knee with failed non-operative treatment; no indication for a uni-compartmental implant or joint-preserving osteotomies; age ranging from 40 to 90 years; American society of anaesthesiologists pre-operative classification grade 1–3; no deformity larger than 20° varus or 15° valgus; no previous bone surgery to the index knee; no previous total joint replacement at the index leg; no post-operative infection of the index knee or thrombosis within the follow-up period.

The patients were randomly assigned into one of the groups. At baseline there were 52 patients in the FB and 48 in the MB group. At 4 years follow-up there was a loss of 7 patients (13.5 %) in the FB group (2 died with no relation to TKA; 5 did not attend the 4 years follow-up) and 6 patients (12.5 %) in the MB group (1 septic implant exchange before 12 months; 3 did not attend the 1 year follow-up; 1 died with no relation to TKA).

The mean age of the patients by entrance in the study was 69.1 ± 7.8 years. The distribution of female and male patients in the sample was 73 and 27, respectively. There was no significant difference between the mean ages of

male and female patients ($p = 0.7$). The significant differences found when comparing the mean body weight ($p = 0.02$) and mean body height ($p < 0.001$) of both genders had no consequences in terms of mean BMI differences ($p = 0.2$). For further demographic data see Table 1.

Since there were no significant differences between the KSS scores in the fixed- and mobile-bearing groups at any measurement time, and no significant differences when comparing the ROM of both groups across the follow-up assessments [26], all patients were pooled into one group for the purpose of this secondary analysis of the data.

Before participating all patients were required to read and sign an informed consent form, in which their permission to anonymously save the navigation data registered during surgery for the purpose of this secondary data analysis was also requested. The medical Ethics Commission of the Federal State of Hamburg approved the research proposal (File #2226). The trial was registered under ClinicalTrial.gov (NCT00822640).

Materials

The computer-assisted navigation system OrthoPilot TKA version 4.2 (BBraun Aesculap, Tuttlingen, Germany) was used to perform all surgeries. The system is based on intra-operatively acquired data. An infrared camera tracks infrared diodes, which have been previously fixed on the femoral and tibia bones, on a hand-held pointer and on the cutting blocks [27]. The optical tracking system used by OrthoPilot is the hybrid Polaris Spectra® (Northern Digital Inc., Waterloo, Ontario, Canada). According to the supplier, the accuracy of the system is 0.25 mm RMS when applying the pyramid measurement volume method [28, 29].

The navigation system defines the mechanical axis of the leg. With navigation-adapted instruments the surgeon performs the femoral and tibial resection cuts under real-time control of the navigation parameters, allowing leg alignment corrections and soft-tissue balance. The reliability of leg alignment when using this system, as well as the reliability of the navigation guided gap technique were tested in the past in experimental settings [30, 31].

The extension and flexion gaps were measured after tibial cutting by the navigation system after introducing a device (Laminar spreader, BBraun Aesculap, Tutlingen, Germany) allowing independent tensioning of the medial and lateral joint gaps. Based on these measurements the femoral component size and position were planned, aiming to minimize gap inequalities and asymmetries as far as possible (tibia first technique). The measurement and calculation of the navigation variables was made on the bases of the

Table 1 Demographic data of the sample by the time of entry in the study

Variables	All	Female	Male	Mean Diff. (p-value) [95 % CI]
Number of Patients	$n = 100$	$n = 73$	$n = 27$	
Age (years)	69.1 ± 7.8	69.3 ± 7.9	68.7 ± 7.4	0.5 ($p = 0.7$) [-4.0 to 2.9]
Body Weight (Kg)	82.6 ± 15.7	80.5 ± 15.5	88.2 ± 14.8	7.7 ($p = 0.02$) [0.8 to 14.6] [*]
Body Height (cm)	167.1 ± 8.4	163.8 ± 6.4	176.0 ± 6.4	12.1 ($p < 0.001$) [9.2 to 15.0] [*]
BMI (Kg/m²)	29.5 ± 5.5	29.9 ± 5.7	28.5 ± 5.0	1.3 ($p = 0.2$) [-3.8 to 1.1]

Values are mean ± SD; [*] = Significant difference

resected bone surfaces. No additional measurements were performed after the implantation of the implant components. Detailed information on the surgical procedure and workflow when using the OrthoPilot system were published previously [32].

Measurements

For the present purpose preoperative and follow-up data acquired at 4- years post-surgery by a trained physician were used.

All surgeries were performed by one of two senior surgeons. Navigation data were recorded during surgery. Some navigation variables were calculated post-surgery based on the data obtained intra-operatively.

The fifteen SMF used in this study are explained in Table 2. Furthermore, the following PSF were used: patient's age by the time of surgery, body weight, body height, BMI, preoperative maximal knee flexion (Pre-OP MKF) and preoperative KSS scores (Pre-OP KSS).

Statistical analysis

Mean and standard deviation were used to describe the data, since all predictor variables are continuous. Normal distribution of the data was confirmed with the Kolmogorov-Smirnov test. Demographic data comparisons between male and female patients in the sample were performed on baseline data with a t-test for independent samples (Table 2).

Multiple regression analyses to estimate the contribution of different independent variables (SMF and PSF) to the explanation of 4-years KSS (dependent variable) were carried out in three phases. In the first phase Pearson's correlation was used to assess the univariate association between each independent variable (potential predictors) and the 4-years KSS scores. A p-value ≤ 0.20 was accepted as the level of significance to ensure that potentially relevant independent variables were not excluded at this stage as recommended in the literature [33]. In the second phase all independent variables that were significantly associated with the 4-years KSS-F

Table 2 Definition of the surgically modifiable factors (SMF)

Name	Abbreviation	Definition	Values
Femoral Joint Line Change max.	FJLCmax	Femoral joint line change from the most prominent condyle	Millimeter
Femoral Joint Line Change min.	FJLCmin	Femoral joint line change from the less prominent condyle	Millimeter
Femoral Component Slope	FS	Femoral component angle in the sagittal plane	Degrees
Tibial Joint Line Change	TJLC	Tibial joint line change from the unworn compartment	Millimeter
Tibial Component Slope	TCS	Tibial component angle in the sagittal plane	Degrees
Extension Gap Size Medial	EGSmed	Medial gap between the femoral and tibial components in extension	Millimeter
Extension Gap Size Lateral	EGSlat	Lateral gap between the femoral and tibial components in extension	Millimeter
Extension Gap Difference Medial-Lateral	EGDM-L	Difference between EGSmed and EGSlat (EG symmetry)	Millimeter
Flexion Gap Size Medial	FGSmed	Medial gap between the femoral and tibial components in 90° flexion	Millimeter
Flexion Gap Size Lateral	FGSlat	Lateral gap between the femoral and tibial components in 90° flexion	Millimeter
Flexion Gap Difference Medial-Lateral	FGDM-L	Difference between FGSmed and FGSlat (FG symmetry)	Millimeter
Flexion Extension Gap Difference	FEGD	Difference between the mean EGS and the mean FGS (Gap equality)	Millimeter
Femoral Offset Changes Medial	FOCmed	Difference between the medial FO before and after femoral component implantation	Millimeter
Femoral Offset Changes Lateral	FOClat	Difference between the lateral FO before and after femoral component implantation	Millimeter
Femoral Rotation	FR	Femoral rotation relative to the posterior condyle line	Degrees

score were entered into two backward multiple regression models. A stepping method criterion with a probability of F to remove ≥ 0.10 was used. The first model included only SMF and the second model included only PSP. Finally, in the third phase, a final model was generated including selected SMF and PSF. The selection of the independent variables for the third model was made based on the results of the two previous procedures, on the literature and on surgeons empirical knowledge. Since the unstandardized regression coefficients (B) communicate the direction (positive or inverse) and the weighting of the independent variable (predictor) relative to the other independent variables in explaining the variation of the dependent variable, only predictors with a unstandardized coefficient, which could be explained according to the existing literature were included in the final model.

The three models met the assumptions of multiple regressions in terms of linearity, homoscedasticity, normality, independence and non-multicollinearity.

All statistical tests were carried out with the use of the IBM SPSS software version 21 for Mac. For all statistical tests the 0.05 level of probability was accepted as the criterion for statistical significance.

Results

The correlation coefficients between the 15 SMF and the 4-years KSS-Function scores are presented in Table 3. Only six had a significant linear relationship with the 4-years KSS-F (Table 3). When considering only the SMF as potential predictors, the prediction model generated contained four of the six variables (FJLCmin, TCS, FGDM-L, FOCmed) and was reached in three steps (Table 4). The model was statistically significant, $F_{(4, 95)} = 3.7$, $p = 0.009$, and accounted for approximately 18 % of the variance of the 4-year KSS-F score ($R^2 = 0.18$, Adj. $R^2 = 0.13$). Three of the four predictors added statistically significantly to the prediction.

The correlation coefficients between PSF and the 4-years KSS-F scores are shown in Table 5. Four of the six PSF (body weight, BMI, age and Pre-OP KSS-F) had a significant linear relationship with the KSS-F score (Table 5). The prediction model generated contained two predictors (age and body weight) and was reached in three steps (Table 4). The model was statistically significant, $F_{(2, 97)} = 5.1$, $p = 0.008$, and explained approximately 11 % of the variance of 4-years KSS-F ($R^2 = .11$, Adj. $R^2 = .08$). Both predictors added statistically significantly to the prediction.

Finally, the combination of BMI, age, Pre-OP KSS-F, TCS and FOCmed significantly predicted 4-years KSS-F, $F_{(5, 94)} = 3.7$, $p = 0.007$, and accounted for approximately 20 % of the variance of 4-years KSS-F ($R^2 = .20$, Adj. $R^2 = .14$). Lower BMI, younger age and

higher KSS-F scores by the time of surgery, together with a positive (posterior) TCS and a good reconstruction (small changes) in FOCmed led to better KSS-F scores at 4-years. Only two of the five predictors added statistically significantly to the prediction (Table 4).

The correlation coefficients between SMF, PSF and the 4-years KSS-Knee scores are presented in Table 6. There were no significant correlations between the SMF and the KSS-Knee score at 4-years for a $p < 0.05$. As described above, a p-value ≤ 0.20 was accepted as the level of significance to ensure that potentially relevant independent variables were not excluded at this stage. Eight potential predictors (see Table 6) were selected and entered into a backward multiple regression model. The models created were not statistically significant. The same procedure was repeated for PSF. Again, no statistically significant models were found. A negative negligible relationship between KSS-K preoperatively and KSS-K at 4-years was statistically significant ($p < 0.05$).

Discussion

The aim of the present study was to investigate, whether it is possible to predict the KSS scores based on PSF and SMF obtained during computer-assisted TKA. The approach used is new. Fifteen potentially relevant SMF were accessed, which in part cannot be measured by radiographic morphometry. To the authors' best knowledge there are no publications available addressing such a high number of SMF. Neither are there any publications available addressing the relationships between PSF, SMF and the KSS ratings.

The key findings of the present study are: (1) PSF could explain 11 % of the 4-years KSS-F scores variability; (2) four SMF could explain 18 % of the 4-years KSS-F variability, however, the unstandardized coefficients (B) of two of the factors considered in the model (FJCmin and FGDM-L) could not be explained, therefore these factors were excluded from the final model; (3) a combination of PSF and SMF could explain the largest proportion (20 %) of the 4-years KSS-F variation.

According to the present results, older age, higher BMI and lower preoperative KSS-F ratings are preconditions that negatively influence the 4-years KSS-Function outcomes.

Several meta-analyses have shown that navigated TKA significantly improves prosthesis alignment, component position and limb alignment [34–36]. Only a few reports have shown that navigation can result in improved functional outcomes in TKA [21, 37].

In a meta-analysis investigating the influence of BMI on the outcomes of primary TKA a trend was reported

Table 3 Correlations between surgically modifiable factors (SMF) and 4-years KSS-F scores

Potential Predictor (Surgically modifiable variables)	KSS-F	FJLCmax	FJLCmin	FS	TJLC	TCS	EGSmed	EGSlat	EGDM-L	FGSmed	FGSlat	FGDM-L	FEGD	FOCmed	FOClat	FR
Femoral Joint Line Change max (FJLCmax)	.25*															
Femoral Joint Line Change min (FJLCmin)	.29*	.52*														
Femoral Component Slope (FS)	-.04	-.06	-.23*													
Tibial Joint Line Change (TJLC)	-.02	-.37*	-.16	-.14												
Tibial Component Slope (TCS)	.22*	.07	-.02	.30*	-.00											
Extension Gap Size Medial (EGSmed)	.05	.07	-.00	.00	-.24*	-.02										
Extension Gap Size Lateral (EGSlat)	.03	.32*	-.17	.17	-.33*	.14	.20									
Extension Gap Difference Med-Lat (EGDM-L)	.08	-.04	.13	-.02	.00	.03	-.22*	.31*								
Flexion Gap Size Medial (FGSmed)	.05	-.29*	-.15	.08	.17	-.09	-.07	-.16	-.11							
Flexion Gap Size Lateral (FGSlat)	-.04	-.30*	-.02	.08	.13	-.12	-.08	-.18	-.03	.71*						
Flexion Gap Difference Med-Lat (FGDM-L)	.16**	.05	.06	-.01	.09	.04	.00	.05	.08	.05	-.41*					
Flexion-Extension Gap Difference (FEGD)	-.02	-.36*	-.02	-.03	.37*	-.07	-.34*	-.53*	-.02	.54*	.62*	-.18				
Femoral Offset Changes Medial (FOCmed)	-.17**	.25*	.11	-.00	-.36*	.05	.26*	.17	-.02	-.29*	-.54*	.31*	-.45*			
Femoral Offset Changes Lateral (FOClat)	-.14**	.33*	.12	-.00	-.33*	.07	.25*	.23*	.03	-.36*	-.50*	.30*	-.45*			
Femoral Rotation (FR)	.05	.16	.07	-.03	.16	-.01	-.08	.05	.09	-.05	.18	-.04	.08	-.33		
Mean ± SD	85.2±15.6	1.5±1.9	0.7±2.3	0.1±1.2	3.0±1.7	3.9±1.1	0.6±1.2	1.7±2.1	1.9±1.4	3.1±1.4	2.8±1.6	0.7±0.9	2.2±1.6	2.6±2.7	0.3±2.5	3.4±1.3

p < .05; (**) p < .20 (Statistically significant linear relationship to 4-Y KSS-F in bold)

Table 4 Multiple regression models for 4-years KSS-F scores

	Dependent variable	Step	Predictors included	Predictors excluded	R^2	Adj. R^2	F	p^*	B	p^{**}
1st Model (only SMF)	4-years KSS-F	1	All six		0.20	0.12	2.6	**0.02**		
		2		FOClat	0.20	0.13	3.1	**0.01**		
		3	FJLCmin	FJLCmax	0.18	0.13	3.7	**0.009**	1.7	**0.02**
			TCS						2.8	**0.04**
			FGDM-L						3.7	**0.03**
			FOCmed						-1.3	0.05
2nd Model (only PSF)	4-years KSS-F	1	All four		0.11	0.07	11.4	**0.04**		
		2		BMI	0.11	0.08	3.5	**0.01**		
		3	Age	Pre-OP KSS-F	0.11	0.08	5.1	**0.008**	-0.2	**0.04**
			Body Weight						-0.6	**0.03**
3rd Model (combination of PSF and SMF)	4-years KSS-F	1	BMI		0.20	0.14	3.4	**0.007**	-0.7	**0.02**
			Age						-0.7	**0.001**
			Pre-OP KSS-F						0.04	0.5
			TCS						2.2	0.1
			FOCmed						-0.7	0.2

p^* = Statistical significance of the model; B = Unstandardized Coefficients; p^{**} = Statistical significance of the predictors included in the final model
Significant p-values in bold; *SMF* Surgically modifiable factors, *PSF* Patient-specific factors

for a lower postoperative KSS in obese (BMI ≥ 30 kg/m^2) patients than in non-obese (BMI < 30 kg/m^2) patients [38]. The present results reinforce this finding.

There is some evidence supporting the hypothesis that SMF, like the PTS and the PCO, influence the maximal knee flexion (MKF) after TKA [14, 39–43]. Since knee flexion is also assessed by the KSS and influences the performance of functional activities, it was hypothesized that these variables could probably predict 4-years KSS-F. According to the expectations and reinforcing the above mentioned studies, the "Tibial Component Slope" (TCS) and the "Femoral Offset Changes Medial" (FOCmed) were considered in the final model, as predictors of the 4-years KSS-F. Higher positive TCS values (which represents the same as higher posterior TCS values) were significant predictors of a higher 4-years KSS-F score. Small or no changes in FOC (the same as PCO), were also significant predictors of

better 4-years KSS-F scores. The present results support the ones of the above referred studies.

For the present sample the strongest predictors of 4-years KSS-F were the TCS, followed by BMI and Age. The present results support early knee replacement surgery once "Age" was significantly negatively correlated with 4-years KSS-F scores. Furthermore the "Pre-OP KSS-F" score was positively correlated with "4-years KSS-F" (Table 5).

Surprisingly, no significant predictors of KSS-K score were found, neither among SMF, nor among PSF. KSS-K is the more objective KSS score, since it is based on the assessor measurements. The authors have no explanation for this finding. Maybe the conversion of the more objective data into to the KSS-K score, with the use an algorithm, is behind this findings.

Due to the fact that this study is a secondary analysis of data, a prospectively performed power analysis wasn't

Table 5 Correlations between patient-specific factors (PSF) and 4-years KSS-F scores

Potential Predictors	**4-years KSS-F**	Body Weight	Body Height	BMI	Age	Pre-OP KSS-F	Pre-OP MKF
Body Weight	-.11**						
Body Height	-.04	.31*					
BMI	-.09**	.86*	-.20*				
Age	-.25*	-.35*	-.13	-.31*			
Pre-OP KSS-F	.08**	-.09	.04	-.12	-.01		
Pre-OP MKF	.03	-.00	.19*	-.09	-.12	.08	
Mean ± SD	85.0 ± 15.1	83.4 ± 15.9	167.1 ± 8.5	29.9 ± 5.6	68.9 ± 7.9	48.5 ± 19.8	110.0 ± 14.2

$^{(*)}$ $p < .05$; $^{(**)}$ $p < .20$; Statistically significant linear relationship to 4-Y KSS-F score in bold. *MKF* maximal knee flexion

Table 6 Correlations between SMF, PSF and 4-years KSS-Knee scores

Potential predictors surgically modifiable variables	KSS-K
Femoral Joint Line Change max (FJLCmax)	.18**
Femoral Joint Line Change min (FJLCmin)	.12**
Femoral Component Slope (FS)	.06
Tibial Joint Line Change (TJLC)	-.06
Tibial Component Slope (TCS)	.18**
Extension Gap Size Medial (EGSmed)	.06
Extension Gap Size Lateral (EGSlat)	.16**
Extension Gap Difference Med-Lat (EGDM-L)	.21**
Flexion Gap Size Medial (FGSmed)	.01
Flexion Gap Size Lateral (FGSlat)	-.09
Flexion Gap Difference Med-Lat (FGDM-L)	-.09
Flexion-Extension Gap Difference (FEGD)	-.16**
Femoral Offset Changes Medial (FOCmed)	-.11**
Femoral Offset Changes Lateral (FOClat)	-.07
Femoral Rotation (FR)	.11**
Patient-specific factors	
Body weight	-.11
Body height	-.04**
BMI	-.09**
Age	.00
KSS-K Preoperatively	-.17*
Maximal knee Flexion (MKF) Preoperatively	-.04
Mean (KSS-K) ± SD	87.2 ± 10.3

Potential predictors with a statistically significant linear relationship for
(*) p< 0.5 or (**) p< .20 in bold

possible. This is a study limitation. Further studies on this issue should be prospectively statistically powered. A second study limitation is related to the fact that co-morbidities were not accessed by the time the patients entered the study. Co-morbidities may significantly predict the results and should be accessed in further studies. A third study limitation concerns the fact that navigation data were obtained based on measurements upon the resected bone surfaces and further calculated by the software of the OrthoPilot system. Future studies on this matter should consider additional measurements after final implantation of the components, since the depth of cement mantle may influence the implant position and consequently the measured gaps.

The results of studies in this area could be used to identify patients at risk of poor outcomes submitting for TKA, as suggested by Lungu et al. [44]. The use of a regression equation prior to surgery to identify patients at risk could help to choose the appropriate course, such as pre-rehabilitation, participation in a weight-loss program before surgery or intensive post-operative rehabilitation.

Conclusions

Computer-navigation is a suitable tool to accurately measure and control a variety of SMF, which seem to affect clinical outcomes after TKA. Two PSF alone accounted for 11 % of the 4-years KSS-F variation. A combination of three PSF and two SMF explained 20 % of the 4-years KSS-F variability. According to the results of the present study, younger age, better preoperative KSS-F scores and lower BMI before surgery, a positive (posterior) Tibial Component Slope (TCS) and small changes in Femoral Offset (FOC) were predictors of better KSS-F scores at 4-years after TKA.

Abbreviations
BMI: body mass index; FB: fixed bearing; HRQL: health related quality of life; KSS: knee society score; KSS-F: knee society function score; MB: mobile bearing; Pre-OP MKF: pre-operatively maximal knee flexion; OA: osteoarthritis; PCO: posterior condylar offset; Pre-OP KSS: pre-operatively knee society score; PSF: patient specific factors; PTS: posterior tibial slope; ROM: range of motion; SMF: surgically modifiable factors (see also Table 2); TKA: total knee arthroplasty.

Competing interests
FL is consultant for B.Braun Aesculap. CJM research-position at the Research Center of the Department of Orthopedics and Joint Replacement at the Schoen Klinik Hamburg Eilbek is sponsored by B.Braun Aesculap. FF, ASS and GM have no financial relationships to disclose in relation to this manuscript.

Authors' contributions
FL and FF designed the study; FF and ASS gathered the data; CJM analyzed the data and wrote the initial draft of the manuscript; FL and CJM ensured the accuracy of the data and analysis; FL and GM reviewed the final version of the manuscript for its intellectual content. FL and FF contributions to the work were equivalent. All authors have read and approved the final version of the manuscript.

Acknowledgements
The authors would like to thank Dr. Bishop for proof reading the final version of the manuscript.

Level of Evidence
Level II, Prognostic study.

Author details
[1]Research Center of the Department of Orthopedics and Joint Replacement at the Schoen Klinik Hamburg Eilbek, Dehnhaide 120, D-22081 Hamburg, Germany. [2]Department of Orthopedics and Joint Replacement at the Schoen Klinik Hamburg Eilbek, Dehnhaide 120, D-22081 Hamburg, Germany. [3]Faculty of Life Sciences at the Hamburg University of Applied Sciences, Lohbrügger Kirchstraße 65, D-21033 Hamburg, Germany. [4]Orthopaedic Department, Jena University Hospital, Campus Eisenberg, Klosterlausnitzer Straße 81, D-07607 Eisenberg, Germany.

References
1. Daigle ME, Weinstein AM, Katz JN, Losina E. The cost-effectiveness of total joint arthroplasty: a systematic review of published literature. Best Pract Res Clin Rheumatol. 2012;26(5):649–58.
2. Krummenauer F, Wolf C, Gunther KP, Kirschner S. Clinical benefit and cost effectiveness of total knee arthroplasty in the older patient. Eur J Med Res. 2009;14:76–84.
3. Losina E, Walensky RP, Kessler CL, Emrani PS, Reichmann WM, Wright EA, et al. Cost-effectiveness of total knee arthroplasty in the United States: patient risk and hospital volume. Arch Intern Med. 2009;169(12):1113–21. discussion 1121-1112.

4. Lingard EA, Katz JN, Wright EA, Sledge CB. Predicting the outcome of total knee arthroplasty. J Bone Joint Surg Am. 2004;86-A(10):2179–86.
5. Alentorn-Geli E, Leal-Blanquet J, Guirro P, Hinarejos P, Pelfort X, Puig-Verdie L. Comparison of quality of life between elderly patients undergoing TKA. Orthopedics. 2013;36(4):e415–9.
6. Brandes M, Ringling M, Winter C, Hillmann A, Rosenbaum D. Changes in physical activity and health-related quality of life during the first year after total knee arthroplasty. Arthritis Care Res. 2011;63(3):328–34.
7. Bruyere O, Ethgen O, Neuprez A, Zegels B, Gillet P, Huskin JP, et al. Health-related quality of life after total knee or hip replacement for osteoarthritis: a 7-year prospective study. Arch Orthop Trauma Surg. 2012;132(11):1583–7.
8. Jones CA, Pohar S. Health-related quality of life after total joint arthroplasty: a scoping review. Clin Geriatr Med. 2012;28(3):395–429.
9. Papakostidou I, Dailiana ZH, Papapolychroniou T, Liaropoulos L, Zintzaras E, Karachalios TS, et al. Factors affecting the quality of life after total knee arthroplasties: a prospective study. BMC Musculoskelet Disord. 2012;13:116.
10. Jacobs CA, Christensen CP. Factors influencing patient satisfaction two to five years after primary total knee arthroplasty. J Arthroplast. 2014;29(6):1189–91.
11. Jacobs CA, Christensen CP, Karthikeyan T. Patient and intraoperative factors influencing satisfaction two to five years after primary total knee arthroplasty. J Arthroplast. 2014;29(8):1576–9.
12. Williams DP, O'Brien S, Doran E, Price AJ, Beard DJ, Murray DW, et al. Early postoperative predictors of satisfaction following total knee arthroplasty. Knee. 2013;20(6):442–6.
13. Bade MJ, Kittelson JM, Kohrt WM, Stevens-Lapsley JE. Predicting functional performance and range of motion outcomes after total knee arthroplasty. Am J Phys Med Rehabil. 2014;93(7):579–85.
14. Malviya A, Lingard EA, Weir DJ, Deehan DJ. Predicting range of movement after knee replacement: the importance of posterior condylar offset and tibial slope. Knee Surg Sports Traumatol Arthrosc. 2009;17(5):491–8.
15. Gadinsky NE, Ehrhardt JK, Urband C, Westrich GH. Effect of body mass index on range of motion and manipulation after total knee arthroplasty. J Arthroplast. 2011;26(8):1194–7.
16. Issa K, Jauregui JJ, Given K, Harwin SF, Mont MA. A prospective, longitudinal study of patient activity levels following total knee arthroplasty stratified by demographic and comorbid factors. J Knee Surg. 2015;28(4):343–7.
17. Pugely AJ, Martin CT, Gao Y, Belatti DA, Callaghan JJ. Comorbidities in patients undergoing total knee arthroplasty: do they influence hospital costs and length of stay? Clin Orthop Relat Res. 2014;472(12):3943–50.
18. Bin SI, Nam TS. Early results of high-flex total knee arthroplasty: comparison study at 1 year after surgery. Knee Surg Sports Traumatol Arthrosc. 2007;15(4):350–5.
19. Huang HT, Su JY, Wang GJ. The early results of high-flex total knee arthroplasty: a minimum of 2 years of follow-up. J Arthroplast. 2005;20(5):674–9.
20. Bae DK, Song SJ. Computer assisted navigation in knee arthroplasty. Clin Orthop Surg. 2011;3(4):259–67.
21. Clayton AW, Cherian JJ, Banerjee S, Kapadia BH, Jauregui JJ, Harwin SF, et al. Does the use of navigation in total knee arthroplasty affect outcomes? J Knee Surg. 2014;27(3):171–5.
22. Fu Y, Wang M, Liu Y, Fu Q. Alignment outcomes in navigated total knee arthroplasty: a meta-analysis. Knee Surg Sports Traumatol Arthrosc. 2012;20(6):1075–82.
23. Hetaimish BM, Khan MM, Simunovic N, Al-Harbi HH, Bhandari M, Zalzal PK. Meta-analysis of navigation vs conventional total knee arthroplasty. J Arthroplast. 2012;27(6):1177–82.
24. Thienpont E, Fennema P, Price A. Can technology improve alignment during knee arthroplasty. Knee. 2013;20 Suppl 1:S21–8.
25. Insall JN, Dorr LD, Scott RD, Scott WN. Rationale of the Knee Society clinical rating system. Clin Orthop Relat Res. 1989;248:13–4.
26. Marques CJ, Daniel S, Sufi-Siavach A, Lampe F. No differences in clinical outcomes between fixed- and mobile-bearing computer-assisted total knee arthroplasties and no correlations between navigation data and clinical scores. Knee Surg Sports Traumatol Arthrosc. 2015;23(6):1660–8.
27. Clemens U, Miehlke RK. Advanced navigation planning including soft tissue management. Orthopedics. 2005;28(10 Suppl):s1259–62.
28. Nothern Digital Incorporation: Polaris Optical Tracking Systems (2015). http://www.ndigital.com/medical/products/polaris-family/#specifications. Accessed 8 December 2015.
29. Wiles AD, Thompsen DG, Frantz DD. Accuracy assessment and interpretation for optical tracking systems. In: Medical Imaging 2004: Visualisation, Image-Guided Procedures and Display: 2004; San Diego, California, USA. 2004. p. 421–32.
30. Han SB, Nha KW, Yoon JR, Lee DH, Chae IJ. The reliability of navigation-guided gap technique in total knee arthroplasty. Orthopedics. 2008; 31(10 Suppl 1).
31. Hauschild O, Konstantinidis L, Strohm PC, Niemeyer P, Suedkamp NP, Helwig P. Reliability of leg alignment using the OrthoPilot system depends on knee position: a cadaveric study. Knee Surg Sports Traumatol Arthrosc. 2009;17(10):1143–51.
32. Lampe F, Hille E. Navigated Implantation of the Columbus Total Knee Arthroplasty with the OrthoPilot System: Version 4.0. In: Navigation and Robotics in Total Joint and Spine Surgery. edn.: Springer Berlin Heidelberg; 2004: 248–253.
33. Katz MH. Multivariate Analysis: A Practical Guide for Clinicians and Public Health Researchers. Cambridge: Cambridge University Press; 2011.
34. Mason JB, Fehring TK, Estok R, Banel D, Fahrbach K. Meta-analysis of alignment outcomes in computer-assisted total knee arthroplasty surgery. J Arthroplast. 2007;22(8):1097–106.
35. Quack VM, Kathrein S, Rath B, Tingart M, Luring C. Computer-assisted navigation in total knee arthroplasty: a review of literature. Biomedizinische Technik Biomedical engineering. 2012;57(4):269–75.
36. Venkatesan M, Mahadevan D, Ashford RU. Computer-assisted navigation in knee arthroplasty: a critical appraisal. J Knee Surg. 2013;26(5):357–61.
37. Moskal JT, Capps SG, Mann JW, Scanelli JA. Navigated versus conventional total knee arthroplasty. J Knee Surg. 2014;27(3):235–48.
38. Si HB, Zeng Y, Shen B, Yang J, Zhou ZK, Kang PD, et al. The influence of body mass index on the outcomes of primary total knee arthroplasty. Knee Surg Sports Traumatol Arthrosc. 2015;23(6):1824–32.
39. Fujimoto E, Sasashige Y, Masuda Y, Hisatome T, Eguchi A, Masuda T, et al. Significant effect of the posterior tibial slope and medial/lateral ligament balance on knee flexion in total knee arthroplasty. Knee Surg Sports Traumatol Arthrosc. 2013;21(12):2704–12.
40. Hohmann E, Bryant A, Reaburn P, Tetsworth K. Does posterior tibial slope influence knee functionality in the anterior cruciate ligament-deficient and anterior cruciate ligament-reconstructed knee? Arthroscopy. 2010;26(11):1496–502.
41. Kim JH. Effect of posterior femoral condylar offset and posterior tibial slope on maximal flexion angle of the knee in posterior cruciate ligament sacrificing total knee arthroplasty. Knee Surg Relat Res. 2013;25(2):54–9.
42. Shi X, Shen B, Kang P, Yang J, Zhou Z, Pei F. The effect of posterior tibial slope on knee flexion in posterior-stabilized total knee arthroplasty. Knee Surg Sports Traumatol Arthrosc. 2013;21(12):2696–703.
43. Singh G, Tan JH, Sng BY, Awiszus F, Lohmann CH, Nathan SS. Restoring the anatomical tibial slope and limb axis may maximise post-operative flexion in posterior-stabilised total knee replacements. Bone Joint J. 2013;95-B(10):1354–8.
44. Lungu E, Desmeules F, Dionne CE, Belzile EL, Vendittoli PA. Prediction of poor outcomes six months following total knee arthroplasty in patients awaiting surgery. BMC Musculoskelet Disord. 2014;15(1):299.

Permissions

All chapters in this book were first published in MD, by BioMed Central; hereby published with permission under the Creative Commons Attribution License or equivalent. Every chapter published in this book has been scrutinized by our experts. Their significance has been extensively debated. The topics covered herein carry significant findings which will fuel the growth of the discipline. They may even be implemented as practical applications or may be referred to as a beginning point for another development.

The contributors of this book come from diverse backgrounds, making this book a truly international effort. This book will bring forth new frontiers with its revolutionizing research information and detailed analysis of the nascent developments around the world.

We would like to thank all the contributing authors for lending their expertise to make the book truly unique. They have played a crucial role in the development of this book. Without their invaluable contributions this book wouldn't have been possible. They have made vital efforts to compile up to date information on the varied aspects of this subject to make this book a valuable addition to the collection of many professionals and students.

This book was conceptualized with the vision of imparting up-to-date information and advanced data in this field. To ensure the same, a matchless editorial board was set up. Every individual on the board went through rigorous rounds of assessment to prove their worth. After which they invested a large part of their time researching and compiling the most relevant data for our readers.

The editorial board has been involved in producing this book since its inception. They have spent rigorous hours researching and exploring the diverse topics which have resulted in the successful publishing of this book. They have passed on their knowledge of decades through this book. To expedite this challenging task, the publisher supported the team at every step. A small team of assistant editors was also appointed to further simplify the editing procedure and attain best results for the readers.

Apart from the editorial board, the designing team has also invested a significant amount of their time in understanding the subject and creating the most relevant covers. They scrutinized every image to scout for the most suitable representation of the subject and create an appropriate cover for the book.

The publishing team has been an ardent support to the editorial, designing and production team. Their endless efforts to recruit the best for this project, has resulted in the accomplishment of this book. They are a veteran in the field of academics and their pool of knowledge is as vast as their experience in printing. Their expertise and guidance has proved useful at every step. Their uncompromising quality standards have made this book an exceptional effort. Their encouragement from time to time has been an inspiration for everyone.

The publisher and the editorial board hope that this book will prove to be a valuable piece of knowledge for researchers, students, practitioners and scholars across the globe.

List of Contributors

Yeying Zhang
Department of Anesthesiology, the Affiliated Hospital of Hangzhou Normal University, 126 Wenzhou Road, Hangzhou, Zhejiang 310015, China

Ming Lu
Department of Cardiology, Second Affiliated Hospital of Zhejiang Chinese M edical University, Hangzhou, Zhejiang 310005, China

Cheng Chang
Department of anesthesiology, School of Medicine, Hangzhou Normal University, the affiliated Hospital of Hangzhou Normal University, 16 Xuelin St, Xiasha Higher Education Campus, Hangzhou, Zhejiang 310036, China

Patrick McAllister
Rebalance MD, 3551 Blanshard St, Victoria, BC V8Z 0B9, Canada

Syed Hamza Mufarrih, Nada Qaisar Qureshi and Azeem Tariq Malik
Aga Khan University, Karachi, Pakistan

Arif Ali and Shahryar Noordin
Aga Khan University Hospital, Karachi, Pakistan

Huda Naim
Dow International Medical College, Karachi, Pakistan

Zhe Du, Bing Yue and You Wang
Department of Bone and Joint Surgery, Renji Hospital, School of Medicine, Shanghai Jiaotong University, 145 Middle Shandong Road, Shanghai 200001, China

Shichang Chen and Mengning Yan
Department of Orthopaedic Surgery, Ninth People's Hospital, Shanghai Jiaotong University School of Medicine, Shanghai, China

Hai-bo Si
Key Laboratory of Transplant Engineering and Immunology, West China Hospital, Sichuan University, No.1 Keyuan 4th Road, Chengdu, Sichuan 610041, China

Department of Orthopedic Surgery, West China Hospital, Sichuan University, 37th Guoxue Road, Chengdu, Sichuan 610041, China

Ti-min Yang, Yi Zeng, Zong-ke Zhou, Fu-xing Pei and Bin Shen
Department of Orthopedic Surgery, West China Hospital, Sichuan University, 37th Guoxue Road, Chengdu, Sichuan 610041, China

Yan-rong Lu and Jing-qiu Cheng
Key Laboratory of Transplant Engineering and Immunology, West China Hospital, Sichuan University, No.1 Keyuan 4th Road, Chengdu, Sichuan 610041, China

Rebecca M. Meiring, Emmanuel Frimpong and Joanne A. McVeigh
Exercise Physiology Laboratory, School of Physiology, Faculty of Health Sciences, University of the Witwatersrand, 7 York Rd, Parktown, Johannesburg, South Africa

Lipalo Mokete, Jurek Pietrzak and Dick Van Der Jagt
Division of Orthopaedics, Faculty of Health Sciences, University of the Witwatersrand, 7 York Rd, Parktown, Johannesburg, South Africa

Mohammed Tikly
Division of Rheumatology, Department of Medicine, Chris Hani Baragwanath Academic Hospital, Faculty of Health Sciences, University of the Witwatersrand, 7 York Rd, Parktown, Johannesburg, South Africa

Mona Badawy
Coastal Hospital, 5253 Hagavik, Norway

Anne M. Fenstad and Christoffer A. Bartz-Johannessen
The Norwegian Arthroplasty Register, Department of Orthopaedic Surgery, Haukeland University Hospital, Bergen, Norway

Kari Indrekvam
Coastal Hospital, 5253 Hagavik, Norway
Department of Clinical Medicine, Institute of Medicine and Dentistry, University of Bergen, Bergen, Norway

Leif I. Havelin and Ove Furnes
The Norwegian Arthroplasty Register, Department of Orthopaedic Surgery, Haukeland University Hospital, Bergen, Norway
Department of Clinical Medicine, Institute of Medicine and Dentistry, University of Bergen, Bergen, Norway

Otto Robertsson and Annette W-Dahl
The Swedish Knee Arthroplasty Register, Lund, Sweden
Department of Clinical Sciences, Lund University Faculty of Medicine, Orthopedics, Lund, Sweden

Antti Eskelinen
The Coxa Hospital for Joint Replacement, Tampere, Finland

Keijo Mäkelä
Department of Orthopaedics and Traumatology, Turku University Hospital, Turku, Finland

Alma B. Pedersen
The Danish Knee Arthroplasty Register, Aarhus, Denmark
Department of Clinical Epidemiology, Aarhus University Hospital, Aarhus, Denmark

Henrik M. Schrøder
Department of Orthopaedic surgery, Næstved Hospital, Næstved, Denmark

Joon Kyu Lee and Ki Tae Kim
Department of Orthopaedic Surgery, Hallym University Sacred Heart Hospital, 22 Gwanpyeong-ro, 170beon-gil, Dongan-gu, Anyang-si, Gyeonggi-do 431-796, Korea

Sahnghoon Lee, Sae Hyung Chun and Myung Chul Lee
Department of Orthopaedic Surgery, Seoul National University Hospital, 101 Daehang-ro, Jongno-gu, Seoul 110-744, Korea

Johannes K. M. Fakler, Cathleen Pönick, Alexander Giselher Brand and Andreas Roth
Department of Orthopaedic Surgery, Traumatology and Plastic Surgery, University Hospital Leipzig, Liebigstrasse 20, D-04103 Leipzig, Germany

Melanie Edel, Robert Möbius, Christoph Josten and Dirk Zajonz
Department of Orthopaedic Surgery, Traumatology and Plastic Surgery, University Hospital Leipzig, Liebigstrasse 20, D-04103 Leipzig, Germany

ZESBO – Center for Research on Musculoskeletal Systems, University of Leipzig, Semmelweisstrasse 14, D-04103 Leipzig, Germany

Jasvinder A. Singh
Medicine Service, VA Medical Center, 700 19th St S, Birmingham, AL 35233, USA
Department of Medicine at School of Medicine, University of Alabama at Birmingham Faculty Office Tower, 805B, 510 20th Street S, Birmingham, AL 35294, USA
Division of Epidemiology at School of Public Health, University of Alabama at Birmingham, 1720 Second Ave. South, Birmingham, AL 35294-0022, USA
Department of Orthopedic Surgery, Mayo Clinic College of Medicine, 200 1st St SW, Rochester, MN 55905, USA

Siamak Noorbaloochi
Center for chronic disease Outcomes Research, Minneapolis Veterans Affairs Health System Center, Minneapolis, MN 55121, USA
Department of Medicine, University of Minnesota, 401 East River Parkway, Minneapolis, MN 55455, USA

Keith L. Knutson
Department of Immunology, Mayo Clinic College of Medicine, 200 1st St SW, Rochester, MN 55905, USA

Kun-hao Hong
Department of Orthopedic Surgery, Guangdong Second Traditional Chinese Medicine Hospital, No. 60 Hengfu Road, Guangzhou, Guangdong 510095, China

Jian-ke Pan, Wei-yi Yang, Ming-hui Luo, Shu-chai Xu and Jun Liu
Department of Orthopedic Surgery, Second School of Clinical Medicine, Guangzhou University of Chinese Medicine, No. 111 Dade Road, Guangzhou, Guangdong 510120, China

Benjamin Panzram, Ines Bertlich, Tobias Reiner, Tilman Walker, Sébastien Hagmann and Tobias Gotterbarm
Clinic of Orthopaedic and Trauma Surgery, University of Heidelberg, Schlierbacher Landstr. 200a, 69118 Heidelberg, Germany

Jens Boldt
Akutklinik Siloah, Worbstrasse 324, CH 3073 Guemligen, Switzerland

Aamir Mahdi and Per Wretenberg
Department of Orthopaedics, Örebro County, Sweden
Faculty of Medicine and Health, School of Medical Sciences, Örebro University, Örebro, Sweden

Maria Hälleberg Nyman
Faculty of Medicine and Health, School of Health Sciences, Örebro University, Örebro, Sweden

P Pinsornsak, S Rojanavijitkul and S Chumchuen
Department of Orthopaedic Surgery, Thammasat University, 99 Moo 18, Khlong Nueng, Khlong Luang, Pathumthani, Thailand 12120

Peng Tian, Gui-jun Xu and Xin-long Ma
Department of Orthopedics, Tianjin Hospital, No. 406, Jiefang Nan Road, Tianjin 300211, People's Republic of China

Wen-bin Liu
Department of Joint Surgery, Tianjin Hospital, No. 406, Jiefang Nan Road, Tianjin 300211, People's Republic of China

Zhi-jun Li
Department of Orthopedics, General Hospital of Tianjin Medical University, No. 154, Anshan Road, Tianjin 300052, People's Republic of China

Yu-ting Huang
Cancer & Immunology Research, Children's Research Institute, Children's National Medical Center, 111 Michigan Avenue, NW, Washington, DC 20010, USA

Jian-ke Pan, Hui Xie, Ming-hui Luo, Da Guo and Jun Liu
Department of Orthopedics, Second Affiliated Hospital of Guangzhou University of Chinese Medicine (Guangdong Provincial Hospital of Chinese Medicine), No. 111 Dade Road, Guangzhou, Guangdong 510120, China

Kun-hao Hong
Department of Orthopedics, Guangdong Second Traditional Chinese Medicine Hospital, No. 60 Hengfu Road, Guangzhou, Guangdong 510095, China

Shajie Dang
Xi'an JiaoTong University, Xi'an 710004, China

Mona Badawy and Kari Indrekvam
Coastal Hospital in Hagavik, 5217 Hagavik, Norway
Department of Clinical Medicine, Institute of Medicine and Dentistry, University of Bergen, 5021 Bergen, Norway

Birgitte Espehaug
Center for Evidence-based Practice, Bergen University College, 5021 Bergen, Norway

Anne Marie Fenstad
The Norwegian Arthroplasty Register, Department of Orthopaedic Surgery, Haukeland University Hospital, 5021 Bergen, Norway

Håvard Dale
Department of Clinical Medicine, Institute of Medicine and Dentistry, University of Bergen, 5021 Bergen, Norway

Leif I. Havelin and Ove Furnes
The Norwegian Arthroplasty Register, Department of Orthopaedic Surgery, Haukeland University Hospital, 5021 Bergen, Norway
Department of Clinical Medicine, Institute of Medicine and Dentistry, University of Bergen, 5021 Bergen, Norway

Piya Pinsornsak and Adisai Chaiwuttisak
Department of Orthopaedics, Faculty of Medicine, Thammasat University, 99 Moo 18, Khlong Nueng, Khlong Luang, Pathum Thani 12120, Thailand

Krit Boontanapibul
Department of Orthopaedics, Chulabhorn International College of Medicine, Thammasat University, 99 Moo 18, Khlong Nueng, Khlong Luang, Pathum Thani 12120, Thailand

Yu-Hao Huang
Graduate Institute of Medical Sciences, National Defense Medical Center, No.161, Min-Chun E. Rd., Sec. 6, Neihu, Taipei 114, Taiwan, Republic of China

Chin Lin, Kwo-Tsao Chiang, Hsien-Feng Chang and Hsueh-Lu Chang
School of Public Health, National Defense Medical Center, No.161, Min-Chun E. Rd., Sec. 6, Neihu, Taipei 114, Taiwan, Republic of China

Jia-Hwa Yang
Graduate Institute of Life Sciences, National Defense Medical Center, No.161, Min-Chun E. Rd., Sec. 6, Neihu, Taipei 114, Taiwan, Republic of China

Leou-Chyr Lin and Chih-Chien Wang
Department of Orthopedics, Tri-Service General Hospital and National Defense Medical Center, No.325, Sec.2, Chenggong Rd., Neihu District, Taipei 114, Taiwan, Republic of China

Chih-Yuan Mou
Department of Aviation Medicine and Physical examination, National Defense Medical Center and Tri-Service General Hospital Songshan Branch, No.131, Jiankang Rd., Songshan District, Taipei 10581, Taiwan, Republic of China

Man-Gang Lee
Department of Surgery, Zuoying Branch of Kaohsiung Armed Forces General Hospital, No.553, Junxiao Rd., Zuoying Dist., Kaohsiung City 813, Taiwan, Republic of China

Wen Su
Department of Nursing, Tri-Service General Hospital, No.161, Min-Chun E. Rd., Sec. 6, Neihu, Taipei 114, Taiwan, Republic of China

Shih-Jen Yeh
Department of Research and Development, Da-Yeh University, No. 168, Xuefu Road, Dacun Township, Changhua County 515, Taiwan, Republic of China

Hung Chang
Department of Physiology and Biophysics, National Defense Medical Center, No.325, Sec. 2, Chenggong Rd., Neihu District, Taipei City 114, Taiwan, Republic of China
Division of Thoracic Surgery, Tri-Service General Hospital, National Defense Medical Center, No.325, Sec. 2, Chenggong Rd., Neihu District, Taipei City 114, Taiwan, Republic of China

Sui-Lung Su
School of Public Health, National Defense Medical Center, No.161, Min-Chun E. Rd., Sec. 6, Neihu, Taipei 114, Taiwan, Republic of China
Graduate Institute of Medical Sciences, National Defense Medical Center, No.161, Min-Chun E. Rd., Sec. 6, Neihu, Taipei 114, Taiwan, Republic of China

Wenbo Wei
Department of Orthopedics, Shaanxi Province People Hospital, Xi'an 710004, China
Xi'an JiaoTong University, Xi'an 710004, China

Department of Anesthesiology, Shaanxi Provincial Cancer Hospital, Xi'an 710001, China

Dapeng Duan
Department of Orthopedics, Shaanxi Province People Hospital, Xi'an 710004, China

Ling Wei
Department of Pain, YangLing Demonstration Zone Hospital, No.15 Kangle street, Yang ling, Xi'an 712100, China

Junichi Nakamura, Takaki Inoue, Toru Suguro, Masahiko Suzuki, Takahisa Sasho, Shigeo Hagiwara, Ryuichiro Akagi, Sumihisa Orita, Kazuhide Inage, Tsutomu Akazawa and Seiji Ohtori
Department of Orthopedic Surgery, Graduate School of Medicine, Chiba University, 1-8-1 Inohana, Chuo-ku, Chiba 260-8677, Japan

Anne Postler, Cornelia Lützner, Franziska Beyer, Eric Tille and Jörg Lützner
University Center of Orthopaedics and Traumatology, University Medicine Carl Gustav Carus Dresden, TU Dresden, Fetscherst. 74, 01307 Dresden, Germany

Stirling Bryan and Ellen Randall
Centre for Clinical Epidemiology & Evaluation, Vancouver Coastal Health Research Institute, West 10th Avenue, Vancouver, BC V5Z 1M9, Canada
School of Population & Public Health, University of British Columbia, 2206 E Mall, Vancouver, BC V6T 1Z3, Canada

Laurie J. Goldsmith
Centre for Clinical Epidemiology & Evaluation, Vancouver Coastal Health Research Institute, West 10th Avenue, Vancouver, BC V5Z 1M9, Canada
Faculty of Health Sciences, Simon Fraser University, 8888 University Drive, Burnaby, BC V5A 1S6, Canada

Jennifer C. Davis
Centre for Clinical Epidemiology & Evaluation, Vancouver Coastal Health Research Institute, West 10th Avenue, Vancouver, BC V5Z 1M9, Canada
Faculty of Management, University of British Columbia – Okanagan Campus, EME 4145 3333 University Way, Kelowna, BC V1V 1V7, Canada

Samar Hejazi
Department of Evaluation & Research Services, Fraser Health Authority, Suite 400, Central City Tower, 13450 102 Avenue, Surrey, BC V3T 0H1, Canada

Valerie MacDonald
Burnaby Hospital & Surgical Network, Fraser Health Authority, 3935 Kincaid St, Burnaby, BC V5G 2X6, Canada

Nitya Suryaprakash
Centre for Clinical Epidemiology & Evaluation, Vancouver Coastal Health Research Institute, West 10th Avenue, Vancouver, BC V5Z 1M9, Canada

Amery D. Wu
Educational and Counselling Psychology and Special Education, University of British Columbia, 2125 Main Mall, Vancouver, BC V6T 1Z4, Canada

Richard Sawatzky
School of Nursing, Trinity Western University, 7600 Glover Rd, Langley, BC V2Y 1Y1, Canada
Centre for Health Evaluation & Outcomes Sciences, Providence Health Care Research Institute, 588 – 1081 Burrard Street, St. Paul's Hospital, Vancouver, BC V6Z 1Y6, Canada

Richard J. Napier, Christopher O'Neill, Seamus O'Brien, Emer Doran, Brian Mockford and David E. Beverland
Orthopaedic Outcomes Assessment Unit, Musgrave Park Hospital, Stockman's Lane, Belfast BT9 7JB, Northern Ireland

Mingmin Shi, Haobo Wu, Yangxin Wang, Wei Wang, Yujie Zhang and Shigui Yan
Department of Orthopaedic Surgery, Second Affiliated Hospital, School of Medicine, Zhejiang University, No.88 Jiefang Road, Hangzhou 310009, People's Republic of China

Lei Chen
Department of Endocrinology and Metabolism, Sir Run Run Shaw Hospital Affiliated with School of Medicine, Zhejiang
University, No. 3 Qingchun Road, Hangzhou 310009, People's Republic of China

Frank Lampe
Research Center of the Department of Orthopedics and Joint Replacement at the Schoen Klinik Hamburg Eilbek, Dehnhaide 120, D-22081 Hamburg, Germany
Faculty of Life Sciences at the Hamburg University of Applied Sciences, Lohbrügger Kirchstraße 65, D-21033 Hamburg, Germany

Franziska Fiedler and Anusch Sufi-Siavach
Department of Orthopedics and Joint Replacement at the Schoen Klinik Hamburg Eilbek, Dehnhaide 120, D-22081 Hamburg, Germany

Carlos J. Marques
Research Center of the Department of Orthopedics and Joint Replacement at the Schoen Klinik Hamburg Eilbek, Dehnhaide 120, D-22081 Hamburg, Germany

Georg Matziolis
Orthopaedic Department, Jena University Hospital, Campus Eisenberg, Klosterlausnitzer Straße 81, D-07607 Eisenberg, Germany

Index

www.ingramcontent.com/pod-product-compliance
Lightning Source LLC
Chambersburg PA
CBHW082033190326
41458CB00010B/3355